# Where Are We Now and Where Is Cell Therapy Headed?

# Where Are We Now and Where Is Cell Therapy Headed?

Guest Editors

**Andrea Papait**
**Paola Chiodelli**

MDPI

Basel • Beijing • Wuhan • Barcelona • Belgrade • Novi Sad • Cluj • Manchester

*Guest Editors*
Andrea Papait
Department of Life Sciences and Public Health
Università Cattolica del Sacro Cuore
Rome
Italy

Paola Chiodelli
Department of Life Sciences and Public Health
Università Cattolica del Sacro Cuore
Rome
Italy

*Editorial Office*
MDPI AG
Grosspeteranlage 5
4052 Basel, Switzerland

This is a reprint of the Special Issue, published open access by the journal *Pharmaceutics* (ISSN 1999-4923), freely accessible at: https://www.mdpi.com/journal/pharmaceutics/special_issues/GLA9VZH6NW.

For citation purposes, cite each article independently as indicated on the article page online and as indicated below:

| Lastname, A.A.; Lastname, B.B. Article Title. *Journal Name* **Year**, *Volume Number*, Page Range. |
|---|

**ISBN 978-3-7258-4945-1 (Hbk)**
**ISBN 978-3-7258-4946-8 (PDF)**
**https://doi.org/10.3390/books978-3-7258-4946-8**

Cover image courtesy of Paola Chiodelli

# Contents

**About the Editors** . . . . . . . . . . . . . . . . . . . . . . . . . . . . . . . . . . . . . . . . . **vii**

**Preface** . . . . . . . . . . . . . . . . . . . . . . . . . . . . . . . . . . . . . . . . . . . . . . . . . . . **ix**

**Andrea Papait and Paola Chiodelli**
An Editorial on the Special Issue "Where Are We Now and Where Is Cell Therapy Headed?"
Reprinted from: *Pharmaceutics* **2025**, *17*, 894, https://doi.org/10.3390/pharmaceutics17070894 . **1**

**Annick Jeannerat, Cédric Peneveyre, Sandra Jaccoud, Virginie Philippe, Corinne Scaletta, Nathalie Hirt-Burri, et al.**
Banked Primary Progenitor Cells for Allogeneic Intervertebral Disc (IVD) Therapy: Preclinical Qualification and Functional Optimization within a Cell Spheroid Formulation Process
Reprinted from: *Pharmaceutics* **2024**, *16*, 1274, https://doi.org/10.3390/pharmaceutics16101274 . **5**

**Annick Jeannerat, Joachim Meuli, Cédric Peneveyre, Sandra Jaccoud, Michèle Chemali, Axelle Thomas, et al.**
Bio-Enhanced Neoligaments Graft Bearing FE002 Primary Progenitor Tenocytes: Allogeneic Tissue Engineering & Surgical Proofs-of-Concept for Hand Ligament Regenerative Medicine
Reprinted from: *Pharmaceutics* **2023**, *15*, 1873, https://doi.org/10.3390/pharmaceutics15071873 . **35**

**Virginie Philippe, Annick Jeannerat, Cédric Peneveyre, Sandra Jaccoud, Corinne Scaletta, Nathalie Hirt-Burri, et al.**
Autologous and Allogeneic Cytotherapies for Large Knee (Osteo)Chondral Defects: Manufacturing Process Benchmarking and Parallel Functional Qualification
Reprinted from: *Pharmaceutics* **2023**, *15*, 2333, https://doi.org/10.3390/pharmaceutics15092333 . **74**

**Xi Chen, Alexis Laurent, Zhifeng Liao, Sandra Jaccoud, Philippe Abdel-Sayed, Marjorie Flahaut, et al.**
Cutaneous Cell Therapy Manufacturing Timeframe Rationalization: Allogeneic Off-the-Freezer Fibroblasts for Dermo-Epidermal Combined Preparations (DE-FE002-SK2) in Burn Care
Reprinted from: *Pharmaceutics* **2023**, *15*, 2334, https://doi.org/10.3390/pharmaceutics15092334 . **107**

**Kevin Y. Wu, Jaskarn K. Dhaliwal, Akash Sasitharan and Ananda Kalevar**
Cell Therapy for Retinal Degenerative Diseases: Progress and Prospects
Reprinted from: *Pharmaceutics* **2024**, *16*, 1299, https://doi.org/10.3390/pharmaceutics16101299 . **132**

**Mei-Ye Li, Wei Ye and Ke-Wang Luo**
Immunotherapies Targeting Tumor-Associated Macrophages (TAMs) in Cancer
Reprinted from: *Pharmaceutics* **2024**, *16*, 865, https://doi.org/10.3390/pharmaceutics16070865 . **162**

**Wei Ye, Meiye Li and Kewang Luo**
Therapies Targeting Immune Cells in Tumor Microenvironment for Non-Small Cell Lung Cancer
Reprinted from: *Pharmaceutics* **2023**, *15*, 1788, https://doi.org/10.3390/pharmaceutics15071788 . **190**

**Paola Chiodelli, Patrizia Bonassi Signoroni, Elisa Scalvini, Serafina Farigu, Elisabetta Giuzzi, Alice Paini, et al.**
Synergistic Effect of Conditioned Medium from Amniotic Membrane Mesenchymal Stromal Cells Combined with Paclitaxel on Ovarian Cancer Cell Viability and Migration in 2D and 3D In Vitro Models
Reprinted from: *Pharmaceutics* **2025**, *17*, 420, https://doi.org/10.3390/pharmaceutics17040420 . **212**

# About the Editors

**Andrea Papait**

Andrea Papait obtained his degree in Biology from the University of Milan Bicocca. During his undergraduate study, he pursued his thesis at the European Institute of Oncology in Milan, where he remained for a one-year fellowship after obtaining his degree. He subsequently obtained his doctorate in Biotechnology in Translational Medicine at the University of Genoa in the laboratory of Professor Ranieri Cancedda, with a thesis on allogeneic platelet derivatives as new tools for the treatment of diabetic foot ulcers.

Since November 2018, Dr. Papait has been enrolled as a Post-Doc Researcher in the Centro di Ricerca E. Menni—Fondazione Poliambulanza (Brescia), directed by Professor Ornella Parolini. His studies have significantly contributed to the understanding of the immunomodulatory properties of mesenchymal stromal cells isolated from placental tissues, and of their derivatives, such as their secretome, and how these contribute to tissue regeneration. Since January 2025 he has been an Assistant Professor (RTT) at the Università Cattolica del Sacro Cuore.

**Paola Chiodelli**

Paola Chiodelli obtained her PhD in Cellular and Molecular Biotechnology applied to Biomedical Science at the University of Brescia (Italy) in 2013, where she investigated the role of glycan structures in endothelial cells during the angiogenic process. After completing her PhD, she pursued her studies at the Laboratory of Experimental Oncology and Immunology at the University of Brescia, with a triennial FIRC fellowship on the role of sialic acid associated with VEGFR2 in VEGF-induced tumor angiogenesis. Since 2016, she has been involved in different projects and has worked independently from a scientific and organizational point of view. In 2020, she was involved as Post-Doc Researcher in the AIRC project "Pro-tumorigenic activity of beta-galactosylceramide: a novel player in cutaneous melanoma". In February 2022, she joined Professor Ornella Parolini's Laboratory at CREM—Fondazione Poliambulanza Brescia, as a postdoc researcher. From February 2023 she has held an RTDA research position at Università Cattolica del Sacro Cuore. Nowadays her studies focus on the impact of mesenchymal stromal cells isolated from the amniotic membrane and their secretome on the tumor microenvironment in pre-clinical models.

# Preface

This Special Issue, "Where Are We Now and Where Is Cell Therapy Headed?", offers a comprehensive snapshot of the evolving field of cell-based therapeutics at a moment of profound conceptual and technological transition. The subject matter spans from traditional applications such as hematopoietic cell transplantation to next-generation engineered immune cells and cell-free derivatives, capturing the field's expansion and diversification. The scope of the Issue is deliberately broad, encompassing both foundational technologies and emerging paradigms.

The primary aim is to map the current state of the field while anticipating its next directions, and contributions were selected to illustrate the shift in central therapeutic principle from cell persistence to signal orchestration. This includes a focus on how paracrine signaling, immune modulation, and the delivery of defined molecular cargo are redefining the utility and identity of therapeutic cells. This collection also brings translational bottlenecks to the forefront—such as product heterogeneity, regulatory uncertainty, and manufacturing challenges—while highlighting the strategies being developed to overcome them.

The motivation for assembling this Special Issue is rooted in the recognition that cell therapy is no longer confined to a regenerative or hematologic niche but is rapidly becoming a modular platform with wide-ranging implications for immunology, oncology, tissue engineering, and beyond. The editorial perspective reinforces a growing consensus that future therapies will operate through transient, highly orchestrated biological effects, rather than permanent cellular integration.

This collection is intended for a multidisciplinary audience that includes researchers, clinicians, translational scientists, and regulatory experts working across regenerative medicine, immunotherapy, bioengineering, and drug delivery.

Ultimately, this Special Issue offers a timely, multifaceted perspective on cell-based and cell-derived therapeutics. It invites the reader to consider not only where the field currently stands, but how a new therapeutic logic—rooted in cellular communication rather than replacement—is reshaping the future of medicine.

**Andrea Papait and Paola Chiodelli**
*Guest Editors*

*pharmaceutics*

MDPI

*Editorial*

# An Editorial on the Special Issue "Where Are We Now and Where Is Cell Therapy Headed?"

**Andrea Papait [1,2,*] and Paola Chiodelli [1,*]**

1 Department of Life Sciences and Public Health, Università Cattolica del Sacro Cuore, 00168 Rome, Italy
2 Fondazione Policlinico Universitario A. Gemelli IRCCS, 00168 Rome, Italy
* Correspondence: andrea.papait@unicatt.it (A.P.); paola.chiodelli@unicatt.it (P.C.)

Cell-based therapies have swiftly transitioned from experimental modalities to core components of modern translational medicine. Initially envisioned as a regenerative tool relying on engraftment and tissue integration, cell therapy has undergone a conceptual shift, and it is becoming increasingly evident that its therapeutic impact is rooted not in cellular persistence, but in the transient orchestration of complex biological responses.

A paradigmatic case is the evolution of mesenchymal stromal cells (MSCs), which have historically been employed for tissue regeneration but are now recognized for their immunomodulatory and paracrine effects [10.1002/sctm.17-0051]. The growing understanding of MSCs as secretory platforms has accelerated interest in cell-free therapeutic strategies, including extracellular vesicles (EVs) and complex secretomes [1–3]. These acellular approaches may mitigate issues related to immune rejection and engraftment failure while offering greater control and standardization.

Nonetheless, certain cell-based interventions remain clinically indispensable. Allogeneic hematopoietic cell transplantation (HCT), for example, is still a foundational therapy for hematological malignancies such as leukemia, lymphoma, and multiple myeloma [4,5]. At the same time, challenges such as graft versus host disease (GvHD) and donor availability have prompted the development of precision genome-editing approaches—most notably, CRISPR-Cas9—to reduce immunogenicity and correct autologous mutations [6].

In oncology, the success of engineered immune effectors—particularly chimeric antigen receptor (CAR) T-cells—has redefined expectations. Initially approved for specific forms of relapsed or refractory B cell malignancies, CAR T-cell therapies represent a new class of "living drugs" capable of sustained, antigen-driven immune activity [7,8]. Their efficacy has spurred efforts to extend the platform to solid tumors and integrate it with other immune-modulatory strategies.

Despite these advances, critical bottlenecks persist. Complex manufacturing pipelines, variability in product quality, nonuniform global regulatory frameworks, and cost-related access disparities all impede clinical scalability [9,10]. The articles in this Special Issue "Where Are We Now and Where Is Cell Therapy Headed?" reflect a translational field that confronts these challenges directly. Collectively, they map a landscape in which cellular and acellular approaches are no longer mutually exclusive but increasingly complementary.

Several contributions focus on the shift from autologous to allogeneic and off-the-shelf strategies. Jeannerat and colleagues demonstrate that FE002-derived progenitor cells retain chondrogenic potential and survive hypoxic and inflammatory stress in intervertebral disc models (Contribution 1). Extending their approach, they develop bioengineered neoligament constructs with FE002-derived tenocytes, achieving rapid fabrication and effective integration (Contribution 2). Philippe and colleagues compare autologous and allogeneic grafts for knee cartilage repair and find that allogeneic products reduce patient variability and enhance scalability without compromising clinical outcomes (Contribution 3). In their paper on burn care, Chen and colleagues describe a hybrid dermo-epidermal graft incorporating both autologous and banked fibroblasts, offering a more agile production timeline with sustained efficacy (Contribution 4).

In parallel, the therapeutic potential of secreted factors is gaining clinical traction. Wu and colleagues provide a comprehensive analysis of ESCs, iPSCs, MSCs, and retinal progenitors for treating degenerative retinal conditions, outlining both opportunities and translational barriers (Contribution 5). Within the cancer immunotherapy space, Li and colleagues. explore cellular strategies to modulate the tumor microenvironment (TME), including the reprogramming of tumor-associated macrophages (Contribution 6) and the enhancement of checkpoint inhibitor responses in non-small cell lung cancer (Contribution 7). Meanwhile, Chiodelli and colleagues demonstrate that conditioned medium from human amniotic MSCs suppresses ovarian cancer proliferation and migration, exhibiting enhanced efficacy in combination with paclitaxel (Contribution 8).

Together, these contributions illustrate a rapidly diversifying field. On the one hand, the development of standardized, bankable cell products reflects a drive toward consistency and broader accessibility. On the other hand, cell-derived EVs and secretomes are emerging as potent therapeutic agents, capable of modulating immune responses, promoting tissue repair, and engaging in cross-tissue signaling.

Regardless, considerable challenges lie ahead. Product heterogeneity remains a critical concern for both cellular and extracellular therapies [11,12], and the lack of universally accepted potency assays and markers of activity further complicates development [13]. Issues of manufacturing scalability [9], cost containment [14–16], and international regulatory alignment [10,17,18] continue to shape—and constrain—the pathway from bench to bedside.

Nevertheless, the field is clearly beginning to gravitate toward therapies that extend beyond the cells themselves. The next generation of interventions is likely to harness not the cell as a unit, but the molecular and vesicular cargo it deploys. This reframing positions cell therapy as a modular, signal-driven platform, which is defined less by cellular identity and more by the biological programs it initiates within the host.

**Author Contributions:** Conceptualization, A.P. and P.C.; writing—original draft preparation, A.P.; writing—review and editing, A.P. and P.C. All authors have read and agreed to the published version of the manuscript.

**Funding:** This research was supported by intramural funds at Università Cattolica del Sacro Cuore, Linea D1 (A.P.).

**Conflicts of Interest:** The authors declare no conflicts of interest.

## Abbreviations

The following abbreviations are used in this manuscript:

| | |
|---|---|
| MSC | Mesenchymal Stromal Cells |
| HCT | Hematopoietic cell transplantation |
| ESC | Embryonic Stem Cells |
| GvHD | Graft Versus Host Disease |
| iPSC | Induced Pluripotent Stem Cells |
| TME | Tumor Microenvironment |
| EV | Extracellular Vesicle |
| CAR | Chimeric Antigen Receptor |

**List of Contributions:**

1. Jeannerat, A.; Peneveyre, C.; Jaccoud, S.; Philippe, V.; Scaletta, C.; Hirt-Burri, N.; Abdel-Sayed, P.; Martin, R.; Applegate, L.A.; Pioletti, D.P.; et al. Banked Primary Progenitor Cells for Allogeneic Intervertebral Disc (IVD) Therapy: Preclinical Qualification and Functional Optimization within a Cell Spheroid Formulation Process. *Pharmaceutics* **2024**, *16*, 1274. https://doi.org/10.3390/pharmaceutics16101274.
2. Jeannerat, A.; Meuli, J.; Peneveyre, C.; Jaccoud, S.; Chemali, M.; Thomas, A.; Liao, Z.; Abdel-Sayed, P.; Scaletta, C.; Hirt-Burri, N.; et al. Bio-Enhanced Neoligaments Graft Bearing FE002 Primary Progenitor Tenocytes: Allogeneic Tissue Engineering & Surgical Proofs-of-Concept for Hand Ligament Regenerative Medicine. *Pharmaceutics* **2023**, *15*, 1873. https://doi.org/10.3390/pharmaceutics15071873.
3. Philippe, V.; Jeannerat, A.; Peneveyre, C.; Jaccoud, S.; Scaletta, C.; Hirt-Burri, N.; Abdel-Sayed, P.; Raffoul, W.; Darwiche, S.; Applegate, L.A.; et al. Autologous and Allogeneic Cytotherapies for Large Knee (Osteo)Chondral Defects: Manufacturing Process Benchmarking and Parallel Functional Qualification. *Pharmaceutics* **2023**, *15*, 2333. https://doi.org/10.3390/pharmaceutics15092333.
4. Chen, X.; Laurent, A.; Liao, Z.; Jaccoud, S.; Abdel-Sayed, P.; Flahaut, M.; Scaletta, C.; Raffoul, W.; Applegate, L.A.; Hirt-Burri, N. Cutaneous Cell Therapy Manufacturing Timeframe Rationalization: Allogeneic Off-the-Freezer Fibroblasts for Dermo-Epidermal Combined Preparations (DE-FE002-SK2) in Burn Care. *Pharmaceutics* **2023**, *15*, 2334. https://doi.org/10.3390/pharmaceutics15092334.
5. Wu, K.Y.; Dhaliwal, J.K.; Sasitharan, A.; Kalevar, A. Cell Therapy for Retinal Degenerative Diseases: Progress and Prospects. *Pharmaceutics* **2024**, *16*, 1299. https://doi.org/10.3390/pharmaceutics16101299.
6. Li, M.-Y.; Ye, W.; Luo, K.-W. Immunotherapies Targeting Tumor-Associated Macrophages (TAMs) in Cancer. *Pharmaceutics* **2024**, *16*, 865. https://doi.org/10.3390/pharmaceutics16070865.
7. Ye, W.; Li, M.; Luo, K. Therapies Targeting Immune Cells in Tumor Microenvironment for Non-Small Cell Lung Cancer. *Pharmaceutics* **2023**, *15*, 1788. https://doi.org/10.3390/pharmaceutics15071788.
8. Chiodelli, P.; Bonassi Signoroni, P.; Scalvini, E.; Farigu, S.; Giuzzi, E.; Paini, A.; Papait, A.; Stefani, F.R.; Silini, A.R.; Parolini, O. Synergistic Effect of Conditioned Medium from Amniotic Membrane Mesenchymal Stromal Cells Combined with Paclitaxel on Ovarian Cancer Cell Viability and Migration in 2D and 3D In Vitro Models. *Pharmaceutics* **2025**, *17*, 420. https://doi.org/10.3390/pharmaceutics17040420.

## References


1. Silini, A.R.; Papait, A.; Cargnoni, A.; Vertua, E.; Romele, P.; Bonassi Signoroni, P.; Magatti, M.; De Munari, S.; Masserdotti, A.; Pasotti, A.; et al. CM from intact hAM: An easily obtained product with relevant implications for translation in regenerative medicine. *Stem Cell Res. Ther.* **2021**, *12*, 540. [CrossRef] [PubMed]
2. Ragni, E.; Papait, A.; Taiana, M.M.; De Luca, P.; Grieco, G.; Vertua, E.; Romele, P.; Colombo, C.; Silini, A.R.; Parolini, O.; et al. Cell culture expansion media choice affects secretory, protective and immuno-modulatory features of adipose mesenchymal stromal cell-derived secretomes for orthopaedic applications. *Regen. Ther.* **2025**, *28*, 481–497. [CrossRef] [PubMed]
3. Kumar, M.A.; Baba, S.K.; Sadida, H.Q.; Marzooqi, S.A.; Jerobin, J.; Altemani, F.H.; Algehainy, N.; Alanazi, M.A.; Abou-Samra, A.B.; Kumar, R.; et al. Extracellular vesicles as tools and targets in therapy for diseases. *Signal Transduct. Target. Ther.* **2024**, *9*, 27. [CrossRef]
4. Prockop, S.; Wachter, F. The current landscape: Allogeneic hematopoietic stem cell transplant for acute lymphoblastic leukemia. *Best Pract. Res. Clin. Haematol.* **2023**, *36*, 101485. [CrossRef] [PubMed]
5. Vuelta, E.; Garcia-Tunon, I.; Hernandez-Carabias, P.; Mendez, L.; Sanchez-Martin, M. Future Approaches for Treating Chronic Myeloid Leukemia: CRISPR Therapy. *Biology* **2021**, *10*, 118. [CrossRef] [PubMed]
6. Bashor, C.J.; Hilton, I.B.; Bandukwala, H.; Smith, D.M.; Veiseh, O. Engineering the next generation of cell-based therapeutics. *Nat. Rev. Drug Discov.* **2022**, *21*, 655–675. [CrossRef] [PubMed]
7. Sterner, R.C.; Sterner, R.M. CAR-T cell therapy: Current limitations and potential strategies. *Blood Cancer J.* **2021**, *11*, 69. [CrossRef] [PubMed]

8. Holzinger, A.; Abken, H. Treatment with Living Drugs: Pharmaceutical Aspects of CAR T Cells. *Pharmacology* **2022**, *107*, 446–463. [CrossRef] [PubMed]
9. Gavan, S.P.; Wright, S.J.; Thistlethwaite, F.; Payne, K. Capturing the Impact of Constraints on the Cost-Effectiveness of Cell and Gene Therapies: A Systematic Review. *Pharmacoeconomics* **2023**, *41*, 675–692. [CrossRef] [PubMed]
10. Joppi, R.; Bertele, V.; Vannini, T.; Garattini, S.; Banzi, R. Food and Drug Administration vs European Medicines Agency: Review times and clinical evidence on novel drugs at the time of approval. *Br. J. Clin. Pharmacol.* **2020**, *86*, 170–174. [CrossRef] [PubMed]
11. Li, J.; Wu, Z.; Zhao, L.; Liu, Y.; Su, Y.; Gong, X.; Liu, F.; Zhang, L. The heterogeneity of mesenchymal stem cells: An important issue to be addressed in cell therapy. *Stem Cell Res. Ther.* **2023**, *14*, 381. [CrossRef] [PubMed]
12. Almeria, C.; Kress, S.; Weber, V.; Egger, D.; Kasper, C. Heterogeneity of mesenchymal stem cell-derived extracellular vesicles is highly impacted by the tissue/cell source and culture conditions. *Cell Biosci.* **2022**, *12*, 51. [CrossRef] [PubMed]
13. Capelli, C.; Cuofano, C.; Pavoni, C.; Frigerio, S.; Lisini, D.; Nava, S.; Quaroni, M.; Colombo, V.; Galli, F.; Bezukladova, S.; et al. Potency assays and biomarkers for cell-based advanced therapy medicinal products. *Front. Immunol.* **2023**, *14*, 1186224. [CrossRef] [PubMed]
14. Majhail, N.S.; Mau, L.W.; Denzen, E.M.; Arneson, T.J. Costs of autologous and allogeneic hematopoietic cell transplantation in the United States: A study using a large national private claims database. *Bone Marrow Transplant.* **2013**, *48*, 294–300. [CrossRef] [PubMed]
15. Ten Ham, R.M.T.; Hovels, A.M.; Hoekman, J.; Frederix, G.W.J.; Leufkens, H.G.M.; Klungel, O.H.; Jedema, I.; Veld, S.A.J.; Nikolic, T.; Van Pel, M.; et al. What does cell therapy manufacturing cost? A framework and methodology to facilitate academic and other small-scale cell therapy manufacturing costings. *Cytotherapy* **2020**, *22*, 388–397. [CrossRef] [PubMed]
16. Khang, M.; Suryaprakash, S.; Kotrappa, M.; Mulyasasmita, W.; Topp, S.; Wu, J. Manufacturing innovation to drive down cell therapy costs. *Trends Biotechnol.* **2023**, *41*, 1216–1219. [CrossRef] [PubMed]
17. Olaghere, J.; Williams, D.A.; Farrar, J.; Buning, H.; Calhoun, C.; Ho, T.; Inamdar, M.S.; Liu, D.; Makani, J.; Nyarko, K.; et al. Scientific Advancements in Gene Therapies: Opportunities for Global Regulatory Convergence. *Biomedicines* **2025**, *13*, 758. [CrossRef] [PubMed]
18. Maryamchik, E.; Ikonomou, L.; Roxland, B.E.; Grignon, F.; Levine, B.L.; Grilley, B.J.; ISCT Committee on the Ethics of Cell and Gene Therapy Expanded Access Working Group. International Society for Cell & Gene Therapy Expanded Access Working Group position paper: Key considerations to support equitable and ethical expanded access to investigational cell- and gene-based interventions. *Cytotherapy* **2025**, *27*, 671–677. [CrossRef] [PubMed]

*pharmaceutics*

MDPI

*Article*

# Banked Primary Progenitor Cells for Allogeneic Intervertebral Disc (IVD) Therapy: Preclinical Qualification and Functional Optimization within a Cell Spheroid Formulation Process

**Annick Jeannerat [1], Cédric Peneveyre [1], Sandra Jaccoud [2,3], Virginie Philippe [2,4], Corinne Scaletta [2], Nathalie Hirt-Burri [2], Philippe Abdel-Sayed [2,5], Robin Martin [4], Lee Ann Applegate [2,6,7], Dominique P. Pioletti [3,*] and Alexis Laurent [1,2,*]**

1 Development Department, LAM Biotechnologies SA, CH-1066 Epalinges, Switzerland; annick.jeannerat@lambiotechnologies.com (A.J.); cedric.peneveyre@lambiotechnologies.com (C.P.)
2 Regenerative Therapy Unit, Plastic, Reconstructive and Hand Surgery Service, Lausanne University Hospital, University of Lausanne, CH-1066 Epalinges, Switzerland; sandra.jaccoud@chuv.ch (S.J.); virginie.philippe@chuv.ch (V.P.); corinne.scaletta@chuv.ch (C.S.); nathalie.burri@chuv.ch (N.H.-B.); philippe.abdel-sayed@chuv.ch (P.A.-S.); lee.laurent-applegate@chuv.ch (L.A.A.)
3 Laboratory of Biomechanical Orthopedics, Federal Polytechnic School of Lausanne, CH-1015 Lausanne, Switzerland
4 Orthopedics and Traumatology Unit, Lausanne University Hospital, University of Lausanne, CH-1011 Lausanne, Switzerland; robin.martin@chuv.ch
5 STI School of Engineering, Federal Polytechnic School of Lausanne, CH-1015 Lausanne, Switzerland
6 Center for Applied Biotechnology and Molecular Medicine, University of Zurich, CH-8057 Zurich, Switzerland
7 Oxford OSCAR Suzhou Center, Oxford University, Suzhou 215123, China
* Correspondence: dominique.pioletti@epfl.ch (D.P.P.); alexis.laurent@lambiotechnologies.com (A.L.); Tel.: +41-21-693-83-41 (D.P.P.); +41-21-546-42-00 (A.L.)

**Abstract: Background/Objectives:** Biological products are emerging as therapeutic management options for intervertebral disc (IVD) degenerative affections and lower back pain. Autologous and allogeneic cell therapy protocols have been clinically implemented for IVD repair. Therein, several manufacturing process design considerations were shown to significantly influence clinical outcomes. The primary objective of this study was to preclinically qualify (chondrogenic potential, safety, resistance to hypoxic and inflammatory stimuli) cryopreserved primary progenitor cells (clinical grade FE002-Disc cells) as a potential cell source in IVD repair/regeneration. The secondary objective of this study was to assess the cell source's delivery potential as cell spheroids (optimization of culture conditions, potential storage solutions). **Methods/Results:** Safety (soft agar transformation, β-galactosidase, telomerase activity) and functionality-related assays (hypoxic and inflammatory challenge) confirmed that the investigated cellular active substance was highly sustainable in defined cell banking workflows, despite possessing a finite in vitro lifespan. Functionality-related assays confirmed that the retained manufacturing process yielded strong collagen II and glycosaminoglycan (GAG) synthesis in the spheroids in 3-week chondrogenic induction. Then, the impacts of various process parameters (induction medium composition, hypoxic incubation, terminal spheroid lyophilization) were studied to gain insights on their criticality. Finally, an optimal set of technical specifications (use of 10 nM dexamethasone for chondrogenic induction, 2% $O_2$ incubation of spheroids) was set forth, based on specific fine tuning of finished product critical functional attributes. **Conclusions:** Generally, this study qualified the considered FE002-Disc progenitor cell source for further preclinical investigation based on safety, quality, and functionality datasets. The novelty and significance of this study resided in the establishment of defined processes for preparing fresh, off-the-freezer, or off-the-shelf IVD spheroids using a preclinically qualified allogeneic human cell source. Overall, this study underscored the importance of using robust product components and optimal manufacturing process variants for maximization of finished cell-based formulation quality attributes.

**Keywords:** allogeneic cytotherapies; back pain; chondrogenesis; cell therapy; hypoxia; intervertebral disc; manufacturing process; spheroids; spine; tissue engineering

## 1. Introduction

Pathological and traumatic affections of the intervertebral disc (IVD) are often the cause of lower back pain (LBP) [1,2]. Importantly, LBP constitutes a widespread health issue, as it is the greatest cause of disability burden worldwide [3]. Specifically, it is expected that more than half of the global population will experience LBP at some point, wherein 5–10% of patients will develop chronic LBP [3–5]. As LBP prevalence increases with age, so do the incured economic impacts (i.e., treatment costs, reduced productivity, loss of income). Of note, the latter have been estimated at over 100 bn USD yearly, with ⅔ of indirect costs (e.g., professional productivity deficits) [6,7]. Notwithstanding, LBP has been identified as the most common cause of disability among young adults in the US and in Europe, wherein LBP prevalence increases are driven by population growth, obesity, and aging [5,8]. Pathophysiologically, IVD affections are implicated in >40% of cases of chronic back pain and constitute the most common non-cancer indication for opioid prescription in the US [9,10].

From an anatomical perspective, the IVD deploys a spacer function between vertebrae in the spine [9]. The inner core of IVDs (i.e., nucleus pulposus [NP]) is constituted by a gelatinous hydrophilic extracellular matrix (ECM), rich in ACAN and COL2 (i.e., a 20:1 ratio). Therein, NP cells are characterized by a chondroid phenotype and generate high ACAN contents, which swell and thus exert sufficient mechanical pressure to maintain appropriate distances between vertebral bodies. The NP is contained in the annulus fibrosus (AF) structure, which is a COL1-rich tissue presenting hyaline cartilaginous endplates [8,9,11]. As a unit, the IVD serves as a shock absorber within the spine, presenting resistance to tensile and torsional forces. As IVDs are mainly avascular and aneural, nutrients and metabolites diffuse from nearby vessels in the endplates and in the outer AF [2,9,12].

From a therapeutic standpoint, conservative LBP treatments primarily aim for pain relief, using physiotherapy, chiropraxie, acupuncture, NSAIDs, opiates, steroids, or muscle relaxants [13]. Surgical approaches (e.g., microdiscectomy, nucleoplasty, annuloplasty, spinal fusion, disc replacement) are indicated when patients do not respond to conservative treatment options. However, spine surgeries often increase the rates of adjacent segment degeneration [14]. Furthermore, patient self-rating of unsuccessful treatment after spinal fusion may exceed 30%, and complications were notably reported in 36% of cases [10,15].

Due to the complex pathophysiological context of IVD degeneration and the limited success of traditional treatment approaches, considerable interest and research have been focused on therapies wielding intradiscal medical device scaffolds and/or biologicals [14,16]. Therein, the objectives are to restore normal IVD functions, notably by enhancing ECM anabolic processes or by reducing the action of catabolic molecules (e.g., MMPs). Therefore, several growth factors (e.g., GDF-5), biologicals (e.g., platelet-rich plasma [PRP]), or cell-based therapeutics are clinically investigated [17–22]. While hyaluronan-based hydrogels and fibrin-based sealants are useful for AF repair or after nucleotomies, bioactive molecules (e.g., glucocorticoids, NSAIDs, anti-TNFs) are often used [23–25]. However, most IVD therapeutic interventions only allow for symptomatic management of pain and present limited efficacy in the long term.

Recently, considerable efforts have been allocated to investigational cell therapies and tissue engineering solutions aiming to regenerate IVDs [3,8,14]. Several autologous cell-based protocols have been developed for IVD treatment, comprising ASCs, B-MSCs, or disc chondrocytes as the cellular active substance [14,26–30]. In an allogeneic setting, juvenile chondrocytes, B-MSCs, discogenic cells (DiscGenics, Salt Lake City, UT, USA), umbilical stem cells, NP particulates (Vivex Biologics, Miami, FL, USA), or mesenchymal precursors (Mesoblast, Melbourne, Australia) have been proposed [3,14,28].

Importantly, in the specific case of cell-based therapies, patient selection methodology was described as highly important for appropriate treatment (i.e., moderate severity in disc degeneration), as mild or advanced lesions may not show measurable improvement [10,26–28]. From a regulatory viewpoint, in order to potentially circumvent some of the reported challenges in cell-based IVD therapies, the use of exosomes has recently been proposed [31]. Such approaches bare the potential to avoid the detrimental effects of harsh IVD environments on implanted cells, adverse tumorigenicity potential, unwanted cell differentiation, or the risk of host immune reaction, which classically limits the application of viable cells [31,32]. However, further research and long-term follow-up are required around such novel biological-derived cell-free protocols.

The primary aim of the present study was to qualify a clinical-grade cryopreserved primary progenitor cell source (FE002-Disc cells) as a potential cellular active substance in IVD therapy. The secondary aim of this study was to assess the formulation potential of FE002-Disc cells in chondrogenically induced spheroids. The primary hypothesis of this study was that the safety and functionality attributes of the considered primary cell source were adapted for the development of investigational cell therapies for IVDs. The secondary hypothesis of this study was that significant functional impacts on the finished products could be induced by modulation of the manufacturing process technical specifications. The significance of this study resided in the establishment of defined processes for preparing fresh, off-the-freezer, or off-the-shelf IVD spheroids using a preclinically qualified allogeneic cell source. Overall, this study confirmed the critical importance of extensively investigating both the cell source and the manufacturing processes in the context of investigational therapeutic product development (i.e., safety and quality enhancement).

## 2. Materials and Methods

### 2.1. Reagents and Consumables

The main reagents and consumables were as follows: DMEM culture medium, L-glutamine, TrypLE™, Opti-MEM™, dexamethasone, BCA assay kits, NuPAGE™ Bis-Tris 4–12% protein gels, β-mercaptoethanol, PMSF, microAmp fast 96-well reaction plates (Thermo Fisher Scientific, Waltham, MA, USA); X-gal powder (Chemie Brunschwig, Basel, Switzerland); papain (Sigma Aldrich, Buchs, Switzerland); FBS, VitCp, low melting point agarose (Merck, Darmstadt, Germany); human platelet lysate (HPL; Stemulate®, Sexton Biotechnologies, Indianapolis, IN, USA); penicillin-streptomycin (Biowest, Nuaillé, France); ITS II 100× (PAN-Biotech, Aidenbach, Germany); TGF-β3 (PeproTech, London, UK); Blyscan-sulfated glycosaminoglycan assay kits (BioColor, Carrickfergus, UK); telomerase activity quantification qPCR assay kits (ScienCell, Carlsbad, CA, USA); saccharose (PanReac AppliChem, Darmstadt, Germany); dextran 40,000 (Pharmacosmos, Wiesbaden, Germany); Lyoprotect bags (Teclen, Oberpframmern, Germany); lyophilization vials (Schott, Mainz, Germany); lyophilization stoppers (Datwyler, Altdorf, Switzerland).

### 2.2. Instruments and Equipment

Cell surface markers were analyzed on a BD Accuri™ C6 Plus FACS system (BD, Franklin Lakes, NJ, USA). Colorimetric and luminescence measurements were performed on a Varioskan LUX multimode plate reader (Thermo Fisher Scientific, Waltham, MA, USA). Telomerase activity assays were run on a QuantStudio 3 PCR Systems instrument (Thermo Fisher Scientific, Waltham, MA, USA). Immunohistochemistry imaging was performed on an inverted IX81 fluorescence microscope (Olympus, Tokyo, Japan). Gel imaging was performed on a Uvitec Mini HD9 gel imager (Cleaver Scientific, Rugby, UK). Sample lyophilization was performed in a LyoBeta Mini pilot freeze-dryer (Telstar, Terrassa, Spain).

### 2.3. Cell Sourcing and Cell Culture Media Composition

The FE002-Disc primary progenitor cell source used for this study consisted of banked primary human diploid cells from a clinical-grade source, as previously described [33]. The considered FE002-Disc primary progenitor cells were procured and produced under the Swiss progenitor cell transplantation program and were made available as cryopreserved stocks (TEC-PHARMA SA, Bercher, Switzerland). Briefly, a regulated organ donation at 14 weeks of gestation (i.e., FE002 donation) served for the establishment of the primary progenitor cell source (i.e., FE002-Disc cell type) used in the investigations presented herein. Full donor informed consent was obtained and confirmed for the organ donation and for the inclusion in the ad hoc progenitor cell transplantation program. In addition to extensive donor medical history screening, cytogenetic analyses, and histopathological investigations of the donated tissues, the donor was serologically tested twice (i.e., at the time of the donation and three months later) for specified pathogens (i.e., CMV, EBV, HBsAg, HBV, HCV, HIV-1, HIV-2, HSV, HTLV-1, HTLV-2, S-West Nile virus, *Toxoplasma gondii, Treponema pallidum*). Among other primary cell sources, primary progenitor IVD cells were isolated in vitro from the FE002 organ donation. The isolated IVD tissue biopsies were mechanically and/or enzymatically processed for the in vitro culture initiation of fibroblastic adherent primary progenitor cells (i.e., FE002-Disc cell types) in good manufacturing practice (GMP)-compliant manufacturing suites. Briefly, the procured IVD tissue samples were thoroughly washed in conserved phosphate-buffered saline (PBS) buffer (Bichsel, Interlaken, Switzerland), further dissected, and appropriately processed and conditioned for adherent primary progenitor cell proliferation initiation.

After the initial addition of adequate proportions of the cell culture medium (i.e., Dulbecco's modified Eagle medium, DMEM, supplemented with 10% *v*/*v* fetal bovine serum, FBS, Gibco™ and Invitrogen™, respectively, Thermo Fisher Scientific [Waltham, MA, USA]), the cell culture vessels were incubated at 37 °C in humidified incubators under 5% *v*/*v* $CO_2$. Following iterative cell culture medium exchange procedures, preliminary progenitor cell cultures were harvested by trypsinization (i.e., 0.05% trypsin-EDTA, Gibco™, Thermo Fisher Scientific, USA) and were further used to perform in vitro monolayer sub-cultures of FE002-Disc cells following the defined ad hoc technical specifications. Following appropriate maintenance and harvest of the primary cell sub-cultures, the obtained biological materials were cryopreserved in individual polymeric vials in a DMSO-containing cryopreservation solution for the establishment of FE002-Disc parental cell banks (PCB) at passage level 1. After appropriate testing, qualification, and quarantine release of the cryopreserved FE002-Disc PCB cellular material lots, these were used as the starting materials in defined serial expansion workflows in order to establish FE002-Disc master cell banks (MCB) and the FE002-Disc working cell banks (WCB).

For the present study, FE002-Disc cells from a WCB were initiated and were serially expanded in complete growth medium (CMtc) consisting of high-glucose DMEM supplemented with 2 mM L-glutamine and 10% *v*/*v* fetal bovine serum (FBS). The FE002-Disc cells were expanded in humidified incubators at 37 °C with 5% $CO_2$ in normoxic (i.e., 21% $O_2$) culture conditions or in hypoxic (i.e., 2% $O_2$) culture conditions. The cultures were maintained until cell monolayers attained confluency, with cell culture medium exchange procedures performed twice weekly. Respective proliferation characteristics (i.e., cellular morphology, population doubling values) were determined between the normoxic and hypoxic culture conditions. The FE002-Disc cells were used between passage levels 5 and 14 in this study, depending on the assay setup. Primary epiphyseal chondroprogenitors (i.e., FE002-Cart.Art cell type) were used as controls, where the cells were maintained in the same way as the FE002-Disc cells and were used between passage levels 6 and 8 in this study [34].

Cryopreserved primary adipose-derived mesenchymal stem cells (i.e., ASC-F cell type, passage level 2, $10^6$ cells/vial) were purchased from ZenBio (Durham, NC, USA). The ASCs were isolated from human subcutaneous abdominal adipose tissue obtained from a competent 34-year-old female Caucasian donor (i.e., BMI 21.3 kg/m$^2$, non-smoker, non-diabetic, non-medicated) undergoing elective surgery. Safety control results from the supplier indicated that the ASCs tested as negative for HIV, hepatitis B, and hepatitis C. Quality control results from the supplier indicated conforming results for cellular viability, trilineage differentiation potential (i.e., adipogenic, chondrogenic, osteogenic), and cell surface markers (i.e., 97.9% positive for CD105, 99.8% positive for CD44, 0.19% positive for CD19, and undetectable for CD31). The stem cells were initiated according to the supplier's specifications and were seeded at $3.0 \times 10^3$ cells/cm$^2$ in T75 flasks. The stem cells were expanded in normoxic culture conditions in specific growth medium (CM-HPL) composed of high-glucose DMEM supplemented with 2 mM L-glutamine and 5% $v/v$ human platelet lysate (HPL). The cultures were maintained until the cell monolayers attained confluency, with medium exchange procedures performed twice weekly. The ASCs were harvested and used for experiments at passage level 4.

The HeLa cell line was obtained from the Musculoskeletal Research Unit at the University of Zurich (Zurich, Switzerland). The cells were expanded in CMtc in normoxic conditions in a quarantine incubator. The cultures were maintained until the cell monolayers attained confluency, with cell culture medium exchange procedures performed twice weekly. The cells were harvested and used for experiments when they reached 100% confluency.

### 2.4. *FE002-Disc Cellular Active Substance Preclinical Characterization Assays*

The FE002-Disc cellular active substance was firstly analyzed in terms of composition, safety attributes, and biological function in order to preliminarily confirm its applicability for therapeutic product formulation. Specifically, the experiments focused on the proteomic composition of the cellular active substance, the in vitro behavior and robustness of the primary cells, and the in vitro exclusion of safety-related concerns (e.g., tumorigenicity or continuous cell line behavior).

#### 2.4.1. Proteomic Composition Screening in Multiplex Analyses

Soluble protein identification and quantification were performed on FE002-Disc cell lysates at Eve Technologies (Calgary, AB, Canada) using multiplex analyses. For sample preparation, $10^7$ cells were harvested from cultures, resuspended in 1 mL PBS, and were thermically lysed using the freeze-thaw method. The samples were then centrifuged at 13,000 rpm at 4 °C for 5 min, and the supernatants were collected. The obtained samples were analyzed by BCA for total protein quantification and were sent on dry ice for multiplex analyses. The retained multiplex kits were as follows: the human angiogenesis array and growth factor 17-plex array, the human cytokine/chemokine 96-plex panel, the human soluble cytokine receptor 14-plex array, the human MMP and TIMP panel for cell cultures, and the cytokine TGF-β 3-plex array. Based on the obtained proteomic data, specific protein concentrations in the samples were calculated by normalization to the total protein contents.

#### 2.4.2. Cell Surface Marker Characterization by Flow Cytometry

From an identity and purity standpoint, the cellular active substance was analyzed for cell surface marker expression. Therefore, cell surface marker characterization was performed by FACS analysis on FE002-Disc cells at passage level 6. The harvested cells were incubated with specific primary antibodies coupled to either FITC or PE fluorophores for 1 h. Selected cell surface marker antibodies were anti-human CD90, CD73, CD105, CD26, CD166, CD44, HLA-ABC, CD19, CD14, CD34, CD45, and HLA-DPQR. Antibody references are presented in Supplementary Methods. The samples were run on a BD Accuri™ C6 Plus FACS system, and data analysis was performed with the BD Accuri™ C6 software, v264.21.

#### 2.4.3. Phenotypic Stability Assessment in Chemical Induction Assays

From an identity and cell type stability standpoint, the cellular active substance was analyzed for potential phenotypic plasticity in chemical induction assays. Therefore,

FE002-Disc cells were analyzed in terms of differentiation potential under adipogenic, osteogenic, and chondrogenic culture conditions. ASCs were included in the assays as positive differentiation controls in adipogenic and osteogenic induction. The effect of in vitro cellular passaging/aging on the differentiation potential of the FE002-Disc cells was evaluated by iteratively performing the experiments in triplicate at passage levels 6–11.

For adipogenic differentiation assays, the cells were seeded in 12-well plates and were maintained in culture in their respective media under normoxic conditions until 80% confluency was attained. The cells were then transferred and maintained in adipogenic induction medium, consisting of proliferation medium supplemented with ITS, 1 μM dexamethasone, 100 μM indomethacin, and 100 μM IBMX. After two weeks of induction, the cells were fixed in 4% formalin and were stained with Oil Red O for the revelation of lipid droplets.

For osteogenic differentiation assays, the cells were seeded in collagen 1-coated 12-well plates and were maintained in culture in their respective media under normoxic conditions until 50% confluency was attained. The cells were then transferred and maintained in osteogenic induction medium, consisting of DMEM with 5% HPL, supplemented with 80 μg/mL VitCp, 5 mM β-glycerophosphate, and 100 nM dexamethasone. After three weeks of induction, the cells were fixed in 4% formalin and stained with Alizarin Red.

For chondrogenic differentiation assays, $5 \times 10^5$ cells were transferred in 15 mL tubes and were centrifuged for 5 min at 500× *g*. The formed cell pellets were then maintained in chondrogenic induction medium, consisting of DMEM supplemented with ITS II 1×, 100 nM dexamethasone, 10 ng/mL TGF-β3, and 82 μg/mL VitCp. The cell pellets were maintained in normoxic conditions for 4 weeks with medium exchanges performed three times per week before fixation in 4% formalin. Following sample inclusion and histology slide preparation, staining with Alcian Blue, anti-ACAN, and anti-collagen 2 antibodies was performed (Musculoskeletal Research Unit, University of Zurich, Zurich, Switzerland).

#### 2.4.4. β-Galactosidase Staining for In Vitro Cell Senescence Assessment

From a first safety evaluation standpoint, the β-galactosidase assay was retained in order to confirm that the FE002-Disc cells possess limited proliferation potential and become senescent over in vitro passaging (i.e., limited proliferation lifespan, excludes tumor cell behavior). Therefore, proliferating cells at passage levels 7 and 14 were fixed for 5 min in fixation solution (i.e., 1.85% formaldehyde with 0.2% glutaraldehyde) and were then rinsed with PBS 1×. Staining was performed at 37 °C with a SA-β-gal staining solution, consisting of 0.1% X-gal, 5 mM potassium ferrocyanide, 5 mM potassium ferricyanide, 150 mM NaCl, and 2 mM $MgCl_2$ in a 40 mM citric acid/sodium phosphate solution at pH 6.0. Following overnight staining, the cells were washed, and the presence of β-galactosidase-positive (i.e., blue staining) cells was observed microscopically. Random field imaging (n = 8) was performed in contrast phase microscopy, and operator enumeration of senescent cells was performed.

#### 2.4.5. Telomerase Activity Quantification for In Vitro Tumorigenicity Assessment

From a second safety evaluation standpoint, an in vitro telomerase activity quantification assay was performed in order to confirm that the FE002-Disc cells present low levels of telomerase activity as compared to the tumorigenic HeLa cells. Therefore, a qPCR telomerase activity quantification kit was used to determine the relative level of telomerase activity in the samples. HeLa cells were used as positive controls, and FE002-Cart.Art cells were used as negative controls. The assay was performed according to the instructions of the manufacturer, wherein frozen dry cell pellets were used as starting materials. Cell lysis was performed by adding lysis buffer supplemented with PMSF and β-mercaptoethanol to the pellets, followed by a 30 min incubation on wet ice. The samples were centrifuged at 12,000× *g* at 4 °C for 20 min, and the supernatants were transferred to new Eppendorf tubes. For telomerase activity detection, the samples, telomerase reaction buffer, and nuclease-free water were mixed and incubated at 37 °C for 3 h. The reaction was quenched by heating the samples at 85 °C for 10 min. The qPCR reactions were prepared by mixing the quenched samples, primers, TaqGreen qPCR master mix, and nuclease-free water. The qPCR run conditions comprised an initial denaturation step of 10 min at 95 °C and 36 amplification cycles (i.e., denaturation over 20 s at 95 °C; annealing over 20 s at 52 °C; extension over 45 s at 72 °C). The samples were run in triplicate. Resulting Ct values > 33 were assessed as being negative. Relative telomerase activity quantification between the HeLa cells and the included primary cells was based on the $2^{-\Delta\Delta Ct}$ calculation method.

#### 2.4.6. Soft Agarose Colony Formation Assay for In Vitro Semi-Quantitative Tumorigenicity Assessment

From a third safety evaluation standpoint, a standard soft agarose cell colony formation assay was used to assess the potential of the FE002-Disc cells to proliferate in non-adherent settings (i.e., a characteristic of tumoral cells). The assays were performed in triplicate in 24-well microplates. The solid agarose layer (i.e., bottom layer) was composed of 0.6% agarose in PBS- and FBS-supplemented growth medium with 1% penicillin-streptomycin. The soft agarose layer (i.e., top layer) was composed of 0.4% agarose and contained the investigated cellular materials (i.e., 500–$10^4$ viable cells/well). The cells had been freshly harvested from confluent cultures. CMtc with 1% penicillin-streptomycin was added on top of the soft agarose layer, and the assay plates were incubated at 37 °C under 5% $CO_2$ (i.e., normoxic and hypoxic conditions) in a humidified incubator for 21 days. The plates were regularly microscopically assessed, and representative imaging was performed (i.e., days 1, 4, 7, 21) to comparatively assess the formation of non-adherent cell colonies.

#### 2.4.7. Timecourse of HIF-1 Induction with Western Blotting Readout

The hypoxic incubation condition retained for this study (i.e., 2% $O_2$ level) was designed to mimick the local hypoxic environment of the IVD structure. In order to assess the impact of incubation condition modification (i.e., from normoxia during the cell amplification phase to hypoxia for the subsequent spheroid manufacturing phase), a HIF-1 induction assay was performed on cell monolayers. Therefore, FE002-Disc cells at passage level 6 were thawed, seeded in 6-cm culture dishes at $3 \times 10^3$ cells/cm$^2$ in CMtc, and maintained in normoxic conditions. When the cells reached 90% confluency, the plates were transferred in hypoxic culture conditions. The cells were then lysed in RIPA lysis buffer supplemented with proteinase inhibitors at different time points and were stored at –20 °C until analysis. Total protein levels in the samples were quantified using a BCA assay. Then, 10 µg of total protein/sample were separated by electrophoresis on 4–12% Bis-tris polyacrylamide gels and were transferred onto a nitrocellulose membrane. The membrane was incubated overnight at 4 °C with primary anti-HIF-1α (BD Biosciences, Franklin Lakes, NJ, USA) and anti-actin (Thermo Fisher Scientific) antibodies. The following day, the membrane was incubated with the corresponding secondary antibody (i.e., anti-mouse-HRP or anti-rabbit-HRP). Revelation was performed with the ECL™ Prime chemiluminescence detection system.

#### 2.4.8. Inflammatory Challenge Assays

In order to assess the behavior and resilience of the FE002-Disc cells in inflammatory environments (e.g., degenerating IVDs), an in vitro inflammatory challenge assay was performed. Therefore, FE002-Disc cells at passage level 5 were seeded at $5 \times 10^3$ cells/cm$^2$ in 24-well plates. The cells were maintained in CMtc in normoxic or hypoxic conditions. After 8 days in culture, the medium was replaced by CMtc supplemented with TNF-α at doses ranging from 0 to 100 ng/mL. The assay plates were incubated again for 24 h. Then, cellular morphology was recorded, and the levels of IL-6 and IL-8 secretion in the assay medium were determined by ELISA (Peprotech, Cranbury, NJ, USA).

### 2.5. FE002-Disc Cell Spheroid Manufacture Optimization and Functional Controls

Therapeutic cell-based products (i.e., cell suspensions or cell spheroids) have been studied for intra-NP delivery in IVD affections. Using the FE002-Disc cellular active substance, finished product prototypes in the form of chondrogenically induced cell spheroids were manufactured, controlled, and optimized for quality and function (e.g., aggrecan deposition and collagen II expression), as described in the following sub-sections.

#### 2.5.1. Cell Spheroid Manufacture under Hypoxia

From a function-oriented manufacturing optimization standpoint, the effects of the chondrogenic induction medium composition and incubation atmosphere on cell spheroid formation were assessed. Therefore, FE002-Disc cells were seeded in cell-repellent 96-well plates using 20–40 $\times$ $10^3$ cells per well and spontaneously formed cell spheroids overnight. The spheroids were maintained in CMtc or in chondrogenic differentiation medium variants (i.e., dexamethasone concentrations of 1–100 nM) and in normoxic or hypoxic conditions. The plates were maintained in culture for three weeks with medium exchanges performed three times per week. Microscopic imaging was performed once a week (i.e., documenting spheroid size evolution over time).

#### 2.5.2. Cell Spheroid Cryopreservation and Lyophilization

In order to potentially obtain off-the-freezer or off-the-shelf spheroid formulations, pilot cryopreservation and lyophilization protocols were investigated. Therefore, large FE002-Disc spheroid batches were prepared with a chondrogenic induction period of three weeks. For the cryopreservation arm, groups of 4 spheroids were suspended in cryotubes in a freezing solution composed of 50% CMtc, 40% FBS, and 10% DMSO. Controlled-rate freezing was performed in a CoolCELL device placed at −80 °C overnight, followed by transfer to liquid nitrogen storage. For the lyophilization arm, groups of 4 spheroids were suspended in 2R clear glass vials in a lyopreservation solution composed of 8% $m/v$ saccharose and 2% $m/v$ dextran 40,000 in a buffered injection-grade solvent. Freezing was performed overnight at −20 °C. Primary drying was performed overnight at a product temperature of 7 °C under 0.08 mbar. Secondary drying was then performed for 6 h at a product temperature of 30 °C under 0.01 mbar. The lyophilized samples were sealed and stored at 4 °C until use.

#### 2.5.3. DMMB Quantification for Assessment of ECM Deposition

From a first chondrogenic function assessment viewpoint, total GAG deposition in the spheroids was quantified using a DMMB kit according to the manufacturer's protocol. Briefly, 4 spheroids were harvested for each condition, washed once with PBS, and were incubated for 3 h in papain digestion buffer until complete lysis. The samples were centrifuged at 10,000 rpm for 10 min, and the supernatants were transferred into new Eppendorf tubes. Total GAG precipitation was obtained by mixing the samples or standard with the dye reagent, followed by 30 min of incubation at ambient temperature. The samples were then centrifuged at 12,000 rpm for 10 min and were carefully inverted to discard all the supernatant. A dissociation reagent was added to the GAG pellets to release the dye, and the samples were vortexed until complete dye dissociation. The samples were centrifuged at 12,000 rpm for 5 min. Finally, 100 µL of standard or sample were transferred to 96-well plates, and the absorbance value was measured at a wavelength of 656 nm. Total GAG contents in the samples were determined using a dye standard curve.

#### 2.5.4. Western Blotting and Immunohistology for Specific ECM Component Visualization

From a second chondrogenic function assessment viewpoint, cartilage oligomeric matrix protein (COMP) expression evaluation in the spheroids was performed by Western blotting. Therefore, 4 spheroids for each condition were pooled, treated with RIPA lysis buffer supplemented with protease inhibitors, and sonicated. The samples were then incubated for 15 min on wet ice, centrifuged at 13,000 rpm for 5 min, and the supernatants were transferred into new Eppendorf tubes. The samples were then separated by electrophoresis on 4–12% Bis-tris polyacrylamide gels and were transferred onto nitrocellulose membranes. The membranes were incubated overnight at 4 °C with the primary anti-COMP (Abcam, Cambridge, UK) and anti-actin (Abcam) antibodies. The following day, the membranes were incubated with the anti-rabbit-HRP secondary antibody. Revelation was performed with the ECL™ Prime chemiluminescence detection system.

From a third chondrogenic function assessment viewpoint, ECM components of the spheroids were evidenced using direct staining and immunohistology. Therefore, at the end of the manufacturing phase, the spheroids were harvested and fixed overnight at 4 °C in a 4% formalin solution. The samples were then rinsed three times with PBS and were transferred to 70% EtOH at 4 °C until inclusion in paraffin. Thin 5-μm sections were cut and stained for ECM components (e.g., ACAN, COL2).

### 2.6. Statistical Analysis and Data Presentation

For the statistical comparison of average values from two sets of data, a paired Student's $t$-test was applied, following an appropriate evaluation of the normal distribution of the data. A $p$-value $< 0.05$ was specified for statistical significance determination. The calculations and data presentation were performed using Microsoft Excel v16.0, Microsoft PowerPoint v16.0 (Microsoft Corporation, Redmond, WA, USA), and GraphPad Prism version 8.0.2 (GraphPad Software, San Diego, CA, USA). Physical descriptions of the spheroid parameters (e.g., circularity, roundness, Feret's diameter) were calculated using the ImageJ software v1.54k (National Institutes of Health, Bethesda, MD, USA).

## 3. Results

### 3.1. Identity and Compositional Attributes of the FE002-Disc Progenitor Cell Source

As the FE002-Disc cell source was not previously extensively characterized, the first area of experimental interest from an identity standpoint consisted in cell surface markers. Therein, FE002-Disc cells presented a panel of cell surface markers similar to that of the previously published FE002-Cart.Art cell source, but also to the FACS profiles described for NPSCs [35,36]. Specifically, FE002-Disc cells were found to be positive for CD73, CD90, CD105, CD26, CD44, CD166, and HLA-ABC markers (Table S1). Furthermore, they were negative for the endothelial cell marker CD34 and for the immune cell markers CD19, CD45, CD14, and HLA-DPQR (Table S1). Of note, no difference in cell surface marker expression was evidenced between cell culture conditions (i.e., normoxic versus hypoxic cell expansions, Table S1). Globally, the obtained FACS data confirmed that the FE002-Disc cells were close to alternative progenitor or stem cell sources in terms of surface marker expression while presenting an appropriate immunological profile for therapeutic allogeneic applications (Table S1) [35,36].

From an active substance composition and function standpoint, the FE002-Disc cell source was investigated using proteomic analyses. Importantly, one of the predominantly described mechanisms of action (MoA) for cell-based therapies is the paracrine effect of the transplanted cells [37–39]. Thus, multiplex analyses were performed on cell lysate soluble fractions in order to identify potentially active proteins/factors to be used as biochemical markers. The samples were analyzed using kits targeting MMPs/TIMPS, angiogenesis and growth factors, TGF-β, cytokines, chemokines, and soluble cytokine receptors. The most abundant proteins belonged to the MMP/TIMPs, growth factors, and soluble receptor families (Table S2). Furthermore, the investigated soluble fractions contained only low amounts of cytokines and chemokines (Table S2). Interestingly, no $\log_{10}$ difference between normoxia and hypoxia culture conditions was evidenced for these proteinic targets (Table S2).

From a more detailed mechanistic breakdown viewpoint, several identified components of the cellular active substance were found to be relevant in an IVD treatment context, as detailed hereafter (Table S2). Notably, increased MMP levels were evidenced in cases of degenerated IVD [12]. Conversely, TIMPs are known to be expressed at low levels in non-degenerated IVD tissue [12]. Thus, the presence of TIMPs in therapeutic biological formulations may participate in the regulation of endogenous MMPs for reduction of ECM degradation. Similarly, the in vivo therapeutic use of HGF was reported to alter matrix catabolism but without promoting anabolism [16]. Of note, IL-6 is upregulated in degenerated IVDs; therefore, downregulation of IL-6 signaling by sgp130 could potentially reduce the degenerative process (Table S2). Furthermore, sTNFR (i.e., natural TNF scavenger) may help to regulate the negative effects (e.g., induced production of MMPs and ILs, cellular apoptosis) of overexpressed TNF in IVD affections [40]. Overall, while proteomic composition is a highly limited functional proxy for cell therapies and tissue engineering products, the presence of factors and proteins with confirmed roles in IVD pathophysiology was interpreted positively from a quality standpoint (e.g., specific active substance functional markers; Table S2).

### 3.2. In Vitro Lifespan of FE002-Disc Progenitor Cells: Quality-Guided Selection of Appropriate Passage Levels

A major advantage of using an allogeneic therapeutic cell source resides in the possibility of preparing standardized products without the need for patient-specific starting material harvest biopsies. The use of primary cells (e.g., FE002-Disc cell source) inherently implies that a defined in vitro cellular lifespan must be characterized and considered for manufacturing (i.e., cell banking, product formulation) technical specification establishment. In detail, primary cells should not be used as an active substance at advanced in vitro passage levels (i.e., end of production passage levels), where loss of quality and functionality attributes may be expected due to the onset of cellular senescence. Thus, a large portion of manufacturing process development was based on iterative quality and functionality assays, performed throughout the in vitro cellular lifespan of the FE002-Disc cells while using culture condition variants.

The critical parameter linking in vitro cellular lifespan and functional stability attributes of the FE002-Disc cell source was phenotypic stability, or the sensitivity of the cells towards chemical induction. Firstly, two-dimentional osteogenic and adipogenic differentiation assays confirmed that FE002-Disc cells behaved consistently throughout serial subculturing (i.e., passage levels 7–11, Figure 1).

In detail, the FE002-Disc cells were shown to produce no mineralized matrix under osteogenic induction, while strong AR staining was observed in ASC controls after 3 weeks of differentiation (Figure 1A,C). Parallelly, mild lipid droplet accumulation within the primary progenitor cells was observed in adipogenic induction, but to a much lower extent than in the ASC controls (Figure 1B,C). This specific behavior (i.e., consistent throughout passages) was potentially linked to the presence of a small and persistent fraction of adipogenic progenitor cells (i.e., low amount, not capable of osteogenesis in this system) in the considered progenitor cell population. Alternatively and more probably, this behavior may be explained by the known properties of NP cells, which intrinsically present some phenotypic plasticity [41]. Importantly, the absence of phenotypic shifts throughout passages in monolayer adipogenic and osteogenic induction conditions confirmed the stability of the cell population toward adherent state differentiation (Figure 1).

Secondly, the chondrogenic differentiation potential of the FE002-Disc cells and the stability thereof were investigated in a three-dimensional (i.e., cell pellets) chemical induction setup. Therein, the chondrogenic potential of the cellular active substance was confirmed (Figure 2).

Specifically, cell pellets maintained in 3D in chondrogenic induction medium presented GAG accumulation (i.e., AB positive staining) and were positive for ACAN and COL2 deposition, which are characteristic NP proteins (Figure 2). Thus, the cells were found to regain chondrogenic differentiation potential and activity in 3D (e.g., induction and deposition of COL2), which is transiently lost during 2D cell expansion. However, a strong impact of in vitro cell aging (i.e., through serial passaging) was observed on the chondrogenic differentiation potential of the cells. In detail, a reduction in pellet size, a reduction in COL2 and ACAN expression, and a reduction in pellet staining homogeneity were recorded after passage level 7 (Figure 2). Thus, while FE002-Disc cells were shown to proliferate homogeneously in vitro in monolayers at least until passage level 11, the investigated functional attributes technically limited their further use to passage levels ≤ 7 (Figures 1 and 2). Finally, it is noted that the retained readouts and specific stains used in the cellular active substance qualification assays corresponded to the current state-of-the-art of characterization and validation of chondrogenic cells for cell and gene therapies (Figure 2) [42].

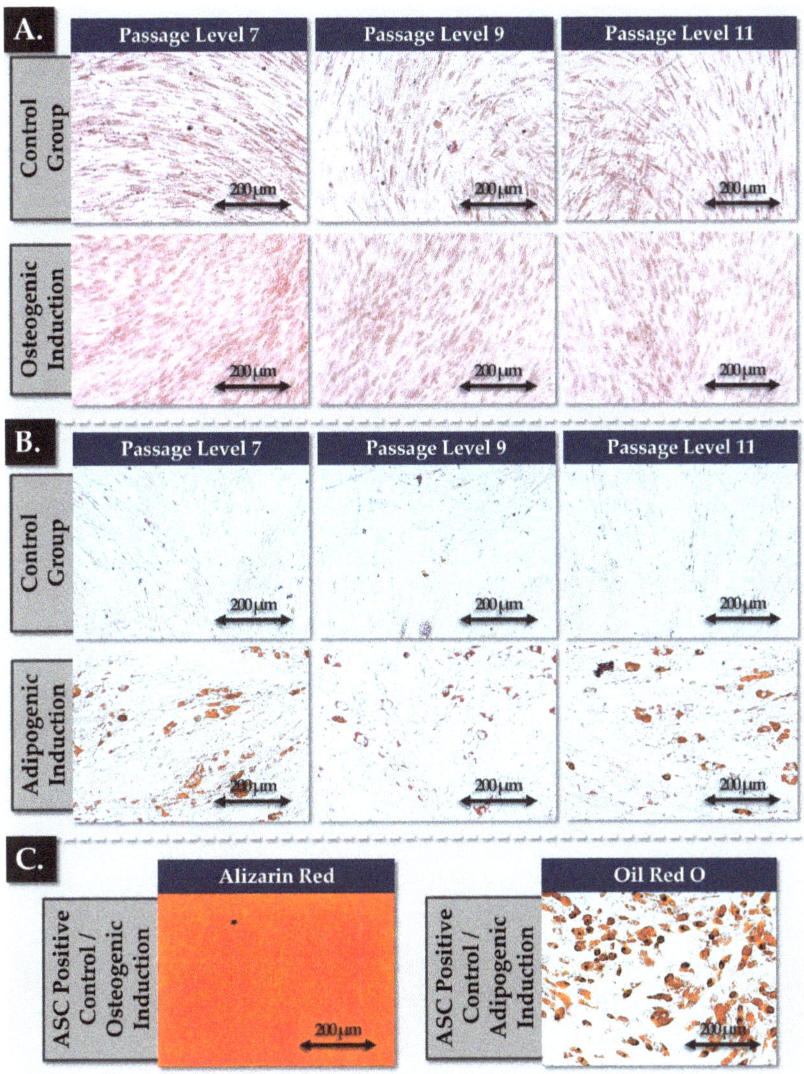


**Figure 1.** Results of iterative FE002-Disc progenitor cell phenotype plasticity assessments in chemical osteogenic and adipogenic induction studies. (**A**) No osteogenic differentiation was observed following Alizarin Red staining. (**B**) Mild adipogenic differentiation (i.e., lipid droplet accumulation upon differentiation in some of the cells in the population but not in all cells) was observed following Oil Red O staining. (**C**) Illustration of positive control groups for osteogenic (Alizarin Red staining, saturated with colorant due to strong cell differentiation) and adipogenic (Oil Red O staining) differentiation, respectively. Positive controls were prepared using ASC cultures, which were submitted to the chemical induction protocols. Scale bars = 200 µm. ASC, adipose stem cells.

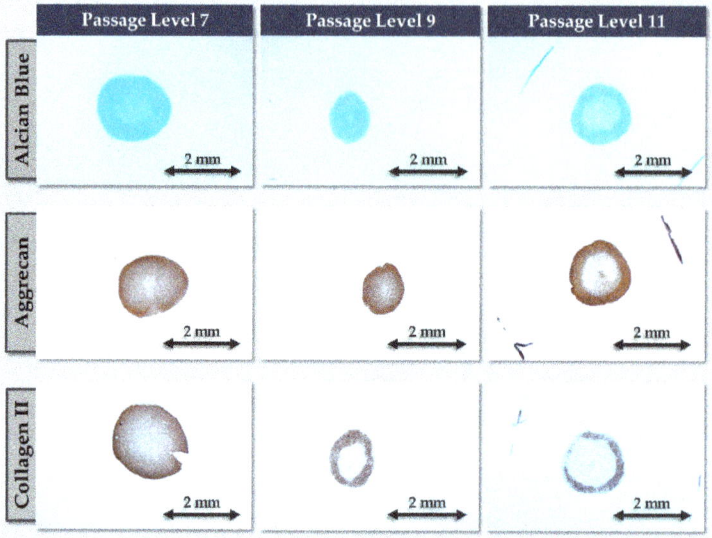


**Figure 2.** Results of iterative FE002-Disc progenitor cell phenotype plasticity assessment in chemical chondrogenic induction studies. The assays were carried out on large cell pellets in order to assess the intrinsic decline in chondrogenic potential over passage levels. Positive chondrogenic differentiation was observed throughout passages following staining of standard markers of cartilage ECM components (i.e., Alcian Blue staining for GAGs or immunohistochemical staining for aggrecan and collagen II). Scale bars = 2 mm. ECM, extracellular matrix; GAG, glycosaminoglycan.

### *3.3. FE002-Disc Progenitor Cell Resilience in Hypoxic and Inflammatory Environments*

The degenerative IVD environment is known to be particularly harsh, with low oxygen and nutrient supplies, inflamed and acidic microenvironments, and important biomechanical constraints [9,24,25]. Therefore, several in vitro experiments were performed in order to assess the resilience of FE002-Disc cells placed in artificially challenging conditions. Such assays aimed to preliminarily determine if the considered progenitor cells were capable of withstanding hypoxic or inflamed environments.

The choice was made to work in a hypoxic environment in the present study in order to approximate the native physiological environment of the IVD cells. Specifically, the human IVD is avascular, resulting in an $O_2$ gradient from the disc exterior region to the disc interior region (i.e., $O_2$ levels reaching down to 1%) [43]. Furthermore, as in vitro hypoxic studies are often conducted between 1–5% $O_2$, the value of 2% $O_2$ was selected herein as a standardized condition in order to mimic a relatively strong hypoxia level that is coherent with physiological tissues [43]. The anticipated effect of hypoxia as regards the behavior of the FE002-Disc cells was initially a reduction of cellular proliferation or function, based on the reduced availability of oxygen, similar to native IVD tissue.

Firstly, the effects of hypoxic incubation conditions on FE002-Disc cell survival and cell proliferation were quantified. Therefore, good monolayer cell adhesion and cellular proliferative morphology were observed in hypoxic culture conditions as compared to normoxic controls (Figure S1). No apparent cell death (i.e., abnormal morphology, cell detachment) or distress was recorded, and cell proliferation was statistically significantly higher in hypoxic environments as compared to normoxia until day 6 of culture (Figures 3A and S1).

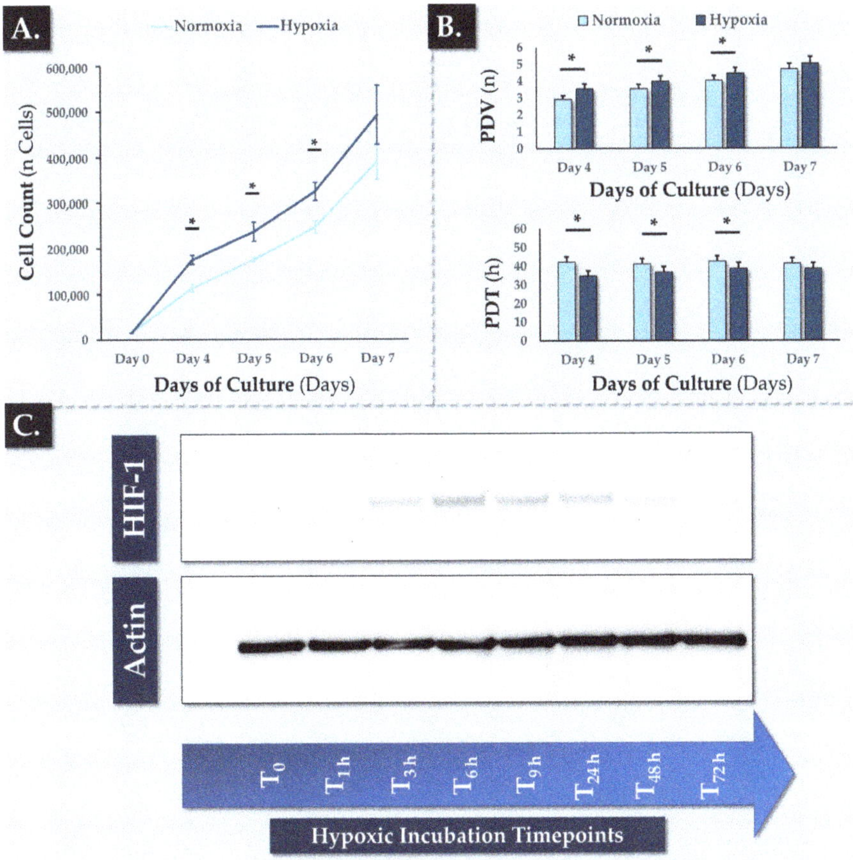


**Figure 3.** Results of FE002-Disc progenitor cell biological responses to hypoxic incubation conditions (i.e., 2% $O_2$). (**A**) Comparative growth curves revealed significantly enhanced cellular proliferation in hypoxic conditions compared to normoxic conditions. (**B**) The significant increase (i.e., $p$-value < 0.05, identified by an asterisk "*") in cellular proliferation under hypoxia was confirmed by analysis of the population doubling values and population doubling times. (**C**) Results of a timecourse HIF-1 detection assay with Western blot revelation. Transient HIF-1 induction was recorded during the first days of primary progenitor cell incubation in a hypoxic environment. Whole-gel imaging is presented in Figure S2. HIF, hypoxia-inducible factor; PDT, population doubling time; PDV, population doubling value.

Of note, no statistically significant differences were found between the groups at the final timepoint of the assay (i.e., day 7 of culture), which was linked to the presence of confluent cells in the hypoxic group (Figure 3A,B). This factor probably inhibited the cellular proliferation for hypoxic cultures, while normoxic cultures were still sub-confluent at the 7-day timepoint. Namely, once the cells reached confluency, their proliferation probably slowed, this event occurring earlier for the hypoxic condition. From a biochemical standpoint, the FE002-Disc cells, which were maintained in normoxia, did not express HIF-1, as expected (Figure 3C). However, cell exposure to hypoxia led to a rapid response by stabilizing the HIF-1$\alpha$ protein and inducing signaling cascades. Consequently, HIF-1 expression was detected as early as 1 h following cell culture transfer from normoxia to hypoxia (Figure 3C). Globally, HIF-1 induction was recorded to be transient, as a progressive reduction in HIF-1 expression was observed after 48 h and 72 h of culture in hypoxia (Figure 3C).

As previously mentioned, inflammation is a hallmark of the degenerative IVD environment [44,45]. Therefore, therapeutic cells of cell-based constructs are mandatorily exposed to such adverse stimuli following transplantation. The resilience and behavior of the FE002-Disc cells were thus experimentally studied in an in vitro model of inflammation. Progenitor FE002-Disc cells were treated with increasing doses of TNF-α (i.e., up to 100 ng/mL) for 24 h and were maintained in normoxic or hypoxic conditions. Cellular morphology was recorded, and the secretion of IL-6 and IL-8 by the cells was quantified by ELISA (Figure 4).

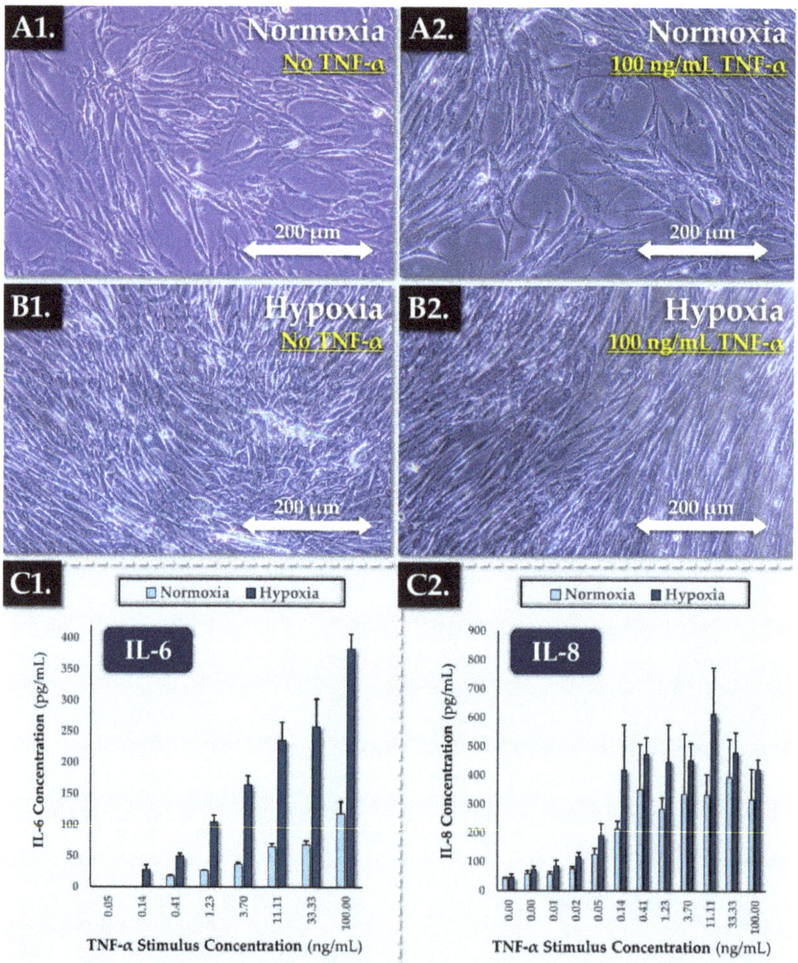


**Figure 4.** Results of FE002-Disc progenitor cell biological responses to a chemical inflammatory stimulus in normoxic and hypoxic culture conditions. (**A1**,**A2**) Normal cellular morphology (i.e., absence of toxicity signs) following expansion in normoxia, with and without TNF-α stimulation. Scale bars = 200 μm. (**B1**,**B2**) Normal cellular morphology (i.e., absence of toxicity signs) following expansion in hypoxia, with and without TNF-α stimulation. Scale bars = 200 μm. (**C1**,**C2**) ELISA-based quantification of total IL-6 and IL-8 following TNF-α stimulation of cells expanded in normoxia and in hypoxia, respectively. IL, interleukin; TNF, tumor necrosis factor.

In detail, the goal of the assay was to determine the cells' behavior upon exposure to TNF, which was retained as a proxy for the hostile environment of the degenerated IVD. Specifically, TNF (i.e., multifunctional pro-inflammatory factor) is an activator of IVD degeneration (e.g., inflammatory response, cellular apoptosis). Indeed, TNF levels are increased in the nucleus pulposus of patients with degenerating IVDs, and it promotes the progression of the disease [46]. Notably, TNF injection in a porcine intervertebral disc model led to degenerative changes in the disc (i.e., decreased disc height, formation of fissures) [46].

Importantly, no changes in cellular morphology and no cellular detachment were observed after 24 h of TNF-α treatment in both incubation conditions, as observed in microscopy images of the cells (Figure 4A,B). In the absence of TNF-α treatment, no IL-6 secretion was observed, while basal IL-8 levels were already detected (Figure 4(C1,C2)). Furthermore, TNF-α stimulation was shown to induce IL-6 and IL-8 secretion in a dose-dependent manner (Figure 4C). In the TNF-α-stimulated groups, no shift in the IL induction curves was observed between normoxic and hypoxic culture conditions (Figure 4C). Of note, the absolute values of IL-6 and IL-8 in the hypoxic condition may have partly resulted from the increased cellular proliferation induced by hypoxia or from cellular potentiation by hypoxia (Figure 4C). Specifically, as the absolute values of secreted IL probably resulted from a complex effect (i.e., presence of more cells in the hypoxic group, presence of metabolically different cells in the hypoxic group), the normalization of IL levels to the cell counts was not performed. Thus, the observed increase in IL-6 and IL-8 levels could not be individually and directly attributed to the use of hypoxic incubation conditions versus the use of normoxic incubation conditions in this experimental setup (Figure 4C). Notwithstanding, TNF stimulation resulted in statistically significant (i.e., $p$-value < 0.05) increases in IL-6 and IL-8 levels in the assay cultures at all tested concentration ranges (Figure 4C).

Finally, even though $EC_{50}$ values could not be experimentally calculated for IL-6 (i.e., the upper plateau was not defined), it was apparent that the IL-8 $EC_{50}$ value was inferior to that of IL-6 (Figure 4C). Globally, the obtained datasets confirmed that the FE002-Disc cells were resilient in models of hypoxic environment and inflammation (Figures 3 and 4). Such attributes were interpreted positively from a physiological function viewpoint for IVD progenitor cells and from a therapeutic standpoint in view of cell implantation in adverse in vivo microenvironments.

### 3.4. FE002-Disc Progenitor Cell Source In Vitro Safety Characterization

The therapeutic use of viable exogeneous cells or cell-based products inherently comports a risk of adverse effects, among which the formation of tumors. Therefore, thorough preclinical safety evaluation of specific cell sources is a prerequisite for any therapeutic product development process, especially for substantially manipulated materials (e.g., culture-expanded cells). For preliminary safety evaluation of the FE002-Disc cell source and following the principle of 3R rules, multiparametric in vitro analyses were performed [47].

Firstly, the FE002-Disc cell source was confirmed to possess a finite in vitro lifespan by experimental verification of cellular senescence attainment over serial passaging. A significant increase in cell PDT was observed between passage levels 6 and 13 (i.e., 92.4 h versus 66.7 h), along with a corresponding decrease in PDV (i.e., 3.60 versus 4.97).

Secondly, β-galactosidase staining demonstrated a statistically significant increase in the presence of senescent cells (i.e., positive blue cells) at high passage levels as compared to lower cell passage levels (i.e., 12.1% positive cells at passage level 6, 44.9% positive cells at passage level 13). Of note, no significant differences were outlined in terms of cellular senescence between the normoxic and the hypoxic culture conditions (Figure S3).

Thirdly, telomerase activity was quantified in FE002-Disc cells and was compared to that of the cancerous HeLa cell line (i.e., positive control) and that of FE002-Cart.Art cells (i.e., negative control). Experimentally, telomerase activity was detected in both of the included progenitor cell types but to a much lower extent than in HeLa cells (Figure S4).

In detail, FE002-Disc cells presented telomerase activity levels higher than those of FE002-Cart.Art cells but similar to those of FE002-Ten primary progenitor tenocytes [34,48]. As no in vivo adverse effects (i.e., specifically with regard to tumor formation) were reported for both the FE002-Cart.Art and the FE002-Ten cells, the obtained telomerase activity data for the FE002-Disc cells was considered to meet expectations from a safety viewpoint [34,48].

Finally, soft agarose colony formation assays were performed in order to experimentally exclude the presence of tumorigenic behavior of the FE002-Disc cells in non-adherent culture conditions. Therein, positive control HeLa cells showed rapid colony formation and colony growth already at day 7 after cell seeding (Figure S5C). Namely, the HeLa cultures were stopped at day 14, as the cell colonies were becoming too large for the retained model. Conversely, no colony formation was observed in the FE002-Disc progenitor cell groups (i.e., normoxia and hypoxia conditions), even though ten times more cells were seeded per well (Figure S5A,B).

Overall, the presented safety-related experiments confirmed that the FE002-Disc cells reached senescence over serial in vitro passaging, presented low levels of telomerase activity, and were incapable of anchorage-independent cellular proliferation. While further in vivo tumorigenicity experiments are warranted to confirm the preclinical safety of the FE002-Disc cell source, the compiled in vitro data reported herein does not exclude such biological materials from further translational research based on safety-related attributes.

### 3.5. FE002-Disc Cell Spheroid Formulation Process and Function-Guided Optimization

Based notably on the use of spheroids/microtissues for the treatment of knee cartilage defects, several similar formulations were studied for IVD applications [49–54]. This approach is notably set forth to protect the transplanted cells in the adverse target implantation environment, as well as to directly supplement the administration site with exogeneous ECM (e.g., ACAN, COL2) [52,55,56]. Therefore, based on the functional and safety data gathered on the FE002-Disc cells in monolayer culture (i.e., cellular active substance), three-dimensional finished product prototypes in the form of cell spheroids were prepared and studied. Experiments were based on the reported effects of medium composition and incubation conditions on the chondrogenic potential of expanded articular chondrocytes [57–62].

Preliminary experiments demonstrated that the FE002-Disc progenitor cells could spontaneously form cell spheroids in low-attachment plates (Figure S6). Therein, the cell spheroids were maintained in culture for 14 days in normoxic or hypoxic environments and in the presence of complete growth medium or chondrogenic induction medium. The most significant increase in spheroid size over time was observed during the second week of culture, when chondrogenic medium and hypoxia culture conditions were combined (Figure S6B). Thus, for all further assays, the use of chondrogenic medium and hypoxic incubation conditions was retained.

Once the basic spheroid formulation process was established, further function-based optimization campaigns were carried out. Firstly, the dexamethasone concentration in the chondrogenic induction medium was optimized. Therein, a macroscopic increase in spheroid size was recorded across all groups between days 6–20, but the 1 nM and 100 nM dexamethasone concentrations tended to yield smaller spheroids (Figure 5A).

From a specific quantitative standpoint, cartilage oligomeric matrix protein (COMP) endpoint expression in the spheroids was strongly reduced when 1 nM dexamethasone was used, but it was otherwise consistent (Figure 5B). Of note, COMP is an ECM glycoprotein originally identified in cartilage and which plays a notable role in chondrogenesis [63]. For a broader quantitative overview of the deposited ECM in the studied spheroids, total GAG quantification was performed. The results showed that GAG contents were influenced by the dexamethasone concentration, where the highest GAG content was observed with 25 nM dexamethasone (Figure 5C). Specifically, the statistical analysis revealed that the GAG contents were significantly higher (i.e., $p$-value $< 0.05$) at 25 nM compared to 100 nM and significantly lower (i.e., $p$-value $< 0.05$) at 1 and 10 nM compared to 100 mM (Figure 5C).

However, reducing the dexamethasone to concentrations as low as 1 nM still resulted in relatively high GAG contents, suggesting that the standard dexamethasone concentration (i.e., 100 nM) could be reduced in the spheroid production process (e.g., 1–25 nM).

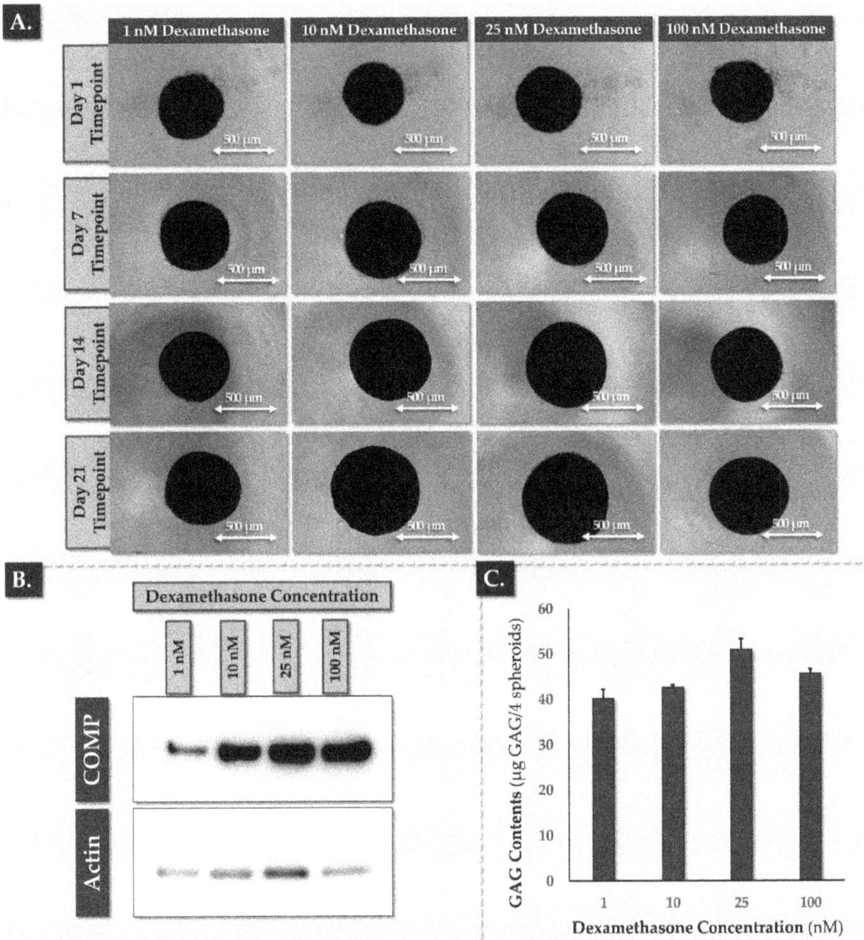


**Figure 5.** Results of FE002-Disc progenitor cell spheroid functional optimization assays, with comparative multiparametric assessment of various dexamethasone concentrations in the chondrogenic induction medium. (**A**) Comparative macroscopic assessment of the effect of dexamethasone concentration on cell spheroid size and morphology at various timepoints. Scale bars = 500 µm. (**B**) Comparative endpoint assessment of the effect of various dexamethasone concentrations on the endpoint expression level of COMP, with Western blot revelation. Whole-gel imaging is presented in Figure S7. (**C**) Comparative endpoint assessment of the effect of various dexamethasone concentrations on the quantity of total GAGs in the cell spheroids. COMP, cartilage oligomeric matrix protein; GAG, glycosaminoglycans.

From a physical characterization viewpoint, analysis of the spheroids produced with 10 and 100 nM dexamethasone (i.e., optimized condition and reference condition, respectively) indicated that the area of the spheroids and their Feret's diameter increased over time in culture and that appropriate circularity and roundness values were consistently obtained (Table 1).

**Table 1.** Physical characterization results of FE002-Disc spheroids produced with 10 nM and 25 nM dexamethasone, as presented in Figure 5.

| Parameter | Circularity | | Feret's Diameter (mm) | | Roundness | |
|---|---|---|---|---|---|---|
| **Dexamethasone Concentration (nM)** | **10 nM** | **100 nM** | **10 nM** | **100 nM** | **10 nM** | **100 nM** |
| D7 Timepoint | 0.47 ± 0.12 | 0.56 ± 0.10 | 0.98 ± 0.05 | 0.97 ± 0.02 | 0.95 ± 0.02 | 0.96 ± 0.01 |
| D14 Timepoint | 0.42 ± 0.16 | 0.46 ± 0.08 | 1.09 ± 0.02 | 1.08 ± 0.05 | 0.96 ± 0.02 | 0.97 ± 0.02 |
| D21 Timepoint | 0.51 ± 0.08 | 0.54 ± 0.08 | 1.19 ± 0.02 | 1.24 ± 0.10 | 0.96 ± 0.01 | 0.88 ± 0.05 |

The results presented in Figure 5 confirmed that the dexamethasone concentration in the chondrogenic induction medium impacted COMP expression and GAG contents, but these quantitative analyses did not allow to evaluate the quality (e.g., homogeneity) of matrix deposition in the considered spheroids. Therefore, histology was performed to observe ECM deposition. Therein, all dexamethasone concentrations resulted in strong endpoint AB and ACAN staining throughout the spheroids (Figure 6).

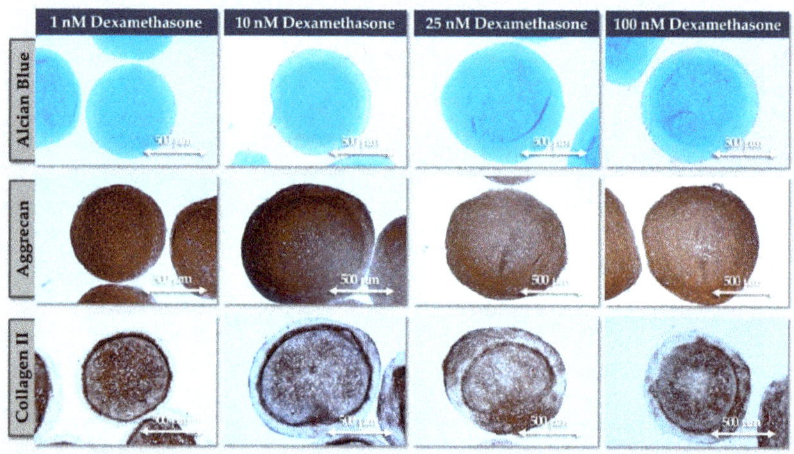


**Figure 6.** Results of FE002-Disc progenitor cell spheroid functional optimization assays, with comparative endpoint histological assessment of various dexamethasone concentrations in the chondrogenic induction medium. Scale bars = 500 µm.

Of note, collagen II was also significantly expressed, but not throughout the spheroids (i.e., formation of an inner matrix-rich core surrounded by a dense cellular outer layer; Figure 6). Importantly, COL2 deposition was affected by the dexamethasone concentration, where a better homogeneity of staining was recorded with reduced concentrations (i.e., 1–10 nM; Figure 6). Based on the compilation of the obtained functional data for FE002-Disc cell spheroid formulation, a relatively low dose of 10 nM dexamethasone was retained in the chondrogenic induction medium. This choice was based on quantitative aspects of ECM component deposition in the spheroids, as well as qualitative aspects of ECM distribution.

Finally, it is noted that despite the absence of systematic verification of cellular viability throughout the spheroid culture period (e.g., ATP-based assays), the presence of metabolically active and functional cells throughout the culture phase was indirectly confirmed. Namely, the consistent increase in the size of the spheroids over time was due to the synthesis of ECM by viable IVD cells, and strong deposition of ECM components throughout the spheroid body over time was recorded (Figures 5 and 6). Such facts presupposed the presence of viable cells in the spheroids, which are the only effectors capable of producing and structuring ECM in the 3D spheroids. Notwithstanding, validation of endpoint cellular viability maintenance in the spheroids is necessary for a finished product, including following transport and storage, yet the scope of the present work was limited to preclinical safety and function qualification, with functional optimization focusing on the cellular active substance and the in vitro process. Full validation campaigns, including ATP-based assays for release and stability testing, may be the focus of the next step of experimental work, as FE002-Disc cells have been preliminarily qualified herein.

### *3.6. FE002-Disc Progenitor Cell Spheroid Stability in Cryopreservation and Lyopreservation*

In order to preliminarily assess the potential of obtaining off-the-freezer or off-the-shelf FE002-Disc spheroids, two stabilization protocols were evaluated. The results indicated that all samples retained macroscopic structural integrity after freezing and lyophilization processing, respectively. Furthermore, histology readouts showed that no loss of ECM was sustained during freezing or lyophilization. Specifically, the spheroids all stained positive for AB, COL2, and ACAN (Figure 7).

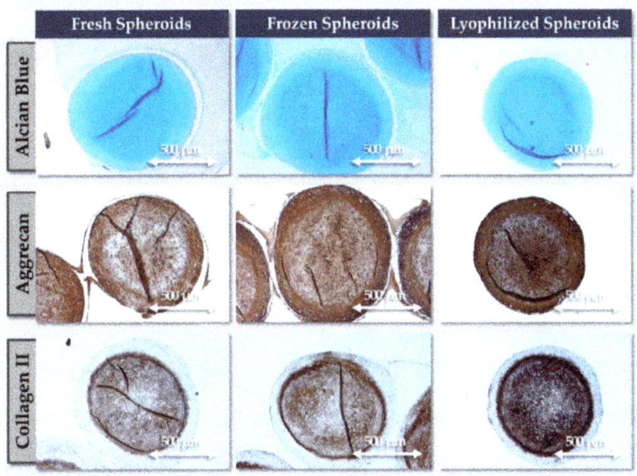


**Figure 7.** Results of FE002-Disc progenitor cell spheroid behavior following cryopreservation and lyopreservation, with histological assessment of critical structural attributes and ECM quality. Cell spheroids were manufactured using 10 nM dexamethasone. Cell spheroids manufactured using 100 nM dexamethasone are represented in Figure S8. Scale bars = 500 µm. ECM, extracellular matrix.

Overall, the functional results obtained with frozen or lyophilized spheroids were interpreted positively from a compositional standpoint (i.e., no deterioration of structure or ECM; Figures 7 and S8). Namely, no adverse effects were recorded in the stabilized groups as regards the quality of the components compared to the freshly harvested spheroids. Such protocols thus bare potential for the formulation of stable and consistent sources of exogeneous ECM components or for the further development of stabilized chondrogenic microtissues. In detail, the conservative nature of the retained pilot stabilization techniques enables us to consider further processing options (e.g., supercritical $CO_2$ decellularization, terminal sterilization) for the investigated biological materials.

## 4. Discussion

### *4.1. Cell Therapies as Promising Contenders for IVD Pathology Management*

The promise of cell-based therapies in IVD degeneration is linked to their multifaceted MoA, which has the potential to address the complexity of disc degeneration [64,65]. Importantly, current conservative treatments help in treating LBP symptoms but do not satisfactorily restore the disc environment, leading to further disc degeneration in the long term. Thus, the goal of cell-based therapies consists in regenerating disc structure or function and reducing LBP in patients. In the available clinical reports, IVD cell therapies were shown to positively impact pain symptoms and reduce disability [66–68]. However, mixed outcomes were reported as regards regenerative aspects (e.g., restoration of IVD height, hydration balance) of the interventions [3,8]. Nonetheless, chondrocytes and IVD cells appear to yield better outcomes for regeneration than alternative biologicals, suggesting that such cell types are better suited for implantation in adverse microenvironments [52–55].

Generally, several hurdles limit the practical identification and benchmarking of optimal cell sources for application in IVD therapies, as the specific MoA are not well-characterized. Selection criteria for therapeutic cellular contenders in investigational IVD treatments are notably based on current in vitro and in vivo data, as follows:

1. Safety attributes: absence of allergic or immunogenic reactions in the host, absence of tumorigenicity,
2. Chondrogenic/discogenic potential: synthesis and deposition of GAGs and collagen II in the implantation environment,
3. Cell sourcing: choice of discogenic cells (e.g., IVD cells, chondrocytes) with potent regeneration capacities and with environment modulatory attributes,
4. Cellular resilience following implantation: in situ resistance to harsh environmental constraints in vivo,
5. Supply chain considerations: allogeneic versus autologous starting biological materials,
6. Adaptability to GMP manufacturing processes: possibility to prepare and formulate therapeutic cells in a clinically deliverable product.

As specifically concerns the option to use allogeneic starting biological materials, more complex qualification steps are required compared to the use of autologous materials (e.g., adventitious agent screening). However, several quality and logistical benefits are procured by the use of allogeneic cell sources, such as reduced variability (i.e., no donor-to-donor influence) and the absence of an invasive harvesting surgery [34]. Based on the criteria and considerations presented hereabove, qualification testing was performed on the FE002-Disc cell source for preliminary demonstration of its applicability in IVD therapeutics.

### 4.2. Adequation of FE002-Disc Progenitor Cells with Cell Therapy Development Schemes

From a cell-based therapeutic product manufacturing standpoint, many elements must be closely considered and documented around the handling of biological materials. These comprise the methodology for qualification of the starting cell source, manufacturing process parameters, technical specifications for the process, and selection of critical materials [33]. Importantly, high scrutiny is allocated toward identifying and managing sources of variability during active substance or drug product manufacture [69]. Design approaches aim to minimize variability and to identify technical alternatives or variants in order to optimize finished product quality and performance [70]. In the respective domains of articular cartilage and IVD cell-based treatments, converging approaches of spheroid implantation in highly demanding host tissues appear most promising [51–54,71–74].

The experimental results gathered herein have notably confirmed the adequation of the FE002-Disc cell source with several requirements of cell therapy translational development. Overall, the investigated functional and safety attributes were assessed as being appropriate for potential formulation and use in IVD applications. Firstly, the sustainability of the cell source (i.e., based on the usable in vitro passage levels) was determined, as the therapeutic use of passage level 6–7 cells would enable to potentially treat thousands of patients. Secondly, the chondrogenic potential of the cells was validated, as effective chondrogenic differentiation (i.e., GAGs and collagen II production) was repeatedly observed (Figures 2 and 6). Furthermore, it was confirmed that the cellular biological activity (i.e., chondrogenic potential) was reduced with in vitro cell aging (Figure 2).

Finally, in vitro cell safety validation was performed using telomerase activity assays, soft agarose assays, and confirmation of the limited lifespan of the primary FE002-Disc cell type. Specifically, the presented safety data were conjointly considered with the previously applied donor qualification panels (e.g., background anamnesis and adventitious agent screens) [33]. Overall, the gathered body of evidence was assessed to qualify the FE002-Disc cell source for further preclinical investigation (e.g., safety and efficacy studies in animal models).

### 4.3. Importance of Therapeutic Cell Resilience in Hypoxic and Inflammatory Environments

Generally, the specific constraints of the IVD implantation environment warrant the technical optimization of the cellular active substance and the finished product form. The degenerative IVD environment is notably hostile, with the absence of perfusion resulting in a hypoxic and glucose-deprived niche. Furthermore, pathological degeneration leads to acidification and inflammatory cytokine release, limiting the potential for exogenous cell survival and engraftment [9,10,75]. From a biological-based formulation viewpoint, integration of anti-inflammatory molecules (e.g., anti-TNF, anti-IL), growth factors, or cell preculture in hypoxia may be considered [76]. A specific difficulty in therapeutic protocol development lies in the sub-optimal modeling of degenerated human IVDs in animal models. Thus, efficiency parameters are often only assessed in human trials. With regard to the composition of the implantation environment, low-glucose and acidic in vitro models may be used to predict in situ cell survival [52,55,56]. Specifically, while the pH in healthy IVDs is neutral (i.e., 6.9–7.2), it drops to 6.0–6.2 in degenerated tissues due to anaerobic glycolysis. It was previously reported that NP stem cells survive better in acidic conditions than ASCs, as acidic conditions reduced cellular proliferation to a greater extent in ASCs [77].

From a more detailed mechanistic and functional viewpoint, nasal chondrocytes were exposed to adverse biochemical cues (i.e., inflammatory and hypoxic conditions) [78]. Therein, IL-1$\beta$ treatment led to catabolic effects, with GAG loss, increased MMP-1 expression, and decreased COL2 [78]. Parallelly, while hypoxic culture conditions did not significantly impact GAGs, increased COL2 levels were evidenced [78]. In further studies, the authors sought an optimal chondrogenic cell source for implantation in IVDs (i.e., maintenance of viability and function in adverse environments) [52]. Therefore, MSCs, articular chondrocytes, and nasal chondrocytes were functionally benchmarked in hypoxic, acidic, inflammatory, and low-glucose conditions. Enhanced survival and ECM deposition of nasal chondrocytes was evidenced in hypoxic/low-glucose conditions, as compared to MSCs and articular chondrocytes [52]. Inflamed environments led to decreased GAG production in MSCs, while this parameter did not negatively impact articular and nasal chondrocytes. In contrast, medium acidification led to a dramatic reduction in GAG production and COL2 induction in all three cell types. Of note, MSCs were more affected than the chondrocytes, as pellets could not form in this environment. Overall, it was shown that MSCs were more vulnerable to harsh environments than articular and nasal chondrocytes, especially regarding chondrogenic properties [52].

Considering the highly specific physiological constraints of degenerative IVDs, various experimental assays were conducted to assess the in situ resilience of the FE002-Disc cells. Experimental designs were based on the references hereabove for articular and nasal chondrocytes. Specifically, it was shown that FE002-Disc cell monolayers were characterized by improved cell proliferation potential in hypoxia compared to normoxia, echoing previous reports on FE002-Ten primary progenitor tenocytes [79]. Furthermore, the present study confirmed that hypoxia (i.e., down to 2% $O_2$) was a positive factor for cellular proliferation and differentiation (Figures 3 and S6). Finally, it was confirmed that FE002-Disc cells were not negatively impacted following exposure to high TNF-$\alpha$ doses (i.e., in normoxia or hypoxia; Figure 4). Overall, this study confirmed that FE002-Disc cells were resilient toward key adverse drivers of IVD microenvironments. In order to further study the resilience of FE002-Disc cells, acidic and glucose-deprived culture conditions could be used to functionally investigate the formation and chondrogenic activity of the cell spheroids, which are expected to present enhanced resistance.

### 4.4. Clinical Advancements of Chondrogenic Cells for IVD Therapy

Due to important scientific interest and high market demand, various therapies and products for IVD treatment have been clinically and commercially brought forward. Notably, these have comprised both autologous and allogeneic therapeutic cell sources, where safety and efficacy data are available. Clinical application of the autologous Novocart DISC Plus product (i.e., expanded cells from herniated disc tissue) aimed to reduce degenerative sequelae following lumbar disk surgery or to prophylactically avoid adjacent disc degeneration [21,66]. The allogeneic MPC-06-ID treatment (i.e., mesenchymal precursor cells, Mesoblast) was reported to be safe and effective in a phase 3 trial with 24 months of follow-up [80]. Specifically, single injections of $6 \times 10^6$ cells resulted in reductions in VAS scores and improved function (i.e., ODI and EQ-5D indexes), most probably through paracrine anti-inflammatory effects.

In another clinical trial on 182 patients, Vivex Biologics investigated the intradiscal delivery (i.e., 20 G spine needle) of allogeneic NP matrix, showing improved VASPI and ODI scores at 12 months (i.e., 54% pain improvement, 53% ODI improvement) [81]. An allogeneic discogenic cell-based approach (i.e., rebonuputemcel, DiscGenics) was tested in early or moderate degenerative IVD cases [68,72]. From a formulation viewpoint, it was shown that fresh and frozen injectable cell-based products could both be effectively used in vivo [67]. Importantly, dosing considerations indicated that lower doses of cells were therapeutically preferrable, possibly due to the adverse impacts of large numbers of apoptotic cells in situ [67]. For rebonuputemcel, phase 3 clinical results were reported in 2023, with improvements in low back pain, function, disc volume, and patient quality of life [82]. Optimal results were obtained with doses of $9 \times 10^6$ cells/mL in hyaluronic acid and cryopreservation excipients, with clinical benefit maintenance after two years [82]. Finally, various alternative clinical-stage examples of cell-based treatments for IVD applications may be set forth, such as CordSTEM-DD (i.e., allogeneic umbilical cord-derived mesenchymal stem cells, CHABiotech), BRTX-100 (i.e., autologous stem cells, BioRestorative), or the RESPINE EU project (i.e., allogeneic BM-MSC) [83–87].

### 4.5. Cell Formulation Optimization for Injectable IVD Treatments

Based on the technical considerations presented hereabove and on the clinical requirements of IVD cases, adaptation of the therapeutic cell formulation attributes may be necessary. Specifically, manufacturing process variants may be used for a given cell source based on the target functional attributes of the implanted materials. The first approach (i.e., technically simpler) consists in the formulation of the expanded cells in suspension form (i.e., with liquid or gel vehicles). Therein, manufacturing processes are notably faster, easier to scale up, and do not require chemical induction. However, this approach is limited by the fact that the cells are dedifferentiated (i.e., no COL2 expression), most sensitive to the harsh implantation environment, and subject to potential cell leakage out of the treated IVD. A potential mitigation measure could consist in the injection of discogenic cells under an appropriate matrix or scaffold, similarly to existing clinical practice in knee articular cartilage chondrotherapy [21,56].

The second approach, which was experimentally retained herein, consists in the generation of chondrogenically matured three-dimensional constructs (i.e., cell spheroids). Specifically, in addition to the selection of a robust therapeutic cell source, such formulation means may be leveraged to further increase the resistance of the cellular payload to harsh implantation environments, as previously described [54,55]. Indeed, it is well known that cells in 2D are much more drug-sensitive than in 3D structures (e.g., spheroids, organoids) [88,89]. Thus, implanted cells are in all probability more protected in 3D structures than in single-cell suspensions. Therein, one of the simplest options is the preparation of cell spheroids with appropriate physical (e.g., size) and functional (e.g., ECM deposition) attributes [53]. In addition to providing physical protection, the 3D structure recapitulates the three-dimensional native cellular environment, which is required for chondrogenic differentiation and the production of GAGs and COL2, both of which are major constituents of the NP. Notably, cell spheroids have been investigated in tissue engineering for the treatment of various tissues (e.g., bone, cartilage, trachea, nerve conduit) [71]. Furthermore, various notable clinical trials using cell spheroids are underway in multiple therapeutic indications (Table 2).

**Table 2.** Selected clinical trials dealing with cell spheroids. ASC, adipose stem cells; IPS, induced pluripotent stem cells; MSC, mesenchymal stem cells.

| Clinical Trial [1] | Spheroids/Cell Type | Therapeutic Indications |
|---|---|---|
| NCT04262167 | Autologous lung stem cells | Idiopathic pulmonary fibrosis |
| NCT04945018 | Allogenic IPS cardiomyocytes | Heart failure |
| NCT05011474 | Autologous matrillin-3 pre-treated ASCs | Disc degeneration |
| NCT05712148 | MSCs | Retinitis pigmentosa |
| NCT04818203 | Autologous dermal fibroblasts | Periorbital wrinkles |

[1] Clinical trial reference numbers are available on https://www.clinicaltrials.gov/, accessed on 2 September 2024.

A notable example of chondrogenic spheroids for spine treatment is the "nose to spine" approach, leveraging the aforementioned nasal chondrocytes [52,53]. Therein, cell spheroids (i.e., $12.5 \times 10^3$ cells/spheroid) were cultured/induced in hypoxia (i.e., 5% $O_2$) for 3–7 days and were formulated for spinal injection (i.e., <600 µm spheroids for use in 22G needles). Specifically, it was shown that these spheroids supported the administration process and were able to fuse with NP spheroids [53]. Furthermore, spheroid formation appears to increase the adhesion properties of the product, thereby reducing cell leakage risks once the spheroids are injected [54]. Interestingly, Kasamkattil et al. directly compared the effects of nasal chondrocyte cell suspensions or spheroid-based formulations in an in vitro degenerative disc disease microtissue NP model [55]. The 3D formulation was shown to increase GAG contents in NP spheroids compared to the cell suspension [55]. Furthermore, a reduction in IL-8 secreted by the NP model was stronger with nasal chondrocyte spheroids in early timepoints [55].

Alternative notable examples of autologous chondrogenic spheroids may be cited, notably for articular chondral defect management [49,51,90]. Therein, products and candidates such as Spherox® or Cartibeads® are prepared in vitro and clinically delivered on the lesion [51,90]. Based on the available evidence on chondrogenic cell spheroids for various therapeutic applications, this formulation approach was retained for the investigated FE002-Disc cells. Of note, a relatively low cell amount/spheroid (i.e., $3 \times 10^4$ cells) was retained based on administration-related spheroid size requirements. It was confirmed herein that the progenitor cells of interest could be effectively formulated as spheroids, with excellent GAG deposition and COL2 induction (Figure 6). However, the need to further understand and optimize the production process (e.g., induction medium composition, hypoxia degree) was clearly evidenced herein. Indeed, the $O_2$ level set at 2% significantly influenced the development of spheroid size, while dexamethasone levels influenced ECM composition (Figures 5, 6 and S6). Thus, additional work is warranted to notably fully understand and characterize the different parameters (i.e., key and critical parameters) for the production of this formulation type. In particular, process transposition towards clinical grade conditions (e.g., qualified consumables and ancillary materials) will require thorough testing and validation.

### *4.6. Study Limitations and Future Perspectives*

The main identified limitations of the present study were related to the number of retained experimental readouts. In particular, the endpoint cellular viability and cell-based functionality (e.g., spheroid fusion assays) attributes were set out of the scope of this study. In detail, for strict consideration of the presented spheroids as a finished product prototype, appropriate formulation, stability, and administration studies would need to be performed. Notwithstanding, the applied functional readouts enabled to indirectly confirm the presence of viable and functional cells in the produced spheroids, which were able to synthesize and deposit ECM components. Furthermore, while the presented datasets did not disqualify the FE002-Disc cell source for quality or safety reasons, further preclinical assessment phases are required (e.g., in vivo work) from a regulatory standpoint [91–94]. Additionally, the present study focused mainly on one therapeutic primary cell type, whereas further validation studies may include additional comparator progenitor cell types and patient-derived adult IVD cell types for appropriate functional benchmarking.

Future research perspectives for this study comprise in-depth functional assessments of the cryopreserved and lyophilized versions of the presented spheroids. In detail, preclinical assays could be designed in order to study the influence of stabilization processes on the function of the spheroids (e.g., ability to fuse to target microtissues). Furthermore, based on the prior application of multiple sources of chondrogenic cells (e.g., nasal chondrocytes or articular chondrocytes) for spheroid-based chondrotherapies and/or IVD therapies, alternative progenitor chondrogenic cells (e.g., FE002-Cart.Art/FE002-Cart cell sources) could be investigated for similar purposes.

## 5. Conclusions

The present study aimed to preclinically qualify FE002-Disc cells and cell spheroids for potential IVD therapeutic applications based on safety and function-oriented assays. The results showed the sustainability of the considered clinical-grade cell source, which was functionally qualified up to passage level 7. Furthermore, this study demonstrated that FE002-Disc cells were well-adapted to growth in adverse environments, as modeled by hypoxia and inflammatory setups. Namely, the in vitro resilience of the considered chondrogenic cells was evidenced, and the critical importance of appropriately establishing the process technical specifications (e.g., incubation atmosphere, dexamethasone concentration) was set forth. Generally, this study enabled to enhance the quality of the obtained FE002-Disc spheroids from a functional viewpoint, with positive pilot indications about finished product storage possibilities (i.e., in frozen or in dry form). Overall, both the applicability of the FE002-Disc cell source and the adequation of the cell spheroid manufacturing process with therapeutic product preclinical development requirements were documented herein. Such elements were considered positively for the further investigation of the therapeutic potential of primary progenitor cell sources in musculoskeletal regenerative medicine.

**Supplementary Materials:** The following supporting information can be downloaded at: https://www.mdpi.com/article/10.3390/pharmaceutics16101274/s1. Supplementary Methods: Antibody reference numbers; Figure S1: Comparative cell proliferation results; Figure S2: Complementary data for HIF-1 Western blotting; Figure S3: Cellular lifespan characterization results; Figure S4: Telomerase activity quantification results; Figure S5: Soft agarose transformation assay results; Figure S6: Cell spheroid manufacturing protocol optimization results; Figure S7: Complementary data for COMP Western blotting; Figure S8: Data on cell spheroid behavior in cryopreservation and lyopreservation studies; Table S1: Results of flow cytometry characterization assays; Table S2: Results of proteomic characterization assays.

**Author Contributions:** Conceptualization, A.J., L.A.A. and A.L.; methodology, A.J., C.P., S.J., V.P., C.S., N.H.-B., L.A.A. and A.L.; software, A.J., C.P., S.J. and A.L.; validation, A.J., C.P., S.J., V.P., C.S., N.H.-B., P.A.-S., R.M., L.A.A., D.P.P. and A.L.; formal analysis, A.J., C.P., S.J., C.S., N.H.-B., L.A.A. and A.L.; investigation, A.J., C.P., S.J., C.S., N.H.-B. and A.L.; resources, L.A.A. and A.L.; data curation, A.J., C.P., S.J., C.S., L.A.A. and A.L.; writing—original draft preparation, A.J., N.H.-B., L.A.A. and A.L.; writing—review and editing, A.J., C.P., S.J., V.P., C.S., N.H.-B., P.A.-S., R.M., L.A.A., D.P.P. and A.L.; visualization, A.J., C.P., N.H.-B. and A.L.; supervision, A.J., L.A.A. and A.L.; project administration, L.A.A. and A.L.; funding acquisition, L.A.A. and A.L. All authors have read and agreed to the published version of the manuscript.

**Funding:** The S.A.N.T.E and Sandoz Foundations have contributed to fund the Swiss progenitor cell transplantation program during the past fifteen years. The funders had no role or involvement in study design, in the collection, analysis, and interpretation of data, in the writing of the report, or in the decision to submit the article for publication. This study was not supported by other specific grants or institutional programs.

**Institutional Review Board Statement:** The procurement of the biological starting materials used for the present study was conducted according to the guidelines of the Declaration of Helsinki, the ICH-GCP, and was approved by the appropriate Cantonal Ethics Committee [95]. The clinical-grade FE002-Disc primary progenitor cell source used in the present study was established from the FE002 organ donation, as approved by the Vaud Cantonal Ethics Committee (University Hospital of Lausanne–CHUV, Ethics Committee Protocol N°62/07, 2007). The FE002 organ donation was registered under a federal cell transplantation program (i.e., Swiss progenitor cell transplantation program).

**Informed Consent Statement:** Appropriate informed consent was obtained from and confirmed by starting material donors at the time of inclusion in the Swiss progenitor cell transplantation program, following specifically devised protocols and procedures, which were validated by the appropriate health authorities.

**Data Availability Statement:** The data presented in this study are available within the article files.

**Acknowledgments:** We would like to thank the S.A.N.T.E and Sandoz Foundations for their unconditional commitments to the Swiss progenitor cell transplantation program through the years. We would like to warmly thank Salim Darwiche, Aymone Lenisa, and Mara Heinold for their technical contributions relative to histology work. Artwork templates were partly created with www.biorender.com, accessed on 20 June 2024.

**Conflicts of Interest:** Authors A.J., C.P. and A.L. were employed by LAM Biotechnologies SA (Epalinges, Switzerland) during the performance of this work. The remaining authors declare no conflict of interest.

## Abbreviations

| | |
|---|---|
| AB | Alcian blue |
| ACAN | aggrecan |
| AF | annulus fibrosus |
| ASC | adipose-derived stem cells |
| ATMP | advanced therapy medicinal product |
| BCA | bicinchoninic acid |
| BMSC | bone marrow stromal cells |
| CD | cluster of differentiation |
| CH | Helvetic Confederation |
| CHUV | Centre hospitalier universitaire vaudois |
| CMtc | complete growth medium |
| COL | collagen |
| COMP | cartilage oligomeric matrix protein |
| CT | cycle threshold |
| DDD | degenerative disc disease |
| DMEM | Dulbecco's modified Eagle medium |
| DMMB | dimethylmethylene blue assay |
| DMSO | dimethyl sulfoxide |
| DNA | deoxyribonucleic acid |
| EC | European Commission |
| ECL | electrochemiluminescence |
| ECM | extracellular matrix |
| FACS | fluorescence activated cell sorting |
| FBS | fetal bovine serum |
| FDA | US Food and Drug Administration |
| FGF | fibroblast growth factor |
| FITC | fluorescein isothiocyanate |
| GAG | glycosaminoglycan |
| GMP | good manufacturing practices |
| h | hour |
| HA | hyaluronic acid |
| HGF | hepatocyte growth factor |
| HIF-1 | hypoxia-inducible factor |
| HLA | human leukocyte antigen |

| | |
|---|---|
| HMGB1 | high mobility group protein B1 |
| HPL | human platelet lysate |
| HRP | horseradish peroxidase |
| IBMX | 3-isobutyl-1-methylxanthine |
| IL | interleukin |
| IPS | induced pluripotent stem cells |
| ITS | insulin, transferrin, selenous acid |
| IVD | intervertebral disc |
| IVDD | intervertebral disc disease |
| LBP | low back pain |
| M-CSF | macrophage colony-stimulating factor |
| min | minute |
| MMPs | matrix metalloproteinases |
| MoA | mechanism of action |
| MSC | mesenchymal stem cells |
| NA | non-applicable |
| NP | nucleus pulposus |
| NSAIDs | non-steroidal anti-inflammatory drugs |
| ODI | Oswestry disability index |
| PBS | phosphate-buffered saline |
| PDT | population doubling time |
| PDV | population doubling value |
| PE | phycoerythrin |
| PMSF | phenylmethylsulfonyl fluoride |
| PRP | platelet rich plasma |
| qPCR | quantitative polymerase chain reaction |
| TGF | transforming growth factor |
| TIMPs | tissue inhibitor of metalloproteinases |
| TNF | tumor necrosis factor |
| sEGFR | soluble epidermal growth factor receptor |
| sTNFRI | soluble tumor necrosis factor receptor I |
| UK | United Kingdom |
| USA | United States of America |
| USD | US dollar |
| VAS | visual analog scale |
| VASPI | visual analog scale pain intensity |
| VitCp | vitamin C 2-phosphate sesquimagnesium salt hydrate |

## References


1. Mohd Isa, I.L.; Teoh, S.L.; Mohd Nor, N.H.; Mokhtar, S.A. Discogenic low back pain: Anatomy, pathophysiology and treatments of intervertebral disc degeneration. *Int. J. Mol. Sci.* **2022**, *24*, 208. [CrossRef] [PubMed]
2. Kim, J.H.; Ham, C.H.; Kwon, W.K. Current knowledge and future therapeutic prospects in symptomatic intervertebral disc degeneration. *Yonsei Med. J.* **2022**, *63*, 199–210. [CrossRef] [PubMed]
3. Soufi, K.H.; Castillo, J.A.; Rogdriguez, F.Y.; DeMesa, C.J.; Ebinu, J.O. Potential role for stem cell regenerative therapy as a treatment for degenerative disc disease and low back pain: A systematic review. *Int. J. Mol. Sci.* **2023**, *24*, 8893. [CrossRef] [PubMed]
4. Meucci, R.D.; Fassa, A.G.; Faria, N.M. Prevalence of chronic low back pain: Systematic review. *Revista Saude Publ.* **2015**, *49*, 1. [CrossRef] [PubMed]
5. Vos, T.; Flaxman, A.D.; Naghavi, M.; Lozano, R.; Michaud, C.; Ezzati, M.; Shibuya, K.; Salomon, J.A.; Abdalla, S.; Aboyans, V.; et al. Years lived with disability (YLDs) for 1160 sequelae of 289 diseases and injuries 1990–2010: A systematic analysis for the Global Burden of Disease Study 2010. *Lancet* **2012**, *380*, 2163–2196. [CrossRef]
6. Knezevic, N.N.; Candido, K.D.; Vlaeyen, J.W.S.; Zundert, J.V.; Cohen, S.P. Low back pain. *Lancet* **2021**, *398*, 78–92. [CrossRef]
7. Dagenais, S.; Caro, J.; Haldeman, S. A systematic review of low back pain cost of illness studies in the United States and internationally. *Spine J.* **2008**, *8*, 8–20. [CrossRef]
8. Binch, A.L.A.; Fitzgerald, J.C.; Growney, E.A.; Barry, F. Cell-based strategies for IVD repair: Clinical progress and translational obstacles. *Nat. Rev. Rheumatol.* **2021**, *17*, 158–175. [CrossRef]
9. Freemont, A.J. The cellular pathobiology of the degenerate intervertebral disc and discogenic back pain. *Rheumatology* **2009**, *48*, 5–10. [CrossRef]

10. Smith, L.J.; Silverman, L.; Sakai, D.; Le Maitre, C.L.; Mauck, R.L.; Malhotra, N.R.; Lotz, J.C.; Buckley, C.T. Advancing cell therapies for intervertebral disc regeneration from the lab to the clinic: Recommendations of the ORS spine section. *JOR Spine* **2018**, *1*, e1036. [CrossRef]
11. Sharifi, S.; Bulstra, S.K.; Grijpma, D.W.; Kuijer, R. Treatment of the degenerated intervertebral disc; closure, repair and regeneration of the annulus fibrosus. *J. Tissue Eng. Regen. Med.* **2015**, *9*, 1120–1132. [CrossRef] [PubMed]
12. Vo, N.V.; Hartman, R.A.; Yurube, T.; Jacobs, L.J.; Sowa, G.A.; Kang, J.D. Expression and regulation of metalloproteinases and their inhibitors in intervertebral disc aging and degeneration. *Spine J.* **2013**, *13*, 331–341. [CrossRef] [PubMed]
13. Nicol, V.; Verdaguer, C.; Daste, C.; Bisseriex, H.; Lapeyre, É.; Lefèvre-Colau, M.M.; Rannou, F.; Rören, A.; Facione, J.; Nguyen, C. Chronic low back pain: A narrative review of recent international guidelines for diagnosis and conservative treatment. *J. Clin. Med.* **2023**, *12*, 1685. [CrossRef] [PubMed]
14. Pennicooke, B.; Moriguchi, Y.; Hussain, I.; Bonssar, L.; Härtl, R. Biological treatment approaches for degenerative disc disease: A review of clinical trials and future directions. *Cureus* **2016**, *8*, e892. [CrossRef]
15. Fritzell, P.; Hägg, O.; Wessberg, P.; Nordwall, A.; Swedish Lumbar Spine Study Group. 2001 Volvo Award Winner in Clinical Studies: Lumbar fusion versus nonsurgical treatment for chronic low back pain: A multicenter randomized controlled trial from the Swedish Lumbar Spine Study Group. *Spine* **2001**, *26*, 2521–2534. [CrossRef]
16. Mowbray, J.; Shen, B.; Diwan, A.D. Intradiscal therapeutics for degenerative disc disease. In *Handbook of Spine Technology*; Springer International Publishing: Cham, Switzerland, 2021; pp. 1091–1110.
17. Clinical Trial N°NCT01124006. A Multicenter, Randomized, Double-Blind, Placebo Controlled, Clinical Trial to Evaluate the Safety, Tolerability and Preliminary Effectiveness of 2 Doses of Intradiscal rhGDF-5 (Single Administration) for the Treatment of Early Stage Lumbar Disc Degeneration. Available online: https://classic.clinicaltrials.gov/ct2/show/NCT01124006 (accessed on 7 May 2024).
18. Clinical Trial N°NCT03122119. Effectiveness of Ultrasound Guided Platelet Rich Plasma Injections in the Sacroiliac Joint. Available online: https://classic.clinicaltrials.gov/ct2/show/NCT03122119 (accessed on 7 May 2024).
19. Zhang, J.; Liu, D.; Gong, Q.; Chen, J.; Wan, L. Intradiscal autologous platelet-rich plasma injection for discogenic low back pain: A clinical trial. *BioMed Res. Int.* **2022**, *2022*, 9563693. [CrossRef]
20. Clinical Trial N°NCT03955315. Study to Evaluate the Safety and Preliminary Efficacy of IDCT, a Treatment for Symptomatic Lumbar Disc Degeneration. Available online: https://classic.clinicaltrials.gov/ct2/show/NCT03955315 (accessed on 7 May 2024).
21. Tschugg, A.; Michnacs, F.; Strowitzki, M.; Meisel, H.J.; Thomé, C. A prospective multicenter phase I/II clinical trial to evaluate safety and efficacy of NOVOCART Disc plus autologous disc chondrocyte transplantation in the treatment of nucleotomized and degenerative lumbar disc to avoid secondary disease: Study protocol for a randomized controlled trial. *Trials* **2016**, *17*, 108. [CrossRef]
22. Amirdelfan, K.; Bae, H.; McJunkin, T.; DePalma, M.; Kim, K.; Beckworth, W.J.; Ghiselli, G.; Bainbridge, J.S.; Dryer, R.; Deer, T.R.; et al. Allogeneic mesenchymal precursor cells treatment for chronic low back pain associated with degenerative disc disease: A prospective randomized, placebo-controlled 36-month study of safety and efficacy. *Spine J.* **2021**, *21*, 212–230. [CrossRef]
23. Gjefsen, E.; Bråten, L.C.H.; Goll, G.L.; Wigemyr, M.; Bolstad, N.; Valberg, M.; Schistad, E.I.; Marchand, G.H.; Granviken, F.; Selmer, K.K.; et al. The effect of infliximab in patients with chronic low back pain and Modic changes (the BackToBasic study): Study protocol of a randomized, double blind, placebo-controlled, multicenter trial. *BMC Musculoskel. Dis.* **2020**, *21*, 698. [CrossRef]
24. Han, F.; Tu, Z.; Zhu, Z.; Liu, D.; Meng, Q.; Yu, Q.; Wang, Y.; Chen, J.; Liu, T.; Han, F.; et al. Targeting endogenous reactive oxygen species removal and regulating regenerative microenvironment at annulus fibrosus defects promote tissue repair. *ACS Nano* **2023**, *17*, 7645–7661. [CrossRef]
25. Wei, Z.; Ye, H.; Li, Y.; Li, X.; Liu, Y.; Chen, Y.; Yu, J.; Wang, J.; Ye, X. Mechanically tough, adhesive, self-healing hydrogel promotes annulus fibrosus repair via autologous cell recruitment and microenvironment regulation. *Acta Biomater.* **2024**, *178*, 50–67. [CrossRef] [PubMed]
26. Herger, N.; Bermudez-Lekerika, P.; Farshad, M.; Albers, C.E.; Distler, O.; Gantenbein, B.; Dudli, S. Should degenerated intervertebral discs of patients with modic type 1 changes be treated with mesenchymal stem cells? *Int. J. Mol. Sci.* **2022**, *23*, 2721. [CrossRef] [PubMed]
27. Sakai, D.; Andersson, G.B. Stem cell therapy for intervertebral disc regeneration: Obstacles and solutions. *Nat. Rev. Rheumatol.* **2015**, *11*, 243–256. [CrossRef] [PubMed]
28. Sakai, D.; Schol, J. Cell therapy for intervertebral disc repair: Clinical perspective. *J. Orthop. Transl.* **2017**, *9*, 8–18. [CrossRef]
29. Meisel, H.J.; Siodla, V.; Ganey, T.; Minkus, Y.; Hutton, W.C.; Alasevic, O.J. Clinical experience in cell-based therapeutics: Disc chondrocyte transplantation. A treatment for degenerated or damaged intervertebral disc. *Biomol. Eng.* **2007**, *24*, 5–21. [CrossRef]
30. Meisel, H.J.; Ganey, T.; Hutton, W.C.; Libera, J.; Minkus, Y.; Alasevic, O. Clinical experience in cell-based therapeutics: Intervention and outcome. *Eur. Spine J.* **2006**, *15*, S397–S405. [CrossRef]
31. Krut, Z.; Pelled, G.; Gazit, D.; Gazit, Z. Stem cells and exosomes: New therapies for intervertebral disc degeneration. *Cells* **2021**, *10*, 2241. [CrossRef]
32. Li, Z.; Wu, Y.; Tan, G.; Xu, Z.; Xue, H. Exosomes and exosomal miRNAs: A new therapy for intervertebral disc degeneration. *Front. Pharmacol.* **2022**, *13*, 992476. [CrossRef]

33. Laurent, A.; Hirt-Burri, N.; Scaletta, C.; Michetti, M.; de Buys Roessingh, A.S.; Raffoul, W.; Applegate, L.A. Holistic approach of Swiss fetal progenitor cell banking: Optimizing safe and sustainable substrates for regenerative medicine and biotechnology. *Front. Bioeng. Biotechnol.* **2020**, *8*, 557758. [CrossRef]
34. Philippe, V.; Jeannerat, A.; Peneveyre, C.; Jaccoud, S.; Scaletta, C.; Hirt-Burri, N.; Abdel-Sayed, P.; Raffoul, W.; Darwiche, S.; Applegate, L.A.; et al. Autologous and allogeneic cytotherapies for large knee (osteo)chondral defects: Manufacturing process benchmarking and parallel functional qualification. *Pharmaceutics* **2023**, *15*, 2333. [CrossRef]
35. Darwiche, S.; Scaletta, C.; Raffoul, W.; Pioletti, D.P.; Applegate, L.A. Epiphyseal chondroprogenitors provide a stable cell source for cartilage cell therapy. *Cell Med.* **2012**, *4*, 23–32. [CrossRef] [PubMed]
36. Wu, H.; Shang, Y.; Yu, J.; Zeng, X.; Lin, J.; Tu, M.; Cheang, L.H.; Zhang, J. Regenerative potential of human nucleus pulposus resident stem/progenitor cells declines with ageing and intervertebral disc degeneration. *Int. J. Mol. Med.* **2018**, *42*, 2193–2202. [CrossRef] [PubMed]
37. Mabotuwana, N.S.; Rech, L.; Lim, J.; Hardy, S.A.; Murtha, L.A.; Rainer, P.P.; Boyle, A.J. Paracrine factors released by stem cells of mesenchymal origin and their effects in cardiovascular disease: A systematic review of pre-clinical studies. *Stem Cell Rev. Rep.* **2022**, *18*, 2606–2628. [CrossRef] [PubMed]
38. Hung, G.; Ashvetiya, T.; Leszczynska, A.; Yang, W.; Hwang, C.W.; Gerstenblith, G.; Barth, A.S.; Johnston, P.V. Paracrine-mediated rejuvenation of aged mesenchymal stem cells is associated with downregulation of the autophagy-lysosomal pathway. *Npj Aging* **2022**, *8*, 10. [CrossRef] [PubMed]
39. Jarrige, M.; Frank, E.; Herardot, E.; Martineau, S.; Darle, A.; Benabides, M.; Domingues, S.; Chose, O.; Habeler, W.; Lorant, J.; et al. The future of regenerative medicine: Cell therapy using pluripotent stem cells and acellular therapies based on extracellular vesicles. *Cells* **2021**, *10*, 240. [CrossRef]
40. Wang, C.; Yu, X.; Yan, Y.; Yang, W.; Zhang, S.; Xiang, Y.; Zhang, J.; Wang, W. Tumor necrosis factor-α: A key contributor to intervertebral disc degeneration. *Acta Biochim. Biophys. Sin.* **2017**, *49*, 1–13. [CrossRef]
41. Croft, A.S.; Guerrero, J.; Oswald, K.A.C.; Häckel, S.; Albers, C.E.; Gantenbein, B. Effect of different cryopreservation media on human nucleus pulposus cells' viability and trilineage potential. *JOR Spine* **2021**, *4*, e1140. [CrossRef]
42. Evenbratt, H.; Andreasson, L.; Bicknell, V.; Brittberg, M.; Mobini, R.; Simonsson, S. Insights into the present and future of cartilage regeneration and joint repair. *Cell Regen.* **2022**, *11*, 3. [CrossRef]
43. Feng, G.; Li, L.; Liu, H.; Song, Y.; Huang, F.; Tu, C.; Shen, B.; Gong, Q.; Li, T.; Liu, L.; et al. Hypoxia differentially regulates human nucleus pulposus and annulus fibrosus cell extracellular matrix production in 3D scaffolds. *Osteoarthr. Cart.* **2013**, *21*, 582–588. [CrossRef]
44. Bitterli, T.; Schmid, D.; Ettinger, L.; Krupkova, O.; Bach, F.C.; Tryfonidou, M.A.; Meij, B.P.; Pozzi, A.; Steffen, F.; Wuertz-Kozak, K.; et al. Targeted screening of inflammatory mediators in spontaneous degenerative disc disease in dogs reveals an upregulation of the tumor necrosis superfamily. *JOR Spine* **2023**, *7*, e1292. [CrossRef]
45. Fan, C.; Wang, W.; Yu, Z.; Wang, J.; Xu, W.; Ji, Z.; He, W.; Hua, D.; Wang, W.; Yao, L.; et al. M1 macrophage-derived exosomes promote intervertebral disc degeneration by enhancing nucleus pulposus cell senescence through LCN2/NF-κB signaling axis. *J. Nanobiotechnol.* **2024**, *22*, 301. [CrossRef] [PubMed]
46. Pan, H.; Li, H.; Guo, S.; Wang, C.; Long, L.; Wang, X.; Shi, H.; Zhang, K.; Chen, H.; Li, S. The mechanisms and functions of TNF-α in intervertebral disc degeneration. *Exp. Gerontol.* **2023**, *174*, 112119. [CrossRef] [PubMed]
47. Díaz, L.; Zambrano, E.; Flores, M.E.; Contreras, M.; Crispín, J.C.; Alemán, G.; Bravo, C.; Armenta, A.; Valdés, V.J.; Tovar, A.; et al. Ethical considerations in animal research: The principle of 3R's. *Rev. Investig. Clin.* **2020**, *73*, 199–209. [CrossRef] [PubMed]
48. Jeannerat, A.; Meuli, J.; Peneveyre, C.; Jaccoud, S.; Chemali, M.; Thomas, A.; Liao, Z.; Abdel-Sayed, P.; Scaletta, C.; Hirt-Burri, N.; et al. Bio-enhanced neoligaments graft bearing FE002 primary progenitor tenocytes: Allogeneic tissue engineering & surgical proofs-of-concept for hand ligament regenerative medicine. *Pharmaceutics* **2023**, *15*, 1873. [CrossRef] [PubMed]
49. Mumme, M.; Barbero, A.; Miot, S.; Wixmerten, A.; Feliciano, S.; Wolf, F.; Asnaghi, A.M.; Baumhoer, D.; Bieri, O.; Kretzcchmar, M.; et al. Nasal chondrocyte-based engineered autologous cartilage tissue for repair of articular cartilage defects: An observational first-in-human trial. *Lancet* **2016**, *388*, 1985–1994. [CrossRef]
50. Almqvist, K.F.; Dhollander, A.A.; Verdonk, P.C.; Forsyth, R.; Verdonk, R.; Verbruggen, G. Treatment of cartilage defects in the knee using alginate beads containing human mature allogenic chondrocytes. *Am. J. Sports Med.* **2009**, *37*, 1920–1929. [CrossRef]
51. Kutaish, H.; Tscholl, P.M.; Cosset, E.; Bengtsson, L.; Braunersreuther, V.; Mor, F.M.; Laedermann, J.; Furfaro, I.; Stafylakis, D.; Hannouche, D.; et al. Articular cartilage repair after implantation of hyaline cartilage beads engineered from adult dedifferentiated chondrocytes: Cartibeads preclinical efficacy study in a large animal model. *Am. J. Sports Med.* **2023**, *51*, 237–249. [CrossRef]
52. Gay, M.H.; Mehrkens, A.; Rittmann, M.; Haug, M.; Barbero, A.; Martin, I.; Schaeren, S. Nose to back: Compatibility of nasal chondrocytes with environmental conditions mimicking a degenerated intervertebral disc. *Eur. Cells Mater.* **2019**, *37*, 214–232. [CrossRef]
53. Gryadunova, A.; Kasamkattil, J.; Gay, M.H.P.; Dasen, B.; Pelttari, K.; Mironov, V.; Martin, I.; Schären, S.; Barbero, A.; Krupkova, O.; et al. Nose to spine: Spheroids generated by human nasal chondrocytes for scaffold-free nucleus pulposus augmentation. *Acta Biomater.* **2021**, *134*, 240–251. [CrossRef]
54. Kasamkattil, J.; Gryadunova, A.; Martin, I.; Barbero, A.; Schären, S.; Krupkova, O.; Mehrkens, A. Spheroid-based tissue engineering strategies for regeneration of the intervertebral disc. *Int. J. Mol. Sci.* **2022**, *23*, 2530. [CrossRef]

55. Kasamkattil, J.; Gryadunova, A.; Schmid, R.; Gay-Dujak, M.H.P.; Dasen, B.; Hilpert, M.; Pelttari, K.; Martin, I.; Schären, S.; Barbero, A.; et al. Human 3D nucleus pulposus microtissue model to evaluate the potential of pre-conditioned nasal chondrocytes for the repair of degenerated intervertebral disc. *Front. Bioeng. Biotechnol.* **2023**, *11*, 1119009. [CrossRef] [PubMed]
56. McDonnell, E.E.; Wilson, N.; Barcellona, M.N.; Ní Néill, T.; Bagnall, J.; Brama, P.A.J.; Cunniffe, G.M.; Darwish, S.L.; Butler, J.S.; Buckley, C.T. Preclinical to clinical translation for intervertebral disc repair: Effects of species-specific scale, metabolism, and matrix synthesis rates on cell-based regeneration. *JOR Spine* **2023**, *6*, e1279. [CrossRef] [PubMed]
57. Martinez, I.; Elvenes, J.; Olsen, R.; Bertheussen, K.; Johansen, O. Redifferentiation of in vitro expanded adult articular chondrocytes by combining the hanging-drop cultivation method with hypoxic environment. *Cell Transplant.* **2008**, *17*, 987–996. [CrossRef] [PubMed]
58. Chijimatsu, R.; Kobayashi, M.; Ebina, K.; Iwahashi, T.; Okuno, Y.; Hirao, M.; Fukuhara, A.; Nakamura, N.; Yoshikawa, H. Impact of dexamethasone concentration on cartilage tissue formation from human synovial derived stem cells in vitro. *Cytotechnology* **2018**, *70*, 819–829. [CrossRef] [PubMed]
59. Demoor, M.; Ollitrault, D.; Gomez-Leduc, T.; Bouyoucef, M.; Hervieu, M.; Fabre, H.; Lafont, J.; Denoix, J.M.; Audigié, F.; Mallein-Gerin, F.; et al. Cartilage tissue engineering: Molecular control of chondrocyte differentiation for proper cartilage matrix reconstruction. *Biochim. Biophys. Acta* **2014**, *1840*, 2414–2440. [CrossRef]
60. Branly, T.; Contentin, R.; Desancé, M.; Jacquel, T.; Bertoni, L.; Jacquet, S.; Mallein-Gerin, F.; Denoix, J.M.; Audigié, F.; Demoor, M.; et al. Improvement of the chondrocyte-specific phenotype upon equine bone marrow mesenchymal stem cell differentiation: Influence of culture time, transforming growth factors and type i collagen siRNAs on the differentiation index. *Int. J. Mol. Sci.* **2018**, *19*, 435. [CrossRef]
61. Gómez-Leduc, T.; Desancé, M.; Hervieu, M.; Legendre, F.; Ollitrault, D.; de Vienne, C.; Herlicoviez, M.; Galéra, P.; Demoor, M. Hypoxia is a critical parameter for chondrogenic differentiation of human umbilical cord blood mesenchymal stem cells in type I/III collagen sponges. *Int. J. Mol. Sci.* **2017**, *18*, 1933. [CrossRef]
62. Enochson, L.; Brittberg, M.; Lindahl, A. Optimization of a chondrogenic medium through the use of factorial design of experiments. *BioRes. Open Access* **2012**, *1*, 306–313. [CrossRef]
63. Kipnes, J.; Carlberg, A.L.; Loredo, G.A.; Lawler, J.; Tuan, R.S.; Hall, D.J. Effect of cartilage oligomeric matrix protein on mesenchymal chondrogenesis in vitro. *Osteoarthr. Cart.* **2003**, *11*, 442–454. [CrossRef]
64. Shi, P.; Chee, A.; Liu, W.; Chou, P.H.; Zhu, J.; An, H.S. Therapeutic effects of cell therapy with neonatal human dermal fibroblasts and rabbit dermal fibroblasts on disc degeneration and inflammation. *Spine J.* **2019**, *19*, 171–181. [CrossRef]
65. Farhang, N.; Silverman, L.; Bowles, R.D. Improving cell therapy survival and anabolism in harsh musculoskeletal disease environments. *Tissue Eng. Part B Rev.* **2020**, *26*, 348–366. [CrossRef] [PubMed]
66. Tschugg, A.; Diepers, M.; Simone, S.; Michnacs, F.; Quirbach, S.; Strowitzki, M.; Meisel, H.J.; Thomé, C. A prospective randomized multicenter phase I/II clinical trial to evaluate safety and efficacy of NOVOCART disk plus autologous disk chondrocyte transplantation in the treatment of nucleotomized and degenerative lumbar disks to avoid secondary disease: Safety results of Phase I—A short report. *Neurosurg. Rev.* **2017**, *40*, 155–162. [CrossRef] [PubMed]
67. Hiraishi, S.; Schol, J.; Sakai, D.; Nukaga, T.; Erickson, I.; Silverman, L.; Foley, K.; Watanabe, M. Discogenic cell transplantation directly from a cryopreserved state in an induced intervertebral disc degeneration canine model. *JOR Spine* **2018**, *1*, e1013. [CrossRef] [PubMed]
68. Silverman, L.I.; Heaton, W.; Farhang, N.; Saxon, L.H.; Dulatova, G.; Rodriguez-Granrose, D.; Flanagan, F.; Foley, K.T. Perspectives on the treatment of lumbar disc degeneration: The value proposition for a cell-based therapy, immunomodulatory properties of discogenic cells and the associated clinical evaluation strategy. *Front. Surg.* **2020**, *7*, 554382. [CrossRef]
69. Silverman, L.I.; Flanagan, F.; Rodriguez-Granrose, D.; Simpson, K.; Saxon, L.H.; Foley, K.T. Identifying and managing sources of variability in cell therapy manufacturing and clinical trials. *Regen. Eng. Transl. Med.* **2019**, *5*, 354–361. [CrossRef]
70. Rodriguez-Granrose, D.; Zurawski, J.; Heaton, W.; Tandeski, T.; Dulatov, G.; Highsmith, A.A.; Conen, M.; Clark, G.; Jones, A.; Loftus, H.; et al. Transition from static culture to stirred tank bioreactor for the allogeneic production of therapeutic discogenic cell spheres. *Stem Cell Res. Ther.* **2021**, *12*, 455. [CrossRef]
71. Chae, S.; Hong, J.; Hwangbo, H.; Kim, G. The utility of biomedical scaffolds laden with spheroids in various tissue engineering applications. *Theranostics* **2021**, *11*, 6818–6832. [CrossRef]
72. Silverman, L.I.; Dulatova, G.; Tandeski, T.; Erickson, I.E.; Lundell, B.; Toplon, D.; Wolff, T.; Howard, A.; Chintalacharuvu, S.; Foley, K.T. In vitro and in vivo evaluation of discogenic cells, an investigational cell therapy for disc degeneration. *Spine J.* **2020**, *20*, 138–149. [CrossRef]
73. Yoon, K.H.; Yoo, J.D.; Choi, C.H.; Lee, J.; Lee, J.Y.; Kim, S.G.; Park, J.Y. Costal chondrocyte-derived pellet-type autologous chondrocyte implantation versus microfracture for repair of articular cartilage defects: A prospective randomized trial. *Cartilage* **2021**, *13*, 1092S–1104S. [CrossRef]
74. Yoon, K.H.; Park, J.Y.; Lee, J.Y.; Lee, E.; Lee, J.; Kim, S.G. Costal chondrocyte-derived pellet-type autologous chondrocyte implantation for treatment of articular cartilage defect. *Am. J. Sports Med.* **2020**, *48*, 1236–1245. [CrossRef]
75. Teixeira, G.Q.; Riegger, J.; Gonçalves, R.M.; Risbud, M.V. Editorial: Intervertebral disc degeneration and osteoarthritis: Mechanisms of disease and functional repair. *Front. Bioeng. Biotechnol.* **2023**, *11*, 1252703. [CrossRef] [PubMed]
76. Tonomura, H.; Nagae, M.; Takatori, R.; Ishibashi, H.; Itsuji, T.; Takahashi, K. The potential role of hepatocyte growth factor in degenerative disorders of the synovial joint and spine. *Int. J. Mol. Sci.* **2020**, *21*, 8717. [CrossRef] [PubMed]

77. Han, B.; Wang, H.C.; Li, H.; Tao, Y.Q.; Liang, C.Z.; Li, F.C.; Chen, G.; Chen, Q.X. Nucleus pulposus mesenchymal stem cells in acidic conditions mimicking degenerative intervertebral discs give better performance than adipose tissue-derived mesenchymal stem cells. *Cells Tissues Org.* **2014**, *199*, 342–352. [CrossRef]
78. Scotti, C.; Osmokrovic, A.; Wolf, F.; Miot, S.; Peretti, G.M.; Barbero, A.; Martin, I. Response of human engineered cartilage based on articular or nasal chondrocytes to interleukin-1β and low oxygen. *Tissue Eng. Part A* **2012**, *18*, 362–372. [CrossRef] [PubMed]
79. Jeannerat, A.; Peneveyre, C.; Armand, F.; Chiappe, D.; Hamelin, R.; Scaletta, C.; Hirt-Burri, N.; de Buys Roessingh, A.; Raffoul, W.; Applegate, L.A.; et al. Hypoxic incubation conditions for optimized manufacture of tenocyte-based active pharmaceutical ingredients of homologous standardized transplant products in tendon regenerative medicine. *Cells* **2021**, *10*, 2872. [CrossRef] [PubMed]
80. Clinical Trial N°NCT02412735. Placebo-Controlled Study to Evaluate Rexlemestrocel-L Alone or Combined with Hyaluronic Acid in Participants with Chronic Low Back Pain (MSB-DR003). Available online: https://clinicaltrials.gov/study/NCT02412735 (accessed on 11 July 2024).
81. Beall, D.P.; Davis, T.; DePalma, M.J.; Amirdelfan, K.; Yoon, E.S.; Wilson, G.L.; Bishop, R.; Tally, W.C.; Gershon, S.L.; Lorio, M.P.; et al. Viable disc tissue allograft supplementation; One- and two-level treatment of degenerated intervertebral discs in patients with chronic discogenic low back pain: One year results of the VAST randomized controlled trial. *Pain Phys.* **2021**, *24*, 465–477.
82. Lorio, M.P.; Tate, J.L.; Myers, T.J.; Block, J.E.; Beall, D.P. Perspective on intradiscal therapies for lumbar discogenic pain: State of the science, knowledge gaps, and imperatives for clinical adoption. *J. Pain Res.* **2024**, *17*, 1171–1182. [CrossRef]
83. Noriega, D.C.; Ardura, F.; Hernández-Ramajo, R.; Martín-Ferrero, M.Á.; Sánchez-Lite, I.; Toribio, B.; Alberca, M.; García, V.; Moraleda, J.M.; González-Vallinas, M.; et al. Treatment of degenerative disc disease with allogeneic mesenchymal stem cells: Long-term follow-up results. *Transplantation* **2021**, *105*, e25–e27. [CrossRef]
84. Clinical Trial N°NCT04530071. Evaluation of Safety, Tolerability, and Efficacy of CordSTEM-DD in Patients with Chronic Low Back Pain. Available online: https://www.clinicaltrials.gov/study/NCT04530071 (accessed on 11 June 2024).
85. Noriega, D.C.; Ardura, F.; Hernández-Ramajo, R.; Martín-Ferrero, M.Á.; Sánchez-Lite, I.; Toribio, B.; Alberca, M.; García, V.; Moraleda, J.M.; Sánchez, A.; et al. Intervertebral disc repair by allogeneic mesenchymal bone marrow cells: A randomized controlled trial. *Transplantation* **2017**, *101*, 1945–1951. [CrossRef]
86. Elabd, C.; Centeno, C.J.; Schultz, J.R.; Lutz, G.; Ichim, T.; Silva, F.J. Intra-discal injection of autologous, hypoxic cultured bone marrow-derived mesenchymal stem cells in five patients with chronic lower back pain: A long-term safety and feasibility study. *J. Transl. Med.* **2016**, *14*, 253. [CrossRef]
87. Horizon 2020 Project. Regenerative Therapy of Intervertebral Disc: A Double Blind Phase 2b Trial of Intradiscal Injection of Mesenchymal Stromal Cells in Degenerative Disc Disease of the Lomber SPINE Unresponsive to Conventional Therapy. Available online: https://cordis.europa.eu/project/id/732163/results (accessed on 11 June 2024).
88. Yan, X.; Zhou, L.; Wu, Z.; Wang, X.; Chen, X.; Yang, F.; Guo, Y.; Wu, M.; Chen, Y.; Li, W.; et al. High throughput scaffold-based 3D micro-tumor array for efficient drug screening and chemosensitivity testing. *Biomaterials* **2019**, *198*, 167–179. [CrossRef] [PubMed]
89. Flampouri, E.; Imar, S.; OConnell, K.; Singh, B. Spheroid-3D and monolayer-2D intestinal electrochemical biosensor for toxicity/viability testing: Applications in drug screening, food safety, and environmental pollutant analysis. *ACS Sens.* **2019**, *4*, 660–669. [CrossRef] [PubMed]
90. Eschen, C.; Kaps, C.; Widuchowski, W.; Fickert, S.; Zinser, W.; Niemeyer, P.; Roël, G. Clinical outcome is significantly better with spheroid-based autologous chondrocyte implantation manufactured with more stringent cell culture criteria. *Osteoarthr. Cart. Open* **2020**, *2*, 100033. [CrossRef] [PubMed]
91. Ikawa, T.; Yano, K.; Watanabe, N.; Masamune, K.; Yamato, M. Non-clinical assessment design of autologous chondrocyte implantation products. *Regen. Ther.* **2015**, *1*, 98–108. [CrossRef] [PubMed]
92. Bukovac, P.K.; Hauser, M.; Lottaz, D.; Marti, A.; Schmitt, I.; Schochat, T. The regulation of cell therapy and gene therapy products in Switzerland. *Adv. Exp. Med. Biol.* **2023**, *1430*, 41–58. [CrossRef]
93. Kim, J.; Park, J.; Song, S.Y.; Kim, E. Advanced therapy medicinal products for autologous chondrocytes and comparison of regulatory systems in target countries. *Regen. Ther.* **2022**, *20*, 126–137. [CrossRef]
94. Nordberg, R.C.; Otarola, G.A.; Wang, D.; Hu, J.C.; Athanasiou, K.A. Navigating regulatory pathways for translation of biologic cartilage repair products. *Sci. Transl. Med.* **2022**, *14*, eabp8163. [CrossRef]
95. World Medical Association. Declaration of Helsinki: Ethical principles for medical research involving human subjects. *JAMA* **2013**, *310*, 2191–2194. [CrossRef]

*pharmaceutics*

*Article*

# Bio-Enhanced Neoligaments Graft Bearing FE002 Primary Progenitor Tenocytes: Allogeneic Tissue Engineering & Surgical Proofs-of-Concept for Hand Ligament Regenerative Medicine

**Annick Jeannerat [1,†], Joachim Meuli [2,†], Cédric Peneveyre [1], Sandra Jaccoud [2,3], Michèle Chemali [2], Axelle Thomas [2], Zhifeng Liao [2], Philippe Abdel-Sayed [2,4], Corinne Scaletta [2], Nathalie Hirt-Burri [2], Lee Ann Applegate [2,5,6], Wassim Raffoul [2,*,‡] and Alexis Laurent [1,2,*,‡]**

1 Preclinical Research Department, LAM Biotechnologies SA, CH-1066 Epalinges, Switzerland; annick.jeannerat@lambiotechnologies.com (A.J.); cedric.peneveyre@lambiotechnologies.com (C.P.)
2 Plastic and Hand Surgery Service, Lausanne University Hospital, University of Lausanne, CH-1011 Lausanne, Switzerland; joachim.meuli@chuv.ch (J.M.); sandra.jaccoud@chuv.ch (S.J.); michele.chemali@chuv.ch (M.C.); axelle.thomas@chuv.ch (A.T.); zhifeng.liao@unil.ch (Z.L.); philippe.abdel-sayed@chuv.ch (P.A.-S.); corinne.scaletta@chuv.ch (C.S.); nathalie.burri@chuv.ch (N.H.-B.); lee.laurent-applegate@chuv.ch (L.A.A.)
3 Laboratory of Biomechanical Orthopedics, Ecole Polytechnique Fédérale de Lausanne, CH-1015 Lausanne, Switzerland
4 DLL Bioengineering, STI School of Engineering, Ecole Polytechnique Fédérale de Lausanne, CH-1015 Lausanne, Switzerland
5 Center for Applied Biotechnology and Molecular Medicine, University of Zurich, CH-8057 Zurich, Switzerland
6 Oxford OSCAR Suzhou Center, Oxford University, Suzhou 215123, China
* Correspondence: wassim.raffoul@chuv.ch (W.R.); alexis.laurent@lambiotechnologies.com (A.L.); Tel.: +41-21-314-25-25 (W.R.); +41-21-546-42-00 (A.L.)
† These authors contributed equally to this work.
‡ These authors also contributed equally to this work.

**Abstract:** Hand tendon/ligament structural ruptures (tears, lacerations) often require surgical reconstruction and grafting, for the restauration of finger mechanical functions. Clinical-grade human primary progenitor tenocytes (FE002 cryopreserved progenitor cell source) have been previously proposed for diversified therapeutic uses within allogeneic tissue engineering and regenerative medicine applications. The aim of this study was to establish bioengineering and surgical proofs-of-concept for an artificial graft (Neoligaments Infinity-Lock 3 device) bearing cultured and viable FE002 primary progenitor tenocytes. Technical optimization and in vitro validation work showed that the combined preparations could be rapidly obtained (dynamic cell seeding of $10^5$ cells/cm of scaffold, 7 days of co-culture). The studied standardized transplants presented homogeneous cellular colonization in vitro (cellular alignment/coating along the scaffold fibers) and other critical functional attributes (tendon extracellular matrix component such as collagen I and aggrecan synthesis/deposition along the scaffold fibers). Notably, major safety- and functionality-related parameters/attributes of the FE002 cells/finished combination products were compiled and set forth (telomerase activity, adhesion and biological coating potentials). A two-part human cadaveric study enabled to establish clinical protocols for hand ligament cell-assisted surgery (ligamento-suspension plasty after trapeziectomy, thumb metacarpo-phalangeal ulnar collateral ligamentoplasty). Importantly, the aggregated experimental results clearly confirmed that functional and clinically usable allogeneic cell-scaffold combination products could be rapidly and robustly prepared for bio-enhanced hand ligament reconstruction. Major advantages of the considered bioengineered graft were discussed in light of existing clinical protocols based on autologous tenocyte transplantation. Overall, this study established proofs-of-concept for the translational development of a functional tissue engineering protocol in allogeneic musculoskeletal regenerative medicine, in view of a pilot clinical trial.

**Keywords:** allogeneic cell therapy; clinical protocols; FE002 primary progenitor tenocytes; hand surgery; ligamentoplasty; proof-of-concept; regenerative medicine; tissue engineering; translational development; standardized transplants

## 1. Introduction

The necessity of functional tendons in the musculoskeletal system and the high incidence of tendon-related disorders are important components of modern socio-economic burdens [1–4]. High diversity is reported in the etiology of tendon disorders, with possible combined promoting and triggering factors (e.g., intrinsic and extrinsic factors, mechanical overuse). Such diverse and combined factors may potentially lead to tendon ruptures [1,5–7]. Then, as the pathological spectrum of tendon disorders is large, various treatment strategies are currently applied and depend on the specific clinical situation [2,3,8–12]. Importantly, symptomatic management of pain and inflammation do not enhance tendon tissue healing capacities, which are inherently poor (i.e., hypocellularity, low vascularization) [1,5,6]. Physiological healing of tendon injuries generally leads to adhesions, scarring, and low overall quality of repair (i.e., mechanically inferior tissues), incurring high morbidity [1,5,13–16]. Notably, injuries to the Achilles tendons are highly prevalent in sports medicine, where 30% of cases require surgical treatment [5,17]. While partial tendon ruptures may be managed by suturing, volumetric tissue defects require surgical grafting [6,18,19]. Therein, autografting of vestigial tendon tissue is clinically preferred. However, its practical availability is inconsistent and incurs additional morbidity (i.e., related to donor-site surgery). These clinical facts have prompted the development of exogeneous tendon grafts or substitutes (e.g., synthetic matrices, biological constructs) [2,9,20–28]. Despite their increased availability and manufacturing process standardization, tendon allografts and xenografts bear an increased risk of tissue inflammation, iatrogenicity, and rejection compared to autografts [3,9,29–32].

Solid scaffold-based solutions for ligament and tendon repair or replacement are well-defined and commercially available [9,20,24]. An ideal ad hoc scaffold should be biocompatible, show in vivo cell adhesion, cell proliferation/migration, and extracellular matrix deposition (i.e., bio-integration) [4,17,21–23,33]. Furthermore, such scaffolds should present good mechanical properties and resist to the physiological strains typically applied to tendons and ligaments [20,21,34]. Therefore, biological (e.g., human or porcine tissues) and synthetic materials have been proposed for tendon surgical reconstruction [9,17,21–26]. While biological scaffolds provide a favorable environment for cells, several manufacturing process-related (i.e., decellularization, sterilization) problematics have been reported (e.g., reduced mechanical attributes or pro-inflammatory effects) [19,21,24]. Conversely, artificial tendon grafts can be standardized, tailored to specific applications, and serially produced with a controlled terminal sterilization step while maintaining appropriate critical quality attributes [9,17,35–37]. However, their biocompatibility is generally found to be lower compared to biological materials (e.g., formation/release of toxic degradation products) [19,22,24]. Therefore, current efforts are directed toward the supplementation of existing tissue suturing or grafting procedures with appropriate biological components (e.g., growth factors, autologous or allogeneic cells, platelet-rich plasma), to potentially optimize tendon healing [38–46].

Notably, growth factors such as platelet-derived growth factor-BB (PDGF-BB) have been preclinically investigated in combination with synthetic scaffolds to promote tendon healing, yielding encouraging results [26,40,41]. As regards the use of platelet-rich plasma (PRP) for tendinopathies, positive symptomatic and functional outcomes have been reported [11,42,47,48]. Recently, various types of therapeutic cell sources were clinically assessed (e.g., mesenchymal stem cells, UVEC, tenocytes) for managing tendon disorders, with positive safety and efficacy outcomes [12,13,49–53]. Among the postulated mechanisms of action of cell therapies, the paracrine modulation of wounded environments by diverse growth factors and cytokines is frequently cited [3,13,38,39]. Of note, autologous cultured tenocyte injections (i.e., Ortho-ATI, Orthocell, Australia) were shown to improve both the function and the MRI tendinopathy scores in chronic lateral epicondylitis at 4.5 years of follow-up [43,52]. In an allogeneic setting, FE002 primary progenitor tenocytes (i.e., clinical grade FE002 progenitor cell source) were proposed as standardized homologous cytotherapeutic materials under the Swiss progenitor cell transplantation program [39,54]. Specifically, FE002 primary progenitor tenocytes were considered for diverse therapeutic tissue engineering purposes or for the optimization of novel injectable medical devices [39,55–58]. Of note, the FE002 primary progenitor tenocytes of interest (i.e., primary cell type) are diploid cells, which are inherently pre-terminally differentiated and possess stable and robust biological attributes. Such characteristics are maintained within large scale in vitro biotechnological manufacture [39,55]. Importantly, FE002 primary progenitor tenocytes are cytocompatible with diverse implantable materials, are immunologically privileged, and are non-tumorigenic [19,39,54]. Therefore, such primary progenitor cells represent an optimal cellular active substance (i.e., the substance responsible for the activity of a medicine). Off-the-freezer preparation of FE002 progenitor cell-seeded allografts (i.e., using synthetic tendon/ligament scaffolds, decellularized biological tendon matrices, or hyaluronan hydrogels) has previously been reported [19,39,54,56]. Therefore, FE002 primary progenitor tenocytes may be applied in diverse musculoskeletal affections, ranging from volumetric tissue substitution to local pain and inflammation management [39]. Specifically, the combination of an appropriate synthetic scaffold and of FE002 primary progenitor tenocytes for tendon or ligament bioengineering bears the potential of leveraging the desirable attributes of both components [39,56].

Therefore, the general aim of the present study was to establish allogeneic tissue engineering and surgical proofs-of-concept for an artificial tendon/ligament graft bearing cultured FE002 primary progenitor tenocytes. In order to pursue this goal, three specific objectives were defined at the time of designing the presented work, namely:

(1) Experimental verification of the compatibility of the FE002 primary progenitor cells and the Neoligaments scaffold at the cellular and proteomic levels;
(2) Technical devising and experimental validation of optimized manufacturing procedures in order to obtain clinically usable combination products;
(3) Clinical devising and experimental validation of surgical procedures and protocols for hand ligament regenerative medicine with the considered implantable and bio-enhanced combination product.

The retained scaffold (i.e., Infinity-Lock 3 Neoligaments device, non-resorbable woven polyester, Xiros, Leeds, UK) was based on the Leeds-Keio (LK) artificial ligament, which was globally clinically applied in various musculoskeletal indications by several groups since 1982 (i.e., extensive clinical follow-up studies available) [59–67]. Designed for passive and gradual integration in patient tissues, the synthetic Infinity-Lock 3 scaffold was incubated with cultured FE002 primary progenitor tenocytes to obtain combination product prototypes [60]. In detail, the objective was to firstly verify the in vitro compatibility of both components, as well as critical and key functional attributes (e.g., cell colonization and extracellular matrix deposition along the scaffold fibers) of the considered combination product, aiming to eventually enhance graft bio-integration in vivo. The second objective was to establish an optimized good manufacturing practice (GMP)-transposable (i.e., adapted for clean room environments) manufacturing process for the combination product, for further translational and clinical applications. The third objective was to validate the applicability of the retained scaffold in two clinical indications of hand ligament surgery within a human cadaveric sub-study, in view of clinical protocol establishment for a pilot clinical trial. Building on the respectively available bodies of knowledge around the considered Neoligaments polymeric scaffold and around the FE002 primary progenitor cell source, tangible data were generated about the considered combinational approach and its applicability in surgical workflows [39,55,56,59–64,67,68]. Overall, this study enabled to set forth tangible proofs-of-concept for the translational development of an allogeneic tissue engineering protocol for bio-enhanced hand ligament surgical reconstructive care.

## 2. Materials and Methods

### 2.1. Reagents and Consumables Used for the In Vitro Studies

The reagents and consumables that were used in this study are summarized hereafter, along with the corresponding manufacturers: purified water, PBS buffer, and NaCl 0.9% solutions (Laboratorium Dr. G. Bichsel, Unterseen, Switzerland); high-glucose DMEM cell culture medium, L-glutamine, D-PBS, TrypLE dissociation reagent, penicillin-streptomycin, BCA assay kits, NuPAGE Bis-Tris 4–12% protein gel, MOPS buffer, loading buffer, DTT, antioxidant, page ruler protein ladder, transfer buffer, MTT, antibodies, and 96-well PCR plates (Thermo Fisher Scientific, Waltham, MA, USA); C-Chip Neubauer hemocytometers (NanoEntek, Seoul, Korea); ethanol, methanol, Tween 20, Telomerase activity assay kits, and HCl (Chemie Brunschwig, Basel, Switzerland); Millipore Stericup with 0.22 μm pores, Trypan blue solution, FBS, collagen I from rat tails, and fibronectin (Merck, Darmstadt, Germany); cell culture vessels and plastic assay surfaces (Greiner BioOne, Frickenhausen, Germany and TPP Techno Plastic Products, Trasadingen, Switzerland); RIPA lysis buffer and antibodies (Abcam, Cambridge, UK); protease inhibitor and CellTiter-Glo kits (Promega, Madison, WI, USA); Live-Dead kits and antibodies (Biotium, Fremont, CA, USA); powdered skim milk (Rapilait, Migros, France); saccharose (PanReac AppliChem, Darmstadt, Germany); dextran 40,000 (Pharmacosmos, Wiesbaden, Germany); Lyoprotect cups and Lyoprotect bags (Teclen, Oberpframmern, Germany); nitrocellulose membranes and ECL (Amersham Protran, Cytiva, Marlborough, MA, USA); BSA (PAN Biotech, Aidenbach, Germany).

### 2.2. Instruments and Equipment Used for the In Vitro Studies

For sample analysis, flat bottom 96-well microtitration plates and Eppendorf tubes were purchased from Greiner (Greiner, Frickenhausen, Germany). Component weighing was performed on a laboratory scale (Ohaus, Parsippany, NJ, USA). Sample centrifugation was performed on a Rotina 420R centrifuge (Hettich, Tuttlingen, Germany). Dynamic cell seeding of scaffolds was performed in a Roto-Therm Plus agitator (Benchmark Scientific, Sayreville, NJ, USA). SDS-Page analyses were performed using a Mini Gel Tank and PowerEase 90W (Thermo Fisher Scientific, Waltham, MA, USA). Gel imaging in white light or in chemiluminescence was performed on a Uvitec Mini HD9 gel imager (Cleaver Scientific, Rugby, UK). Colorimetric and luminescence measurements were performed on a Varioskan LUX multimode plate reader (Thermo Fisher Scientific, Waltham, MA, USA). Immunohistochemistry and Live-Dead imaging were performed on an inverted IX81 fluorescence microscope (Olympus, Tokyo, Japan). Telomerase activity PCR analyses were run on a StepOne Real-time PCR Systems instrument (Thermo Fisher Scientific, Waltham, MA, USA). Sample lyophilization was performed in a LyoBeta Mini freeze-dryer (Telstar, Terrassa, Spain). Sample terminal sterilization by γ-irradiation was performed by Ionisos, Dagneux, France.

### 2.3. Surgical and Grafting Materials Used for the Ex Vivo Studies

For the needs of the in vitro and ex vivo work (i.e., human cadaveric model), the artificial ligaments and surgical instruments (i.e., medical devices) were provided by Xiros, Leeds, UK. The provided artificial ligaments (i.e., woven polyester tapes) were 3 mm-wide Neoligaments Infinity-Lock 3 devices (i.e., two different manufacturing process-related options) and Jewel ACL devices. The provided surgical instruments were from a FlexPasser Tendon Retrieval Kit. Standard hand surgery instruments, materials, and consumables were provided by the Plastic and Hand Surgery Service at the CHUV Lausanne University Hospital, Lausanne, Switzerland.

### 2.4. FE002 Primary Progenitor Tenocyte Cell Sourcing and In Vitro Cellular Active Substance Lot Manufacture

The FE002 primary progenitor tenocyte source used for the in vitro experiments of this study consisted of banked primary human diploid cells (i.e., clinical grade FE002 progenitor cell source). The considered FE002 progenitor cells were procured and produced under the Swiss progenitor cell transplantation program and were made available for the present study as cryopreserved stocks, as previously described elsewhere [55]. All of the FE002 primary progenitor tenocytes used in the present study were characterized by in vitro passage levels of 6–8. Briefly, frozen vials of FE002 cells were used as cellular seeding materials for the in vitro expansions necessary to generate the cellular active substance lots. Rapid thawing of the vials was performed and the cells were suspended in warmed complete cell culture medium (i.e., DMEM; 10% $v/v$ FBS; 5.97 mM L-glutamine). The cell suspension titers and the relative cellular viability were determined by hemocytometer counts using Trypan blue exclusion dye. The cell suspensions were then used to homogeneously seed an appropriate amount of culture vessels using a $1.5 \times 10^3$ cells/cm$^2$ relative seeding density. The seeded cell culture vessels were incubated at 37 °C in humidified incubators under 5% $v/v$ $CO_2$. Cellular adherence checks were performed the following day and the cell culture medium was exchanged twice weekly. The cell culture vessels were examined at each medium exchange procedure, for confirmation of cell proliferation, adequate proliferative cellular morphology maintenance (i.e., characteristic spindle-shape morphology), and absence of observable extraneous agent contamination. Once optimal cell monolayer confluency was attained (i.e., >95%), the cells were harvested. The cell suspension titers and the relative cellular viability were determined. These cell suspensions were defined as a "fresh cellular active substance lot", for cell type characterization/qualification studies or for seeding onto synthetic Neoligaments scaffolds for finished combination product preparation. Alternatively, "cryopreserved cellular active substance lots" were used for synthetic scaffold seeding. Therefore, the cell suspensions were used directly after thawing, following the cell enumeration control step. For the needs of the present study, a cellular active substance lot was therefore composed of one of the following:

- "Fresh cellular active substance lot": Suspension of FE002 primary progenitor tenocytes (i.e., homogeneous cellular suspension in an appropriate solvent/medium, e.g., DMEM-based medium), expanded once in vitro in monolayer culture, harvested, and controlled before further use;
- "Cryopreserved cellular active substance lot": Cryopreserved FE002 primary progenitor tenocytes (i.e., homogeneous cellular suspension in an appropriate solvent/medium), conditioned in cryopreservation vials, extemporaneously thawed/rinsed, and controlled before further use.

### 2.5. Patient Primary Tenocyte Cell Sourcing and In Vitro Cell Lot Manufacture

The patient primary tenocyte source used for the in vitro experiments of this study consisted of banked primary human diploid cells (i.e., Ad001-Ten standardized cell source). All of the patient tenocytes used in the present study were characterized by in vitro passage levels of 6–8. Patient tenocytes were obtained from the Biobank of the Department of Musculoskeletal Medicine in the CHUV Lausanne University Hospital, Lausanne, Switzerland, in the form of cryopreserved vial lots. Biological material sourcing and primary cell type establishment had been performed from a hand digit flexor tendon (i.e., medical waste) of a 74-year-old female patient. The patient tenocytes were manufactured using serial in vitro cellular expansion rounds, following the same technical specifications as the considered FE002 primary progenitor tenocytes. The patient tenocytes were used for the in vitro experiments of this study, either in "fresh cellular active substance lot" form or in "cryopreserved cellular active substance lot" form.

### 2.6. FE002 Primary Progenitor Tenocyte Cellular Active Substance Characterization Assays

The assays presented hereafter were performed in order to complement the existing body of knowledge around FE002 primary progenitor tenocytes, as previously reported for this cellular active substance or cellular starting material [39,55–58].

2.6.1. Quality and Potency-Related Characterization and Qualification Assays

Firstly, mass spectrometry proteomic characterization assays were performed to gain insights into the major constituents of the cellular active substance of interest. The comparative proteomic analyses were performed using quantitative mass spectrometry, following the protocol reported by Jeannerat et al. (2021) [55]. Briefly, FE002 primary progenitor tenocytes and patient primary tenocyte samples were lysed and the protein contents were digested using an adapted filter-aided sample preparation (FASP) protocol. The obtained peptides were labelled and were analyzed by LC-MS/MS. Mass spectrometry proteomic data were deposited at the ProteomeXchange Consortium (http://www.proteomexchange.org/, accessed on 23 May 2023) via the PRIDE partner repository with the dataset identifier PXD028359 [55]. Specific data processing then enabled to obtain relative protein levels in the various samples, for comparative consideration. Relatively abundant proteins were retained for further analysis within both experimental groups (i.e., progenitor or patient tenocytes) and were compared to literature reference sources [69].

Secondly, in order to verify that the considered FE002 cellular active substance is capable of adhering on tendon extracellular matrix (ECM) components, an in vitro cellular adhesion assay was performed. Briefly, 96-well ELISA microplates were coated overnight with 50 µg/mL collagen I, 100% FBS, or 5 µg/mL fibronectin. The microplates were then washed with PBS and blocked for 1 h using PBS with 1% BSA. Freshly harvested FE002 primary progenitor tenocytes or primary patient tenocytes were suspended in DMEM with 1% BSA at a final concentration of $2 \times 10^5$ cells/mL. Volumes of 100 µL of cell suspension were dispensed in each well and the microplates were incubated for 1 h at 37 °C. The plates were then gently washed using DMEM with 1% BSA and pictures of the wells were taken on an inverted microscope, for the comparative assessment of cellular adhesion.

2.6.2. Quality and Safety-Related Characterization and Qualification Assays

Firstly, a β-galactosidase staining assay was performed, in order to confirm that the considered FE002 primary progenitor tenocytes were a cell type (i.e., and not a cell line) with a finite in vitro lifespan and reached senescence in culture at high passage levels under standard conditions. Cells at in vitro passage levels known to be characterized by significantly reduced proliferation capacities in the retained manufacturing system (i.e., passage levels > 8) were used for the assays. Briefly, FE002 primary progenitor tenocytes were seeded in T25 cell culture flasks at $1.5 \times 10^3$ cells/cm$^2$ and were expanded until reaching 70% confluency. The cells were then fixed for 5 min in 10 mL of fixation solution containing 1.85% formaldehyde with 0.2% glutaraldehyde. The cells were then rinsed twice using PBS. The cells were stained overnight at 37 °C with a SA-β-gal staining solution containing 0.1% X-gal, 5 mM potassium ferrocyanide, 5 mM potassium ferricyanide, 150 mM NaCl, and 2 mM $MgCl_2$ in a 40 mM citric acid/sodium phosphate solution at pH 6.0. The cells were washed twice with PBS and once with DMSO to remove the staining solution. The presence of β-galactosidase-positive (i.e., stained in blue) cells was assessed microscopically. Staining for the senescence marker β-galactosidase was performed between in vitro passage levels 8 and 10.

Secondly, a telomerase activity assay was performed using the Telomerase activity quantification qPCR assay kit in order to confirm the non-tumorigenic potential of the considered FE002 primary progenitor tenocytes (i.e., absence of significant levels of telomerase activity). Telomerase activity quantification was performed using frozen cellular dry pellets (i.e., passage level 8 for the FE002 cells). HeLa cells were obtained from the Musculoskeletal Research Unit at the University of Zurich (Zurich, Switzerland) and were used as positive controls in the telomerase assay. For cell lysate preparation, cellular dry pellets (i.e., 2–5 $\times 10^6$ cells/tube) were retrieved from −80 °C storage. Cells lysis was performed by mixing the cells with 20 µL of lysis buffer (i.e., supplemented with PMSF and β-mercaptoethanol before use) per million cells before a 30-min incubation period on ice. The samples were then centrifuged at 12,000 rpm for 20 min at 4 °C. The supernatants were transferred to new Eppendorf tubes. For the telomerase-mediated reaction, 0.5 µL of sample, 4 μL of 5× telomerase reaction buffer, and 15.5 μL of nuclease-free water were mixed and incubated for 3 h at 37 °C. The reaction was quenched by heating the samples for 10 min at 85 °C. The samples were centrifuged at 1500× *g* for 10 s and were stored on ice. The wells necessary for the qPCR reactions were prepared in triplicate in qPCR plates by mixing 1 μL of the prepared sample, 2 μL of primers, 10 μL of TaqGreen qPCR master mix, and 7 μL of nuclease-free water. The qPCR plates were sealed and centrifuged at 1500× *g* for 15 s. The samples were run on a StepOne Real-time PCR Systems instrument. The qPCR run conditions comprised an initial denaturation step of 10 min at 95 °C and 36 amplification cycles (i.e., denaturation over 20 s at 95 °C; annealing over 20 s at 52 °C; extension over 45 s at 72 °C). Samples with a Ct >33 in value were considered as being negative. Relative telomerase activity quantification between two samples was based on the $2^{-\Delta Ct}$ calculation method.

### *2.7. FE002 Primary Progenitor Tenocyte-Seeded Neoligaments Graft: Manufacturing Process Development Phase*

#### 2.7.1. Progenitor Cell Seeding and Combination Product Incubation Processes

In order to establish an initial proof-of-concept for scaffold-based FE002 progenitor cell-bearing construct bioengineering, conservative parameters and technical specifications were used. Two synthetic scaffold cell seeding strategies were experimentally investigated. Firstly, a static cell seeding protocol was used. Neoligaments Infinity-Lock 3 scaffold pieces of 1 cm in length were placed in 12-well microplates and volumes of 250 μL of cell suspension (i.e., fresh FE002 cellular active substance in complete cell culture medium, at various final cellular concentrations ranging from 25 × $10^3$ to $10^5$ cells/scaffold) were homogeneously dispensed in order to completely soak the scaffolds. Cell recovery quality control plates (i.e., 6-well microplates) were prepared at that time, with the same technical specifications as for FE002 primary progenitor tenocyte manufacturing activities. The sample-bearing microplates were incubated for 1 h at 37 °C, to enable initial cellular attachment. Then, volumes of 500 μL of complete cell culture medium (i.e., with 1% penicillin-streptomycin) were dispensed in each well and the microplates were incubated again. The cell-seeded scaffolds were maintained in culture for 14 days with medium exchange procedures performed twice per week before endpoint harvest.

Secondly, a dynamic cell seeding protocol was used. Fresh 1 cm-pieces of Infinity-Lock 3 scaffold were placed in 2 mL Eppendorf tubes and 1 mL of cell suspension (i.e., fresh FE002 cellular active substance in complete cell culture medium, at various final cellular concentrations) was dispensed in each tube. Cell recovery quality control plates were prepared at that time, as described hereabove. The tubes were incubated at 37 °C overnight under rotational agitation (i.e., 13 rpm, monoaxial rotation), to enable initial cellular attachment. Then, the scaffolds were transferred to 15 mL centrifugation tubes and were covered with 1 mL of fresh complete cell culture medium (i.e., with 1% penicillin-streptomycin). The volumes of 1 mL of spent culture medium (i.e., used for overnight dynamic cell seeding) were conserved and were used to prepare secondary cell recovery quality control plates. The cell-seeded scaffolds were maintained in culture for 14 days with medium exchange procedures performed twice per week before endpoint harvest. The dynamic cell seeding protocol was then repeated using fresh patient tenocyte suspensions (i.e., in "fresh cellular active substance lot" form), for cytocompatibility comparison with the FE002 primary progenitor tenocytes and for validation of the ability of patient cells to adhere to the synthetic scaffolds. The dynamic cell seeding protocol was then repeated again using two sub-types of Infinity-Lock 3 scaffolds (i.e., plasma-treated and non-plasma treated scaffolds), for assessment of the impact of the additional scaffold processing step on cytocompatibility and cellular functionality parameters.

For endpoint cell-seeded construct harvesting, the spent cell culture medium was removed from the 3D culture vessels. The constructs were rinsed thrice by immersion in warm PBS and were made available for further in vitro studies or for conditioning in finished product transport medium. At each step of the construct incubation process, the recovery quality control microplates were assessed (i.e., cell adherence on the culture surface and low cellular detachment, appropriate adherent cell morphology, positive cell confluency evolution, appropriate cellular metabolic activity) as part of in-process controls (IPC). Appropriate post-process controls (PPC) were implemented as appropriate.

#### 2.7.2. CellTiter-Glo Assay for Endpoint Assessment of Cellular Metabolic Activity within the Combination Products

A CellTiter-Glo assay was used to assess the metabolic activity of the cells on the constructs following the incubation period. Briefly, the constructs were harvested, rinsed, and placed in 24-well microplates. Volumes of 200 μL of PBS and 200 μL of CellTiter-Glo reagent were dispensed in each well. Micropipette tips were then used to lightly crush the immerged constructs. The plates were incubated for 10 min at ambient temperature. Finally, 200 μL of supernatant were isolated from each well and luminescence was measured.

#### 2.7.3. MTT Assay for Endpoint Assessment of Cellular Metabolic Activity and Cell Distribution throughout the Combination Products

An MTT assay was used to assess the cytocompatibility of the FE002 primary progenitor tenocytes and the Neoligaments scaffolds (i.e., Infinity-Lock 3 and Jewel ACL devices). Specifically, the MTT assay was used to confirm (i) the adherence of the cells throughout the scaffolds, (ii) the maintenance of cellular metabolic activity on the scaffolds, and (iii) the quality of cellular colonization of the scaffolds (i.e., homogeneous repartition of the cells on the available fiber surfaces). Furthermore, MTT assays were performed at various timepoints (i.e., between 1 day and 3 weeks) of the incubation phase of the cell-seeded constructs and enabled to assess the 3D in vitro cellular proliferation and migration on the scaffolds. For endpoint analysis, the constructs were harvested and incubated for 2 h at 37 °C in a 5 mg/mL MTT solution. Following rinsing of the constructs, photographic imaging was performed. For the further quantification of the MTT dye in the considered constructs, the dye was extracted using a 0.04 N HCl ethanolic solubilization solution. Then, volumes of 150 μL of the MTT extracts were transferred to 96-well microplates. Sample absorbance values were determined at a wavelength of 570 nm.

#### 2.7.4. Live-Dead Assay for Endpoint Assessment of Cellular Viability and Distribution throughout the Combination Products

A Live-Dead assay (i.e., viability and toxicity assay kit) was used to assess cellular viability, cellular adhesion, and cellular morphology directly on the constructs, according to the manufacturer's instructions. Briefly, the Live-Dead staining solution was prepared by mixing 10 mL of D-PBS, 5 μL calcein, and 20 μL ethidium homodimer III. The cell-seeded scaffolds were harvested, rinsed with D-PBS, and incubated with the Live-Dead staining solution for 30 min at ambient temperature. The samples were then washed to remove any excess reagents and were imaged on an Olympus IX81 microscope using the appropriate channels.

#### 2.7.5. Western Blotting for Endpoint Assessment of Extracellular Matrix Component Synthesis and Deposition within the Combination Products

Western blotting analysis was used in order to assess the synthesis and deposition of selected tendon-related ECM proteins (e.g., collagen I, decorin) within the incubated constructs. Briefly, the cell-seeded scaffolds were harvested, washed with PBS, and incubated for 15 min on ice in 300 μL of RIPA lysis buffer supplemented with protease inhibitors. The samples were centrifuged at 3000× $g$ for 5 min at 4 °C and the supernatants were stored at −20 °C until analysis. The samples were separated by electrophoresis on NuPAGE 4–12% Bis-tris polyacrylamide gels before being transferred onto nitrocellulose membranes. The membranes were blocked in 0.05% PBS-Tween 20 supplemented with 4% skimmed milk for 15 min at ambient temperature and were then incubated overnight at 4 °C in the primary antibody solution (i.e., anti-collagen I, anti-decorin, or anti-actin). The following day, the membranes were washed in PBS-Tween 20 buffer and were incubated for 1 h at ambient temperature in the corresponding HRP-secondary antibody. Revelation was performed using the ECL Prime chemiluminescence detection system. For all of the presented Western blotting assays, the following antibodies were used:

- Primary anti-collagen I antibody: Abcam Ref. N°ab34710 (1:1000 dilution)
- Primary anti-decorin antibody: Abcam Ref. N°ab277636 (1:1000 dilution)
- Primary anti-actin antibody: Thermo Fisher Ref. N°PA1-21167 (1:200 dilution)
- Secondary anti-rabbit HRP antibody: Biotium Ref. N°20403 (1:2000 dilution)
- Secondary anti-mouse HRP antibody: Biotium Ref. N°20401 (1:2000 dilution)

#### 2.7.6. Immunofluorescence Imaging for Endpoint Assessment of Extracellular Matrix Component Synthesis and Deposition throughout the Combination Products

Direct immunofluorescence staining was used to assess cellular adhesion, cellular morphology, and tendon-related extracellular matrix protein (e.g., collagen I, aggrecan, decorin) deposition throughout the incubated constructs. Briefly, the cell-seeded scaffolds were harvested, washed with PBS, and fixed overnight in PAF at 4 °C. An antigen retrieval step was then performed for 10 min at 37 °C in an antigen retrieval buffered solution (i.e., 0.05 M Tris-HCl; 0.1% $CaCl_2$; 0.15 M NaCl) supplemented with 2 mg/mL hyaluronidase. Then, the samples were blocked for 1 h at ambient temperature in a 0.05% PBS-Tween 20 solution supplemented with 1% BSA. The samples were incubated overnight at 4 °C in a primary antibody solution (i.e., phalloidin-iFluor594, anti-collagen I, anti-aggrecan). Except for phalloidin staining, revelation was eventually performed by incubating the constructs in the corresponding secondary antibodies coupled to Alexa Fluor 488. The samples were imaged on an Olympus IX81 microscope. For all of the presented immunofluorescence assays, the following antibodies were used:

- Primary anti-phalloidin-iFluor594 antibody: Abcam Ref. N°ab176757 (1:1000 dilution)
- Primary anti-decorin antibody: Abcam Ref. N°ab175404 (1:100 dilution)
- Primary anti-collagen I antibody: Abcam Ref. N°ab138492 (1:100 dilution)
- Primary anti-aggrecan antibody: Abcam Ref. N°ab3778 (1:100 dilution)
- Primary anti-tenomodulin antibody: Thermo Fisher Ref. N°PA5-112767 (1:100 dilution)
- Rabbit IgG isotype control antibody: Abcam Ref. N°ab172730 (1:100 dilution)
- Mouse isotype control antibody: Abcam Ref. N°ab170190 (1:100 dilution)
- Secondary anti-rabbit Alexa 488 antibody: Abcam Ref. N°ab150081 (1:250 dilution)
- Secondary anti-mouse Alexa 488 antibody: Abcam Ref. N°ab150113 (1:250 dilution)

### *2.8. FE002 Primary Progenitor Tenocyte-Seeded Neoligaments Graft: Manufacturing Process Optimization Phase*

#### 2.8.1. Optimized Cell Seeding and Combination Product Incubation Processes

In order to establish a combination product manufacturing process characterized by enhanced scalability and ease of transposition to GMP manufacturing settings, several modifications to the initial technical specifications were implemented. The main objective at this point was to reduce the overall manufacturing period for the cell-seeded constructs and to separate the cellular active substance manufacturing phase from the combination product manufacturing phase, while conserving the endpoint quality attributes of the constructs. Therefore, high cell seeding densities were used (i.e., $10^5$ cells/cm of scaffold) and the construct incubation period was reduced from 14 days to 6 $\pm$ 2 days. Endpoint characterization assays were performed (i.e., MTT, Live-Dead, immunofluorescence) to comparatively assess the quality attributes of the combination products in both experimental conditions (i.e., conservative vs. optimized manufacturing workflow). The results of these assessments were summarized in ad hoc parametric grading tables.

#### 2.8.2. Pilot Assessment of Combination Product Lyophilization & Sterilization Processes

In order to initiate a preliminary evaluation for the feasibility of obtaining temperature-stable and terminally-sterilized FE002 primary progenitor tenocyte-seeded constructs, pilot lyophilization and sterilization studies were performed. Firstly, cell-seeded constructs were prepared using fresh FE002 progenitor cellular active substance materials with a 3-week incubation period. Following endpoint harvest, the constructs were immerged in lyopreservation solution composed of 8% saccharose and 2% dextran 40,000 in diluted PBS buffer. The samples were initially frozen at −20 °C. Following loading in the freeze-dryer, annealing was performed between −20 °C and −30 °C. Primary drying was performed over 48 h under a partial vacuum of 0.08 mbar and with a shelf temperature of −22 °C. Secondary drying was performed over 14 h under a partial vacuum of 0.008 mbar and with a shelf temperature of 25 °C. The resulting freeze-dried samples were then conditioned in airtight boxes and were stored at 4 °C until further use. A sublot of samples was processed by $^{60}$Co gamma irradiation at a dose of 25–30 kGy. For comparative sample analysis, the contents of the boxes were rehydrated with the appropriate amount of distilled water and were left to soak for 5 min. Endpoint characterization assays were performed (i.e., Live-Dead, immunofluorescence imaging) in order to assess the quality attributes in both of the experimental conditions (i.e., lyophilized samples and lyophilized/irradiated samples). The results of these assessments were compared to those obtained on freshly harvested constructs and were summarized in ad hoc parametric grading tables.

### 2.9. *Human Ex Vivo Surgical Study for Clinical Protocol Establishment in Hand Ligament Regenerative Medicine*

#### 2.9.1. Ex Vivo Human Anatomy Material Procurement and Surgical Processing

For the needs of the ex vivo part of the study, human anatomical body limbs were provided by the Unit of Anatomy and Morphology of the University of Lausanne (Lausanne, Switzerland). All of the ex vivo work was performed on the premises of the Unit of Anatomy and Morphology of the University of Lausanne. The retained ex vivo anatomical model consisted of a left arm from an elderly female patient, sectioned mid-humerus. The arm was frozen but was not chemically preserved before the study. The arm was thawed and was stored at 4 °C until use in the study. In order to optimize the use of human cadaveric samples, the arm was used in a perforator flaps training after completion of this study. To this goal, intra-arterial infusion with 60 mL of commercial latex milk mixed with green acrylic colorant was performed 24 h before the ex vivo study, in order to optimally visualize the microvascular structures. At the end of both studies, all biological materials were disposed of following the applicable regulations and waste management workflows within the Unit of Anatomy and Morphology of the University of Lausanne.

#### 2.9.2. Ex Vivo Neoligaments Graft Implantation Procedure for Ligamento-Suspension Plasty after Trapeziectomy

For the needs of the procedure, the arm was prepared and was placed through an operating field. An initial incision was performed on the dorsal aspect of the trapeziometacarpal joint. Subcutaneous dissection followed, preserving the dorsal branch of the radial nerve. After opening of the articular capsule, the trapezium was fully removed and the flexor carpi radialis (FCR) tendon was exposed. The FlexPasser device was then used to reach under the FCR and to set the ad hoc polymeric sheath in place. Using the sheath, the Infinity-Lock 3 device was passed under the FCR. Excess Infinity-Lock 3 materials were excised and both ends of the device were fixed using osteosutures with Supramid 3-0 (B. Braun, Melsungen, Germany) threads on the basis of the metacarpal bone. Sufficient tension was set to achieve an effective suspension of the thumb upon testing.

#### 2.9.3. Ex Vivo Neoligaments Graft Implantation Procedure for Thumb Metacarpo-Phalangeal Ulnar Collateral Ligamentoplasty

For the needs of the procedure, an initial incision was performed to gain access to the ulnar collateral ligament (UCL). The UCL was sectioned and a 1 cm-portion of the ligament was removed in order to artificially create the equivalent of a complete rupture. Testing of the articulation confirmed an excessive laxity following the section. The Infinity-Lock 3 device was installed and was sutured in place distally first, using Supramid 3-0. Excess Infinity-Lock 3 materials were excised and the free end of the device was sutured proximally using the same thread. Testing of the articulation confirmed that the lateral stability of the joint was restored. If the remaining portions of the artificial ligament were to be insufficient for direct suturing, direct fixation into the bone could be performed using an anchor such as Micro-Mitek (DePuys Synthes, Comté de Bristol, MA, USA). The artificial grafts showed some filamentory fragmentation after being cut. This was assessed as being similar to what can be clinically observed in native tendons and did not impact the stability of the construct.

### 2.10. Statistical Analysis of the Data and Presentation of the Results

For the statistical comparison of average values from two sets of data, a paired Student's $t$-test was applied, following appropriate evaluation of the normal distribution of data, wherein a $p$-value $< 0.05$ was retained as a base for statistical significance determination. The calculations and data presentation were performed using Microsoft Excel (Microsoft Corporation, Redmond, WA, USA), Microsoft PowerPoint, and GraphPad Prism version 8.0.2 (GraphPad Software, San Diego, CA, USA).

## 3. Results

### 3.1. FE002 Primary Progenitor Tenocytes Possess Quality and Safety Attributes Compatible with Translational and Clinical Musculoskeletal Tissue Engineering

In order to confirm and to further document the quality- and safety-related attributes of the considered FE002 primary progenitor tenocytes, several cellular active substance characterization and qualification studies were performed in vitro. For facilitated reading of the results, a general overview of the design of the study, presenting the major phases, is presented in Figures S1A and S1B. Firstly, a comparative proteomic analysis revealed that the considered FE002 primary progenitor tenocytes contained major proteinic constituents known to compose native human tendons (e.g., ECM proteoglycans, collagens, ECM glycoproteins), which were also found in the considered patient primary tenocyte group (Table 1).

**Table 1.** Results of the comparative proteomic analysis for the determination of the major constituents in FE002 primary progenitor tenocyte and patient tenocyte samples (i.e., from cells expanded in vitro in monolayers). Relative quantitative data were expressed as fold change logarithms (i.e., base 2 log), with a significance threshold value specified at 0.9 for upregulation and an FDR threshold value specified at ≤0.01. The data are reported for three selected protein classes, namely collagens, ECM glycoproteins, and ECM proteoglycans. ECM, extracellular matrix; FC, fold change; FDR, false discovery rate.

| Protein Class | Protein Name | Short Protein Name | Patient Tenocytes vs. FE002 Progenitor Tenocytes logFC Value | FDR Value |
| --- | --- | --- | --- | --- |
| 1. ECM Proteoglycans | Basement membrane-specific heparan sulfate proteoglycan core protein | HSPG2 | −0.2981 | ≤0.01 |
| | Versican core protein | VCAN | −0.4311 | ≤0.01 |
| | Aggrecan core protein | ACAN | −0.8185 | ≤0.01 |
| | Decorin | DCN | 1.5648 | ≤0.01 |
| | Biglycan | BGN | 0.3762 | ≤0.01 |
| | Prolargin | PRELP | 0.3975 | ≤0.01 |
| | Testican-1 | SPOCK1 | 0.3765 | ≤0.01 |
| | Podocan | PODN | 1.1864 | ≤0.01 |
| | Mimecan | OGN | −1.5874 | ≤0.01 |

**Table 1.** *Cont.*

| Protein Class | Protein Name | Short Protein Name | Patient Tenocytes vs. FE002 Progenitor Tenocytes logFC Value | FDR Value |
|---|---|---|---|---|
| 2. Collagens | Collagen alpha-3(VI) chain | COL6A3 | 0.2684 | ≤0.01 |
| | Collagen alpha-1(XII) chain | COL12A1 | −0.4344 | ≤0.01 |
| | Collagen alpha-2(I) chain | COL1A2 | −0.9689 | ≤0.01 |
| | Collagen alpha-1(I) chain | COL1A1 | −1.2075 | ≤0.01 |
| | Collagen alpha-1(XIV) chain | COL14A1 | −2.0388 | ≤0.01 |
| | Collagen alpha-2(VI) chain | COL6A2 | 0.1635 | ≤0.01 |
| | Collagen alpha-1(III) chain | COL3A1 | −0.8283 | ≤0.01 |
| | Isoform 2 of Collagen alpha-1(V) chain | COL5A1 | −1.3237 | ≤0.01 |
| | Collagen alpha-1(XVIII) chain | COL18A1 | −0.1641 | ≤0.01 |
| | Collagen alpha-2(V) chain | COL5A2 | −1.4452 | ≤0.01 |
| | Collagen alpha-1(II) chain | COL2A1 | 0.6062 | ≤0.01 |
| | Collagen alpha-1(XVI) chain | COL16A1 | −0.3993 | ≤0.01 |
| | Collagen alpha-1(IV) chain | COL4A1 | −0.6277 | ≤0.01 |
| | Collagen alpha-1(VIII) chain | COL8A1 | 0.7691 | ≤0.01 |
| | Collagen alpha-1(XI) chain | COL11A1 | −0.4923 | ≤0.01 |
| 3. ECM Glycoproteins | Fibronectin | FN1 | 0.9885 | ≤0.01 |
| | Laminin subunit beta-2 | LAMB2 | −0.6965 | ≤0.01 |
| | Tenascin | TNC | 0.1536 | ≤0.01 |
| | Laminin subunit alpha-4 | LAMA4 | −0.2982 | ≤0.01 |
| | Laminin subunit gamma-1 | LAMC1 | −0.1818 | ≤0.01 |
| | Peroxidasin homolog | PXDN | −0.1384 | ≤0.01 |
| | von Willebrand factor A domain-containing protein 5A | VWA5A | 0.6092 | ≤0.01 |
| | Transforming growth factor-beta-induced protein ig-h3 | TGFBI | 0.3414 | ≤0.01 |
| | Thrombospondin-1 | THBS1 | −0.4929 | ≤0.01 |
| | Tenascin-X | TN-X | 0.9108 | ≤0.01 |
| | Laminin subunit beta-1 | LAMB1 | 0.1839 | ≤0.01 |
| | Lactadherin | MFGE8 | −0.2366 | ≤0.01 |
| | EGF-like repeat and discoidin I-like domain-containing protein 3 | EDIL3 | 0.3395 | ≤0.01 |
| | Procollagen C-endopeptidase enhancer 1 | PCOLCE | −0.4078 | ≤0.01 |
| | Laminin subunit alpha-3 | LAMA3 | −0.1923 | ≤0.01 |
| | Extracellular matrix protein 1 | ECM1 | 1.2584 | ≤0.01 |
| | Fibulin-2 | FBLN2 | −0.5234 | ≤0.01 |
| | Thrombospondin-2 | THBS2 | 0.1871 | ≤0.01 |
| | Latent-transforming growth factor beta-binding protein 1 | LTBP1 | −0.2777 | ≤0.01 |
| | Collagen triple helix repeat-containing protein 1 | CTHRC1 | −2.3638 | ≤0.01 |
| | Fibulin-1 | FBLN1 | 0.5411 | ≤0.01 |
| | Latent-transforming growth factor beta-binding protein 3 | LTBP3 | −0.3839 | ≤0.01 |
| | Insulin-like growth factor-binding protein 7 | IGFBP7 | 0.2386 | ≤0.01 |
| | CCN family member 1 | CYR61 | 0.8094 | ≤0.01 |
| | Cysteine-rich with EGF-like domain protein 2 | CRELD2 | −0.6177 | ≤0.01 |
| | Netrin-G1 | NTNG1 | −0.5626 | ≤0.01 |
| | Latent-transforming growth factor beta-binding protein 2 | LTBP2 | 0.9153 | ≤0.01 |

**Table 1.** *Cont.*

| Protein Class | Protein Name | Short Protein Name | Patient Tenocytes vs. FE002 Progenitor Tenocytes logFC Value | FDR Value |
|---|---|---|---|---|
| | Cartilage oligomeric matrix protein | COMP | −0.3154 | ≤0.01 |
| | Cysteine-rich with EGF-like domain protein 1 | CRELD1 | −0.5640 | ≤0.01 |
| | Insulin-like growth factor-binding protein 5 | IGFBP5 | −1.4395 | ≤0.01 |
| | Adipocyte enhancer-binding protein 1 | AEBP1 | 1.0318 | ≤0.01 |
| | Insulin-like growth factor binding protein 3 isoform b | IGFBP3 | 0.9616 | ≤0.01 |
| | Microfibril-associated glycoprotein 4 | MFAP4 | −2.3113 | ≤0.01 |
| | Fibrillin-2 | FBN2 | −0.6129 | ≤0.01 |
| | Slit homolog 3 protein | SLIT3 | −0.3010 | ≤0.01 |
| | Laminin subunit alpha-1 | LAMA1 | 0.6983 | ≤0.01 |
| | Slit homolog 2 protein | SLIT2 | 0.5349 | ≤0.01 |
| | Thrombospondin-3 | THBS3 | −0.5152 | ≤0.01 |
| | Target of Nesh-SH3 | ABI3BP | 0.5272 | ≤0.01 |
| | Laminin subunit alpha-5 | LAMA5 | −0.7307 | ≤0.01 |
| | Netrin-4 | NTN4 | −0.5776 | ≤0.01 |
| | Matrix-remodeling-associated protein 5 | MXRA5 | −0.3548 | ≤0.01 |

Secondly, an in vitro cellular adhesion assay was performed using patient primary tenocytes and FE002 primary progenitor tenocytes, to comparatively assess their respective adhesion potentials on ubiquitous ECM components (e.g., collagen I, fibronectin, i.e., found in abundant amounts in tendinous tissues). The results indicated that both of the considered primary cell types were capable of similar and rapid adhesive behaviors on collagen I-, fibronectin-, and FBS-coated surfaces (Figure S2). Of note, FBS is known to contain vitronectin, which is among the molecules most probably responsible for the considered cellular adhesive properties. Thirdly, a β-galactosidase staining assay confirmed that FE002 primary progenitor tenocytes reached senescence at high in vitro passage levels (e.g., passage level N°10), thereby confirming the finite nature of the cell type's lifespan (Figure S3). Finally, a comparative telomerase activity quantification assay enabled to confirm that FE002 primary progenitor tenocytes possess telomerase activity levels which are two orders of decimal magnitude below those of known tumoral cell lines (i.e., HeLa cells, Table S1). Generally, the obtained in vitro original data complemented the previously published biological characteristics/attributes of FE002 primary progenitor tenocytes [39,55]. Overall, the obtained data enabled to set forth important quality- and functionality-related attributes of FE002 primary progenitor tenocytes (i.e., capacity to adhere to known components of tendons and ligaments) and important safety-related attributes (i.e., low propensity for presenting tumorigenic behaviors) of this cellular active substance.

### *3.2. Allogeneic FE002 Primary Progenitor Tenocytes May Be Rapidly Combined with Neoligaments Devices to Form Biologically-Enhanced Grafts*

The sound development of a cell-scaffold finished combination product implies that the chosen scaffold should be perfectly biocompatible with the therapeutic cellular active substance of interest. Specifically, the cells need to be able to bind to the scaffold's fibers/surfaces and remain viable up until the time of finished product clinical administration. In addition, the cell seeding process must be efficient, to reduce the proportion of non-binding cells. The synthetic material composing the Neoligaments Infinity-Lock 3 scaffold is known to passively allow cell and tissue ingrowth following clinical application. Therefore, the initial focus point of the present study, in view of establishing allogeneic musculoskeletal tissue engineering protocols, consisted in the validation of cytocompatibility aspects between Neoligaments scaffolds and FE002 primary progenitor tenocytes. For material rationalization purposes, the in vitro studies were performed on Infinity-Lock 3 or Jewel ACL scaffold subunits of 1 cm, obtained by fractionation of whole device units. Various cell seeding strategies were investigated, using two cell seeding modalities (i.e., static vs. dynamic), various cell seeding relative doses, and various construct incubation time-periods. The results confirmed the cytocompatibility between the considered Neoligaments scaffolds and the FE002 primary progenitor tenocytes. Furthermore, significant differences between the two cell seeding strategies were evidenced, favoring the exclusive subsequent use of dynamic cell seeding protocols for the in vitro assays of the study (Figure 1(A1,A2)).

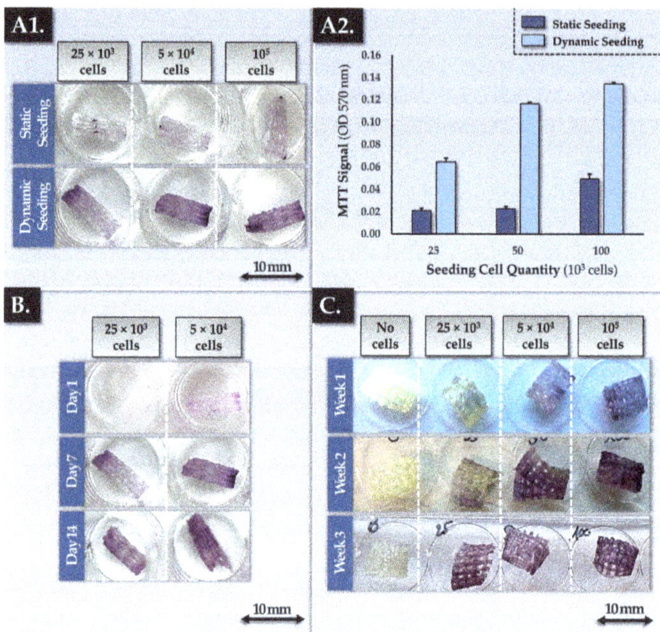


**Figure 1.** Results of biocompatibility and tissue engineering process development studies aiming to establish the cell seeding density, the cell seeding type (i.e., static or dynamic cell seeding), and the combination product incubation period. The results outlined that in optimal conditions, the FE002 progenitor cells adhere on the scaffolds, are capable of 3D proliferation, and stay metabolically active (i.e., positive MTT readout). (**A1**,**A2**) Dynamic seeding of FE002 primary progenitor tenocytes on the Infinity-Lock 3 scaffolds resulted in superior colonization (i.e., increased efficiency) compared to static cell seeding, as assessed by MTT staining (i.e., cell viability and localization on the scaffold). A dose-dependent relationship was evidenced between the cell seeding density and the scaffold colonization capacity. Imaging was performed 7 days after cell seeding of plasma-treated scaffolds. (**B**) Results indicated that the dynamically seeded FE002 cells were capable of proliferation on the scaffolds. An assessment of various combination product incubation periods revealed that significant scaffold colonization and homogeneous cellular proliferation were attained with a dose of $5 \times 10^4$ cells/scaffold at the 7-day and 14-day timepoints. The observed significant increase in MTT signals was confirmed by quantitative analysis (data not shown). (**C**) Similar results of scaffold colonization by FE002 cells were obtained with Jewel ACL scaffolds (i.e., with dynamic cell seeding), as assessed by MTT staining. These results indicated that such scaffolds could potentially be used with a high degree of versatility for musculoskeletal bioengineering, depending on the anatomical location of the affection. Overall, the use of higher cell seeding densities enables reaching of high cell quantities within the combination products in shortened incubation time-periods. OD, optic density.

Specifically, after cell seeding and construct incubation, MTT staining and the subsequent MTT dye quantification firstly demonstrated the presence of metabolically active cells binding to the scaffolds. Secondly, while the cell seeding density had a significant impact on scaffold colonization capacity by the cells at early construct incubation time-points, samples at late time-points (i.e., two or three weeks of incubation) displayed comparable cellular colonization (Figure 1B,C). These results generally indicated that the Infinity-Lock 3 and Jewel ACL scaffolds were comparable in terms of wettability/cytocompatibility and that the FE002 primary progenitor tenocytes were capable of homogeneous 3D proliferation throughout both scaffolds (Figure 1). Furthermore, it was shown that a dynamic cell seeding protocol was required to enable significant cellular adhesion to the scaffold fibers and that some sort of saturation occurred after homogeneous scaffold colonization was achieved by the cells (Figure 1).

The obtained cytocompatibility data gathered using the MTT readout was confirmed by the Live-Dead readout, showing the presence of adherent and viable cells along the scaffold fibers following incubation (Figure S4). Scaffold autofluorescence had been previously experimentally excluded. In endpoint, most of the present FE002 primary progenitor tenocytes were assessed as being alive (i.e., green staining), while only a few dead cells (i.e., red staining) could be observed on the scaffolds. Furthermore, Live-Dead cell staining allowed to specifically observe the spreading and alignment of the cells along the scaffold fibers (Figure S4). Overall, while the MTT readout enabled the rapid global evaluation of cellular adhesion, scaffold colonization quality, and cellular metabolic activity maintenance, the Live-Dead readout provided complementary information (i.e., relative viable cellular proportion, cell conformation along the fibers). Finally, additional potency-related data were gathered in endpoint on the Infinity-Lock 3 scaffolds bearing FE002 primary progenitor tenocytes, by using immunofluorescence readouts (Figure S5). These results confirmed the presence and the structural organization along the scaffold fibers of ECM components which are naturally present in tendons (i.e., decorin, tenomodulin, aggrecan, phalloidin), confirming the ability of the cultured FE002 primary progenitor tenocytes to deploy their functions in appropriate 3D environments (Figure S5).

Successful tendinous or ligament tissue replacement using a synthetic scaffold requires a form of progressive in vivo graft colonization by the tissues and cells of the patient. While the cytocompatibility and the cellular adhesion potentials of the considered FE002 primary progenitor tenocytes were already assessed, the cytocompatibility of the scaffold with patient primary tenocytes required characterization work (Figures 1 and S2). Specifically, preliminary assays showed that patient primary tenocytes were capable of excellent cellular adhesion on major tendon ECM components (i.e., biological surfaces, e.g., collagen I, fibronectin) in vitro (Figure S2). Then, the MTT-based cytocompatibility assay, previously described for the FE002 primary progenitor cell source, was performed again on cell-seeded constructs bearing patient primary tenocytes. Qualitative and quantitative results of these assays confirmed similar behaviors between the FE002 primary progenitor cells and the patient cells on the Infinity-Lock 3 scaffold, with enhanced metabolic activity recorded in the patient tenocyte groups (Figure 2(A1,A2)).

Such similar behaviors between the two considered primary cell types were further confirmed in Live-Dead assays, in immunofluorescence assays (e.g., phalloidin, aggrecan revelation), and in MTT-based histology assays on the patient tenocyte-seeded samples (Figures S4, S6 and S7). Furthermore, MTT-based timepoint analyses performed on constructs bearing patient tenocytes demonstrated the cellular proliferation and the scaffold colonization potentials of the latter (Figure S7). Then, a Western blot analysis confirmed that total protein quantities on the scaffolds and specific protein (i.e., aggrecan, decorin, collagen I, actin) quantities on the scaffolds were significantly increased at the 3-week timepoint compared to the 1-week timepoint (full data not shown). Importantly, the gathered experimental data enabled to confirm in vitro that the artificial scaffolds behaved as intended in the presence of patient primary tenocytes (i.e., isolated from hand tendon tissue), namely with the physical provision/presence of an appropriate 3D environment allowing (i.e., passively) biological material ingrowth.

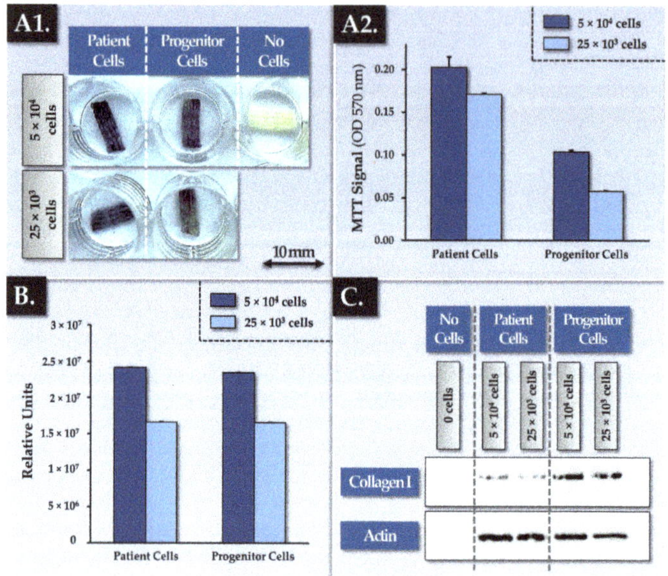


**Figure 2.** Results of comparative assessments for Infinity-Lock 3 scaffold colonization capacities by patient primary tenocytes and by FE002 primary progenitor tenocytes. (**A1**) Both cell types were shown to be able to bind and proliferate throughout the scaffolds. Imaging was performed 13 days after dynamic cell seeding of plasma-treated scaffolds. (**A2**) Patient primary tenocytes were shown to possess similar scaffold colonization capacities compared to FE002 primary progenitor tenocytes, as assessed by MTT staining. A dose-dependent relationship was evidenced between the cell seeding density and scaffold colonization capacity. Superior metabolic activity levels were recorded in the patient tenocyte group. Analyses were performed 6 days after dynamic cell seeding of plasma-treated scaffolds. (**B**) CellTiter-Glo quantification data from the same scaffold lots (i.e., 6 days of incubation) showed similar results compared to the MTT quantification data. (**C**) Western blotting results revealed a dose-dependent and enhanced human collagen I synthesis and deposition within the scaffolds by the FE002 primary progenitor tenocytes compared to the patient primary tenocytes. Whole gel imaging for collagen I and actin is presented in Figure S8. OD, optical density.

In view of optimizing the quantitative in-process controls for scaffold cellular colonization assessment, a CellTiter-Glo readout was used to comparatively characterize constructs bearing FE002 primary progenitor tenocytes or patient primary tenocytes (Figure 2B). The results were in line with the data obtained using the MTT-based readouts (i.e., presence of a dose-response relationship and slightly superior absolute values for the patient primary tenocyte groups, Figure 2(A1,A2),B). While the CellTiter-Glo readout is more sensitive and can be performed rapidly to obtain quantitative results, as compared to the MTT-based readout, the qualitative assessment of scaffold colonization (i.e., cellular adhesion and distribution) is however not possible. It should be noted that as both quantitative readouts are based on metabolic reactions, their use for the quantitative comparison of different cell types is not directly possible without prior normalization. In addition to the comparative and quantitative assessments of scaffold colonization potentials at a cellular level (i.e., MTT-based and CellTiter-Glo readouts), immunology-based readouts revealed that the constructs bearing FE002 primary progenitor tenocytes contained more synthesized and deposited ECM components (e.g., collagen I) compared to the patient primary tenocyte groups (Figure 2C). Close consideration of these potency-related results indicated that multiparametric controls (i.e., at least at cellular and proteomic levels) were necessary for appropriate endpoint construct or finished combination product assessment.

As regards the type of Infinity-Lock 3 scaffolds to potentially be used in musculoskeletal tissue engineering, two technical processing options exist. The first option corresponds to the CE-marked scaffold (i.e., non-plasma treated scaffold). The second option corresponds to a plasma-treated scaffold, developed for enhanced wettability and cellular/tissular colonization properties [70]. Comparative multiparametric assessment (i.e., MTT- and immunology-based assays) of plasma-treated vs. non-plasma-treated scaffolds firstly revealed no significant differences between the groups, as all of the considered samples performed well in terms of functionality parameters (Figure 3).

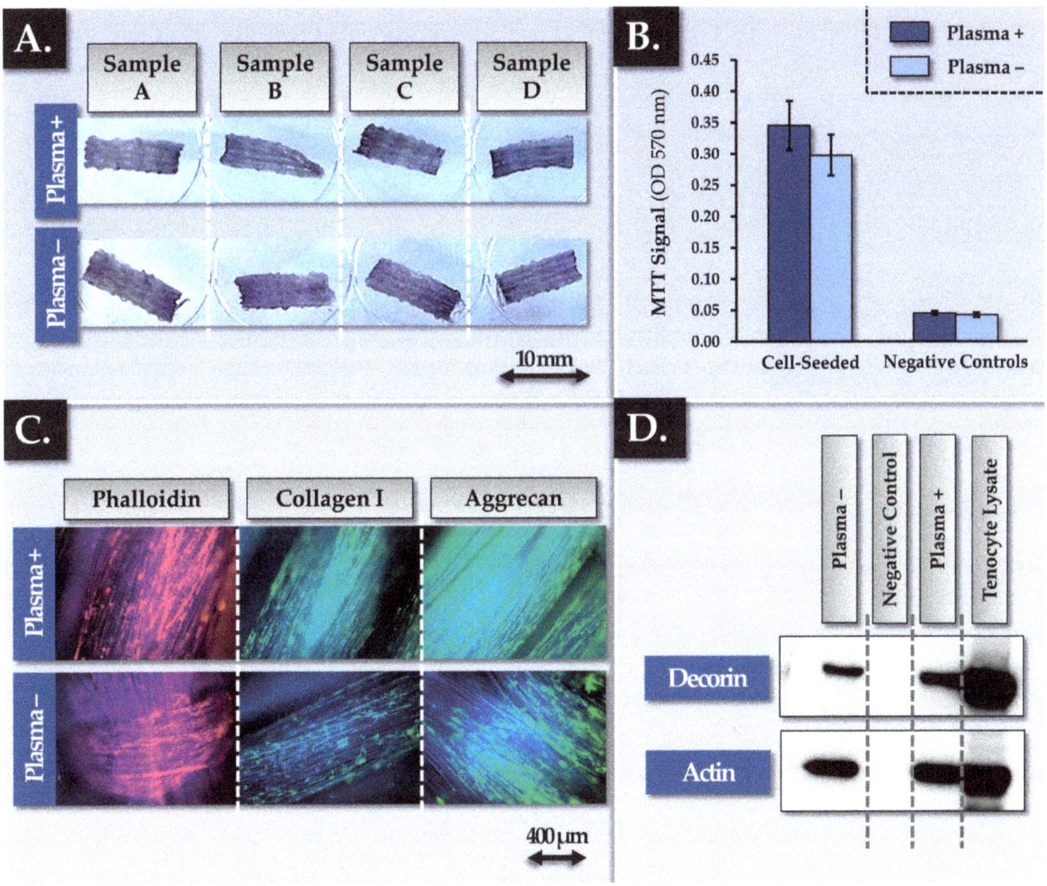


**Figure 3.** Results of the parallel qualification studies for plasma-treated and non-plasma-treated Infinity-Lock 3 scaffolds following FE002 primary progenitor tenocyte seeding and incubation for three weeks. (**A**,**B**) Results revealed no observable or statistically significant difference (i.e., $p$-value = 0.11) in the scaffold colonization potential of dynamically-seeded FE002 primary progenitor tenocytes between the two groups, as assessed by MTT staining and subsequent dye quantification. (**C**) Similar behaviors (i.e., phalloidin, collagen I, aggrecan synthesis and deposition) were evidenced for the two scaffold groups by immunofluorescence. (**D**) Similar behaviors in terms of decorin synthesis and deposition within the scaffolds were evidenced for the two considered groups by Western blotting. Whole gel imaging for decorin and actin is presented in Figure S9. OD, optical density.

Specifically, FE002 primary progenitor tenocyte adhesion on the scaffolds was not found to be influenced by scaffold plasma pre-treatment (Figure 3A,B). The whole construct surface was indeed covered with cells and ECM proteins such as actin, collagen I, aggrecan, and decorin (Figure 3C). The observed equivalence between the plasma-treated and the non-plasma-treated Infinity-Lock 3 scaffolds was further investigated in endpoint using comparative grading of efficacy/potency-related parameters of the cellular component of the combined finished product (Table 2).

**Table 2.** Grading table for the assessment of equivalence between plasma-treated and non-plasma-treated Infinity-Lock 3 scaffolds within the finished product manufacturing workflows. Equivalence was assessed for finished product efficacy-related parameters/attributes only (i.e., cellular components). ECM, extracellular matrix; 3D, three dimensions.

| Efficacy Parameter Type | Controls/Assays | Targets & Acceptance Criteria | Endpoint Construct Gradings [1] | |
|---|---|---|---|---|
| | | | Non-Plasma-Treated | Plasma-Treated |
| Cellular Viability Maintenance in 3D | MTT; Live-Dead | Presence of viable cells throughout the constructs | +++ | +++ |
| Cellular Quantity in 3D | MTT; Live-Dead | Presence of cells throughout the constructs; In amounts comparable to historical data | +++ | +++ |
| Cellular Adhesion & Cellular Morphology in 3D | Live-Dead | Presence of adherent cells throughout the constructs; Cellular alignment along the scaffold fibers | ++ | +++ |
| Cellular Proliferation Capacity in 3D | CellTiter-Glo; Live-Dead | Presence of cells throughout the constructs in larger amounts than after cell seeding | +++ | +++ |
| Cellular Colonization Homogeneity in 3D | MTT; Live-Dead | Presence of homogeneously distributed cells throughout the constructs | +++ | +++ |
| Extracellular Matrix Synthesis & Deposition in 3D | Immunofluorescence; Immunohistochemistry | Presence of adherent ECM components along the fibers within the constructs | ++ | +++ |
| Extracellular Matrix Deposition Homogeneity in 3D | Immunofluorescence | Presence of homogeneously distributed ECM throughout the constructs | +++ | +++ |

[1] Gradings were attributed as follows: (+++) = conforming, excellent performance; (++) = conforming, good performance; (+) = conforming; (±) = unclear, additional data required; (–) = non-conforming.

Therein, the results confirmed that all of the considered samples were characterized by good performance for all of the investigated parameters (Table 2). At this point of the study, the available knowledge and data about cellular colonization of the Infinity-Lock 3 scaffold and ECM component synthesis/deposition throughout the scaffold enabled the establishment of a theoretical model describing the various steps and functionality-related mechanisms at play during construct cell-seeding and incubation (Figure S10). At this point, the protocol for obtaining the Infinity-Lock 3 constructs bearing allogeneic FE002 primary progenitor tenocytes was assessed as being established and validated, with multiparametric characterization of the obtained bio-enhanced grafts (Figures 1 and 3, Table 2).

### 3.3. Bio-Enhanced Constructs Bearing Viable FE002 Primary Progenitor Tenocytes May Potentially Be Converted into Temperature-Stable & Devitalized Cell-Based Therapeutic Products

A proof-of-concept sub-study was then carried out in order to investigate the potential for further processing (i.e., stabilization by lyophilization, $\gamma$-irradiation terminal sterilization) of the obtained FE002 progenitor cell-bearing constructs. The result indicated that construct lyophilization resulted in the obtention of temperature-stabilized grafts, within a devitalized cellular therapeutic product setting (Figures S11 and S12, Table 3).

**Table 3.** Grading table for the assessment of lyophilized and lyophilized/irradiated constructs (i.e., cellular components) within exploratory finished product manufacturing optimization studies. ECM, extracellular matrix; 3D, three dimensions.

| Efficacy Parameter Type | Controls/Assays | Targets & Acceptance Criteria | Endpoint Construct Gradings [1] | |
|---|---|---|---|---|
| | | | Lyophilized | Lyophilized/Irradiated |
| Cellular Quantity in 3D | Live-Dead | Presence of cells throughout the constructs in amounts comparable to historical data | ++ | + |
| Cellular Adhesion & Cellular Morphology in 3D | Live-Dead | Presence of adherent cells throughout the constructs; Cellular alignment along the scaffold fibers | ++ | ± |
| Cellular Colonization Homogeneity in 3D | MTT; Live-Dead | Presence of homogeneously distributed cells throughout the constructs | +++ | ± |
| Extracellular Matrix Synthesis & Deposition in 3D | Immunofluorescence | Presence of adherent ECM components along the fibers within the constructs | ++ | + |
| Extracellular Matrix Deposition Homogeneity in 3D | Immunofluorescence | Presence of homogeneously distributed ECM throughout the constructs | +++ | ± |

[1] Gradings were attributed as follows: (+++) = conforming, excellent performance; (++) = conforming, good performance; (+) = conforming; (±) = unclear, additional data required; (–) = non-conforming.

Furthermore, while lyophilized construct terminal sterilization was not technically excluded at this point (i.e., significant residual presence of cellular materials and ECM components within the irradiated samples), it was assessed that extensive further formulation work and processing optimization was required, in order to potentially obtain appropriate devitalized cellular or cell-free constructs (Figures S11 and S12, Table 3).

### 3.4. Bio-Enhanced Constructs Bearing FE002 Primary Progenitor Tenocytes May Be Obtained Using an Optimized and GMP-Transposable Manufacturing Process

The specific bases for allogeneic musculoskeletal tissue engineering using FE002 primary progenitor tenocytes and Infinity-Lock 3 scaffolds were set forth in the previous sections. In order to further establish an optimized and GMP-transposable process for cell-seeded construct manufacture, further in vitro studies were performed. Specifically, the first technical aspect of optimization to be investigated pertained to the state of the FE002 progenitor cell seeding materials (i.e., cellular active substance form) at the start of the finished combination product manufacturing phase. Specifically, all of the in vitro assays presented in the previous sections of the study were performed with fresh cellular active substance materials. Therefore, the first objective of the optimization phase was to use cryopreserved cellular active substance materials instead (i.e., for scaffold seeding), with extemporaneous thawing of the cell seeding lot (i.e., for temporal decoupling of the 2D cell expansion phase and the 3D construct manufacturing process). The second objective of the optimization phase was to establish a temporally condensed construct incubation process, for overall manufacturing resource and therapeutic pathway rationalization. Therefore, parametrically controlled cellular active substance and scaffold-based cell-bearing construct manufacturing processes were established, based on existing practices in musculoskeletal cell-based therapeutic approaches (Figures S13 and S14).

Experimentally, cryopreserved FE002 primary progenitor tenocyte cellular active substance lots were directly prepared and used to dynamically seed Infinity-Lock 3 scaffolds (i.e., high seeding cell dose of $10^5$ cells/cm of scaffold) and the constructs were incubated as described previously for a time-period of 7 days. Cell recovery controls were performed in 2D culture to assess the cellular adhesion and proliferation potentials/behaviors after thawing. The results of the optimization studies firstly confirmed the quality-related attributes (i.e., in vitro adhesion, proliferation) of the cellular active substance following extemporaneous thawing as equivalent to the same attributes of the fresh cellular active substance (Figure 4(A1,A2)).

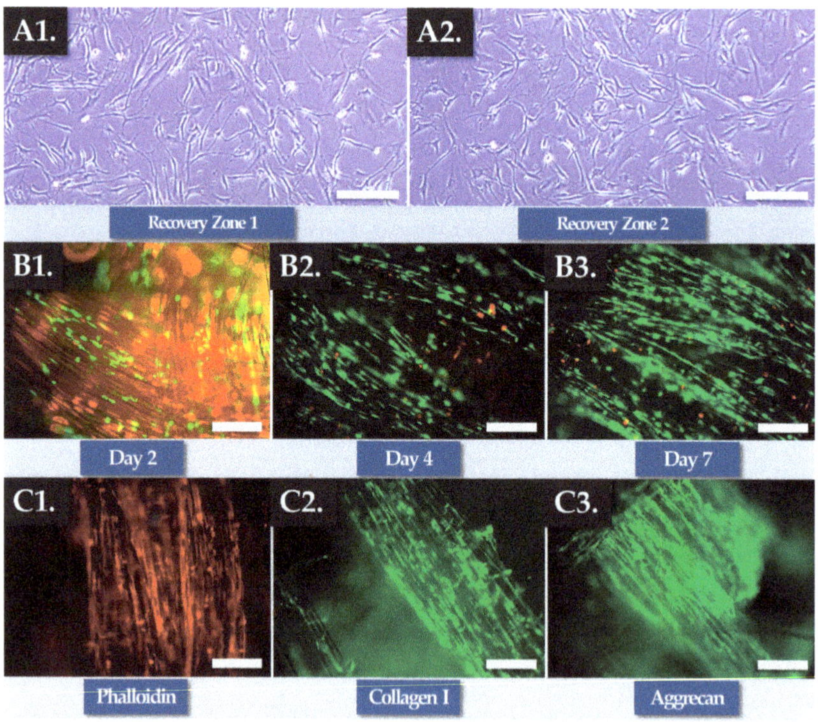


**Figure 4.** Results of finished product manufacturing process optimization work, using FE002 primary progenitor tenocytes and Infinity-Lock 3 scaffolds in culture for 7 days. (**A1**,**A2**) Cell recovery assays confirmed that the seeded cells conserved in vitro adhesion and proliferation capacities following direct initiation from cryostorage. Scale bars = 75 µm. (**B1**–**B3**) Iterative Live-Dead assays showed that the cells adhered throughout the scaffold, aligned themselves along the fibers, and spread along the fibers during proliferation. Several dead cells (i.e., in red fluorescence) could be observed, yet most of the cells were found to be viable (i.e., in green fluorescence). Overall, the proportion of viable cells was found to be more important at the 4-day and the 7-day timepoints. (**C1**–**C3**) Endpoint immunostainings were found to be positive for phalloidin, collagen 1, and aggrecan, confirming cellular alignment and extracellular matrix synthesis and deposition along the scaffold fibers after 7 days of incubation.

Secondly, the results confirmed the functionality-related attributes of the FE002 primary progenitor tenocytes during and after construct incubation (i.e., cellular adhesion and proliferation along the scaffold fibers, Figure 4(B1–B3)). Specifically, Live-Dead data confirmed cellular viability maintenance and proliferation within the construct, especially at the two later timepoints (Figure 4(B1–B3)). Importantly, a minoritarian yet significant amount of non-viable cells (i.e., in red fluorescence) were recorded at the 2-day timepoint, while only small amounts of non-viable cells were recorded at later timepoints (Figures 4(B1–B3) and S15). Such results confirmed the need for a minimal in vitro incubation period of the cell-seeded constructs of at least 4 days, in order to maximize in situ cellular viability and function. Specific endpoint Live-Dead assays showed adherent, viable, and highly organized FE002 primary progenitor tenocyte networks throughout the scaffolds (Figure S16). Thirdly, the results confirmed the functionality-related aspects of the FE002 primary progenitor tenocytes following construct incubation (e.g., ECM component synthesis and deposition along the scaffold fibers, Figures 4(C1–C3), S17 and S18). Specifically, immunohistology performed at the 7-day timepoint showed that the scaffold fibers were coated with actin, phalloidin, collagen I, and aggrecan (Figure 4(C1–C3)). Overall, no significant differences were observed in terms of quality, purity, and potency-related parameters between the standard combined finished product manufacturing protocol (i.e., low cell seeding dose, 14 days of incubation) and the optimized protocol (i.e., high cell seeding dose, 7 days of incubation, Table 4).

**Table 4.** Grading table for the assessment of equivalence between the standard protocol and the accelerated protocol within combined finished product manufacturing. Equivalence was assessed for finished product efficacy-related parameters/attributes only (i.e., cellular components) using the non-plasma-treated Infinity-Lock 3 scaffold. ECM, extracellular matrix; 3D, three dimensions.

| Parameter Class | Parameter Type | Controls | Targets & Acceptance Criteria | Endpoint Construct Gradings [1] | |
|---|---|---|---|---|---|
| | | | | Standard Protocol 14 Days | Optimized Protocol 7 Days |
| Quality | Cellular Adherence/Viability in 2D | Recovery plates | Presence of viable & adherent cells in recovery plates | +++ | +++ |
| Quality | Cellular Quantity/Proliferation Capacity in 2D | Recovery plates | Presence of actively proliferating cells in recovery plates | +++ | +++ |
| Purity | Cellular Population Identity & Non-Contamination in 2D | Recovery plates | Specific cellular morphology comparable to historical data; Monomodal cellular population | +++ | +++ |
| Potency | Cellular Viability in 3D | MTT; Live-Dead | Presence of a majority of viable cells | +++ | +++ |
| Potency | Cellular Quantity/Proliferation Capacity in 3D | CellTiter-Glo; Live-Dead | Presence of actively proliferating cells on the constructs | +++ | +++ |
| Potency | Cellular Adhesion & Morphology in 3D | Live-Dead | Presence of cells throughout the constructs; Alignment of cells along the construct fibers | +++ | +++ |

**Table 4.** *Cont.*

| Parameter Class | Parameter Type | Controls | Targets & Acceptance Criteria | Endpoint Construct Gradings [1] | |
|---|---|---|---|---|---|
| | | | | **Standard Protocol 14 Days** | **Optimized Protocol 7 Days** |
| Potency | Cellular Colonization Homogeneity in 3D | MTT; Live-Dead | Homogeneous presence of cells throughout the constructs | +++ | ++ |
| Potency | Extracellular Matrix Synthesis & Deposition | Immunohistochemistry; Immunofluorescence | Presence of adherent ECM components along the scaffold fibers | +++ | +++ |
| Potency | Extracellular Matrix Deposition Homogeneity in 3D | Immunofluorescence | Homogeneous ECM presence throughout the constructs | +++ | +++ |

[1] Gradings were attributed as follows: (+++) = conforming, excellent performance; (++) = conforming, good performance; (+) = conforming; (±) = unclear, additional data required; (–) = non-conforming.

Of note, both the plasma-treated and the non-plasma-treated Infinity-Lock 3 scaffolds were used within the optimized cell-seeded construct manufacturing protocol. Therein, no significant differences were evidenced between both scaffold types (Figures S15–S18). At this point of the study, the optimized protocol for obtaining clinically usable constructs bearing allogeneic FE002 primary progenitor tenocytes was assessed as being established and validated, in conformity with the corresponding controlled and parametrically defined manufacturing processes (Figures S13 and S14, Tables S2–S5). Overall, it was shown that the combined finished products, displaying appropriate critical and key quality attributes, could be rapidly manufactured using a simple GMP-transposable process, starting with cryopreserved FE002 cellular active substance materials.

### *3.5. Infinity-Lock 3 Constructs May Be Applied in Several Indications of Cell-Assisted Hand Ligament Regenerative Medicine*

The intended therapeutic uses of the FE002 primary progenitor tenocyte-seeded constructs comprise several applications in the surgical management of hand tendon/ligament reconstructive interventions. In order to specifically verify the applicability of the Infinity-Lock 3 scaffold in two of the considered therapeutic indications, an ex vivo anatomical model was used. The first part of the ex vivo study enabled to confirm the applicability of the Infinity-Lock 3 construct for ligamento-suspension plasty after trapeziectomy (Figure 5).

Specifically, it was confirmed that the structural and physical roles of such grafts were satisfactorily filled by the Infinity-Lock 3 construct, based on the surgical assessments of the authors. This application was considered of particular interest for patients presenting severe local osteoarthritis symptoms. Notably, it was noted that the length of the Infinity-Lock 3 construct was substantially reduced, following suturing and resection of excess synthetic graft materials, confirming the need for the production of excess graft material lengths (i.e., to comply with handling and surgical implantation needs, Figure 5J–L). The second part of the ex vivo study enabled to confirm the applicability of the Infinity-Lock 3 construct for thumb metacarpo-phalangeal ulnar collateral ligamentoplasty (Figure 6).

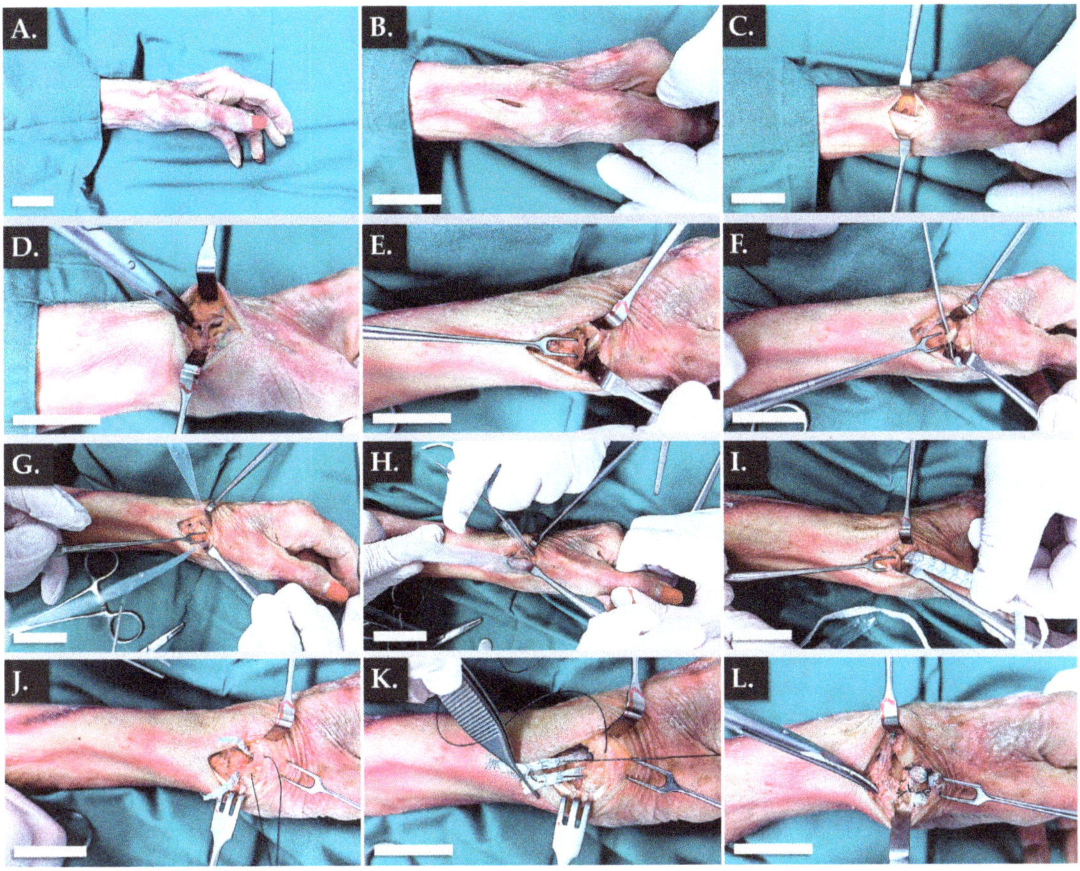


**Figure 5.** Illustrated step-by-step surgical overview of the ligamento-suspension plasty after trapeziectomy procedure using the Infinity-Lock 3 construct. (**A**) Initial setup. (**B**) Incision. (**C**) Exposure of APL and EPB tendons. (**D**) Exposure of the dorsal branch of the radial nerve. (**E**) FCR exposure. (**F**) FlexPasser installation. (**G**) Sheath installation. (**H**,**I**) Installation of the Infinity-Lock 3 construct using the sheath. (**J**) Removal of excess synthetic graft material. (**K**,**L**) Suturing of the Infinity-Lock 3 construct to the bone. Scale bars = 2.5 cm. APL, abductor pollicis longus; EPB, extensor pollicis brevis; FCR, flexor carpi radialis.

It was confirmed once more that the structural and physical roles of such grafts were satisfactorily filled by the Infinity-Lock 3 construct, based on the surgical assessments of the authors (Video A, Video B). This application was considered of particular interest for patients presenting acute UCL ruptures, also known as "skiers' thumb". Specifically, it was confirmed from a surgical point-of-view that the construct was adapted for the considered use and that the intervention resulted in the obtention or restoration of appropriate thumb mobility (Video A, Video B). Overall, the presented ex vivo results enabled to establish surgical proofs-of-concept and surgical protocols for hand ligament regenerative medicine, in view of the further translational and clinical studies to be performed with the considered allogeneic bioengineered grafts.

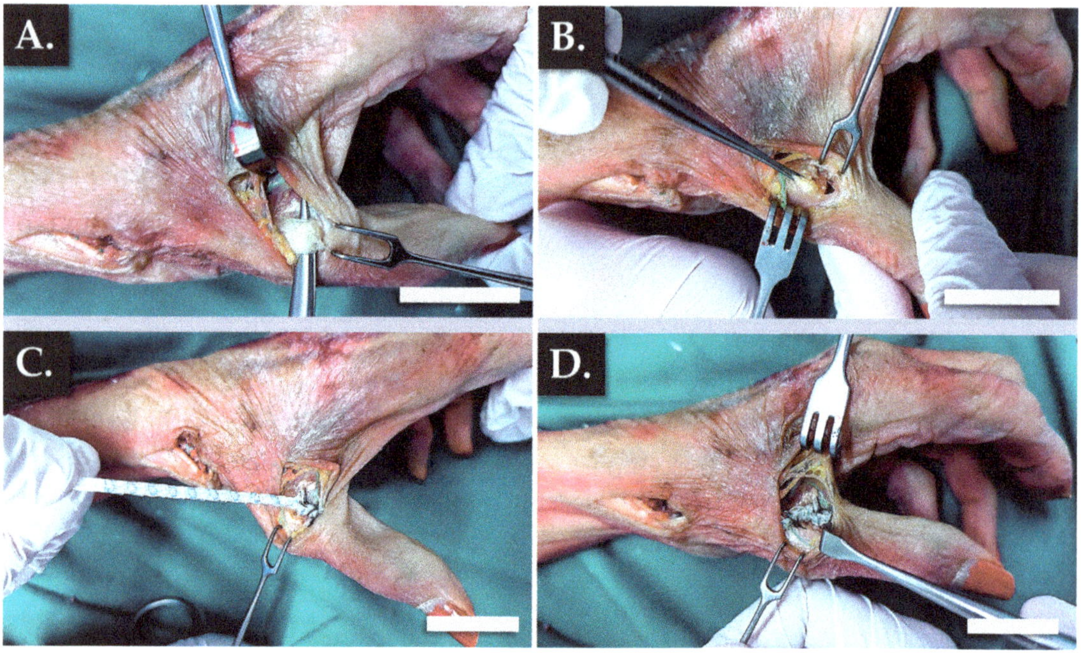


**Figure 6.** Illustrated step-by-step surgical overview of the thumb metacarpo-phalangeal ulnar collateral ligamentoplasty. (**A**) Exposure of the thumb UCL. (**B**) Ablation of a portion of the thumb UCL. (**C**) Distal suture of the Infinity-Lock 3 construct. (**D**) Proximal suture of the Infinity-Lock 3 construct. Scale bars = 2.5 cm. UCL, ulnar collateral ligament.

## 4. Discussion

### *4.1. Quality and Efficacy Parameters/Attributes: Cytocompatibility, Cellular Function, and Proteomic Constituents in the FE002 Primary Progenitor Tenocyte-Bearing Constructs*

The general approach to musculoskeletal tissue engineering adopted within this study was firstly oriented toward finished product quality attribute maximization and secondly toward technical simplification, for the eventual obtention of overall manufacturing efficiency (Figures S1A and S1B). As is required by legal and normative documentation relative to novel cell-based or cell-containing products, the study focused on two main successive phases, namely the FE002 cellular active substance production and then the scaffold-based cell-bearing combined finished product production. As concerns the former, an extensive body of knowledge around the FE002 primary progenitor tenocyte clinical grade cell source predated the present study and was largely reported in the literature [19,39,55–58,71]. Specifically, multiple aspects of FE002 primary progenitor cell type characterization and qualification have been investigated, up to and including an in vivo GLP study in rabbits [39,71]. Furthermore, extensive validation work pertaining to primary progenitor cell type manufacturing in multi-tiered biobanking systems enabled to confirm the stability and the sustainability of the therapeutic cell source, based on in-house experience with GMP-produced and clinically applied alternative FE002 primary progenitor cells (e.g., FE002 dermal progenitor fibroblasts) [39,72].

Generally, an important concern regarding the in vivo implantation of viable exogeneous cells for therapeutic purposes is the risk of tumor formation. Notwithstanding the available data (i.e., in vitro, in ovo, and in vivo) relative to FE002 primary progenitor tenocyte safety (i.e., iterative karyotyping, soft agar tumorigenicity assay, CAM model, rabbit model), additional documentation of cellular active substance safety attributes was required [39,71]. Therefore, cell type lifespan characterization assays (e.g., in vitro senescence confirmation by evolutive population doubling value assessment and β-galactosidase activity determination) enabled to unequivocally confirm the primary nature of diploid FE002 primary progenitor tenocytes (Figure S3). Secondly, the results of the determination of telomerase activity within the FE002 primary progenitor cellular active substance fell in line with the data gathered the in soft agar and in vivo assays, namely the inability of the FE002 primary progenitor tenocytes to develop tumoral growth/behaviors in the retained experimental settings (Table S1) [39]. Specifically, the telomerase activity quantification assays enabled to provide a quantitative assessment for an important parameter related to safety attributes of the cellular active substance, contrasting with the soft agar and in vivo assays (i.e., descriptive or semi-quantitative, Table S1) [39].

Of note, telomeres protect chromosome ends against chromosomal fusion, recombination, or terminal DNA degradation [73]. Telomeres progressively shorten during processes of DNA replication and cell division in primary cell types (i.e., non-continuous cells), eventually leading to a progressive stop in replication and therefore resulting in cell senescence [73]. Telomerase is a reverse transcriptase enzyme capable of adding telomeric repeats to chromosome ends. In somatic human cells, telomerase activity is decreased after birth resulting in telomere length shortening with each cell division [73]. In contrast, cancer cells have high telomerase activity resulting in telomere maintenance and cell immortality [73]. The original data gathered on FE002 primary progenitor tenocytes, when compared to that of known cancerous cell lines (i.e., HeLa and HCT-116 positive controls), confirmed the appropriate level of function of telomerase in the cellular active substance of interest (Table S1).

Overall, the aggregated safety-related data around the FE002 primary progenitor tenocyte source was assessed as appropriate and conforming to the further considered therapeutic use of such cells in human regenerative medicine [39]. Specifically, the telomerase assay results were interpreted positively in light of the fact that at least one continuous cell line (i.e., immortalized cells) has been safely and effectively used in large-scale orthopedic clinical trials, with no reported safety concerns linked to inherent cellular active substance safety parameters (i.e., Invossa, Kolon TissueGene, Rockville, MD, USA) [74]. Therefore, while classical approaches to safety evaluation of novel cell-based therapies remain of critical importance before initiating clinical investigational use, recent developments and the available clinical data should also be factored in the corresponding risk analyses.

With regards to functionality-oriented aspects of FE002 primary progenitor cell type characterization, the original in vitro data presented in this study (e.g., cellular adhesion on ECM-coated surfaces) confirmed the biocompatibility data previously gathered using ex vivo decellularized equine tendon tissues (Figure S2) [19]. Furthermore, detailed investigation into the interactions between the FE002 primary progenitor tenocytes and the synthetic Infinity-Lock 3 scaffold have confirmed the compatibility and the function at cellular and proteinic levels (Figures 1 and 4). From a mechanistic point-of-view, the rationale for combining therapeutic FE002 primary progenitor tenocytes on synthetic scaffolds may be considered as multifaceted. Firstly, within the context of hand ligament reconstructive surgery, the scaffold itself passively exerts the principal (i.e., necessary and sufficient) mode of action (i.e., structural tissular repair/replacement). Thus, the mode of action of the biological constituents (i.e., allogeneic FE002 cells and materials produced by them) is ancillary to that of the scaffold, when considering the finished combination product (Figure S10). Secondly, it is known that patient tissues and cells colonize the passive scaffold, in a manner or rate dependent upon the structural specificities of the synthetic device, based on existing in vivo preclinical and clinical reports (Tables S6–S8) [60,68]. Therefore, the use of a biologically-enhanced construct bearing allogeneic FE002 progenitor materials has the potential to qualitatively enhance graft bio-integration following implantation (e.g., scaffold colonization by host cells, avoidance of tissue adhesions, regulation of inflammation, modulation of implantation tissular environment) [75,76].

Specifically, the FE002 progenitor cell-bearing Infinity-Lock 3 constructs are known to be covered in biological materials (i.e., allogeneic progenitor cells, ECM constituents), which can potentially additionally or actively (i.e., in contrast to the passive nature of the barren scaffold itself in that regard) enable colonization of the graft by endogenous host tissues and cells. It was shown that scaffold colonization with FE002 primary progenitor tenocytes resulted in fiber coating with collagen I, decorin, and aggrecan, which are known tendon/ligament ECM proteins. Therefore, ECM deposition should create a different kind of localized favorable environment for integration by the surrounding patient tissues, through biological enhancement (e.g., biological priming) of the scaffold. Indeed, one major identified problem of tendinous tissue healing is the reduced quality of repair, leading to important rates of tissue re-tear [5–7,15]. Modern strategies to improve tendon healing outcomes are oriented toward biological-enhanced (e.g., growth factors, PRP, or various therapeutic cell sources) devices, with encouraging results (Table S9) [3,12]. Therein, the effects of bio-supplementation in tendon and ligament surgery have notably been investigated for several decades [75,76]. It was specifically shown that the combination of artificial LK scaffolds with a strip of fascia lata or infrapatellar fat pad accelerated tissue induction and increased the remodeling processes in vivo [75,76]. Such elements strongly support the considered use of FE002 primary progenitor materials for Infinity-Lock 3 scaffold bio-enhancement from a mechanistic viewpoint, aiming to provide biological cues for holistically optimized tissular repair/regeneration.

At the proteomic level, the experimental data has shown that the considered FE002 progenitor cellular active substance was composed of collagens, ECM glycoproteins, and ECM proteoglycans (Table 1) [55]. Data analyses revealed that the reported protein panel for the FE002 primary progenitor cells was highly similar to that of the patient primary tenocytes considered in this study and additional cross-referencing was made to reported proteomic analyses of human tendons (i.e., relative comparison possible) [69]. Importantly, this analysis demonstrated that FE002 primary progenitor tenocytes maintain the expression of critical human tendon ECM proteins after in vitro monolayer expansion and cell banking (Table 1). While collagen represents 60–85% of tendon dry mass and collagen I is the most abundant form of collagen in tendon tissue, additional minor ECM proteins have been identified in the FE002 progenitor cellular active substance and are important for tendon function and tendon health (Table 1) [77]. In the collagen family, the identified COL1, COL3, but also COL5, COL6, and COL12 proteins are known for their role in fibrillogenesis, and FE002 primary progenitor tenocytes also express a panel of ECM-associated glycoproteins (e.g., COMP, fibronectin, tenascin-C, Table 1). Furthermore, large proteoglycans (e.g., aggrecan) and SLRPs proteoglycans (e.g., decorin, biglycan) were identified and are involved in several aspects of tendon biology (i.e., fibrillogenesis, modulation of cell proliferation, migration, or differentiation) (Table 1) [69,77]. Overall, it was confirmed that the considered FE002 primary progenitor tenocytes contained proteinic constituents that are characteristic of human tendinous tissues and that could be of functional interest within the presented scaffold-based progenitor cell-bearing combination product, for bio-enhancement by synthetic fiber coating (Table 1) [69]. Concomitantly to ECM protein deposition throughout the Infinity-Lock 3 scaffolds, the FE002 primary progenitor tenocytes are also a source of additional biological factors (e.g., FGF-2 or HGF growth factors), which can locally assist and potentially promote the complex processes of tissue healing, in a similar way as PRP or MSC injections/grafting [78–88]. Therein, the use of standardized therapeutic primary cell sources (e.g., clinical grade FE002 primary progenitor cell sources) may be considered as advantageous over the use of genetically manipulated materials, from a technical simplicity and an in vivo safety standpoint [89–95]. Importantly, while new tendon/ligament tissue is forming and migrating within the implanted construct, the scaffold itself possesses, by design, the physical properties allowing to withstand the mechanical constraints applied onto the articulation [60,76]. From a technical and processing point-of-view, the present study set forth several proofs-of-concept for combination product preparation, stabilization, and sterilization. While finished product terminal irradiating sterilization was not technically excluded based on the available functional readouts, it was assessed that significant further studies were required in order to obtain acceptable off-the-shelf combination constructs. It is important to note that process parameters and product attributes are specific to the applied process and that the requirements for the final form of the product notably depend on the intended clinical use.

Generally, the reasoning and rationale for cell-seeded construct use in musculoskeletal regenerative medicine is based on existing experience with chondrocyte therapy, wherein biological enhancement of matrices has been studied [96]. This approach aims to prime the implanted grafts and to provide stimulatory signals to the surrounding environment in order to optimize tissular repair [96]. Extensive characterization work and clinical hindsight are available in this domain, notably for autologous chondrocytes cultured on synthetic scaffolds (e.g., Chondro-Gide, Optimaix) in vitro [96]. By analogy, the obtained functionality-related data gathered on the FE002 primary progenitor tenocyte cellular active substance of interest confirmed that despite "substantial manipulation" of the cells in serial monolayer culture, cellular quality attributes and functionality are conserved. Such considerations are based on widely known and regulatorily accepted manufacturing and control parameters in the field of cartilage tissue engineering (i.e., comprising a cell culture expansion phase) [96]. Therein, demonstration of the ability of the therapeutic cells to readopt a chondrogenic behavior in 3D culture (i.e., following the 2D expansion phase, characterized by a transient loss of chondrogenicity) constitutes the basis of in vitro product potency characterization and qualification. By extension, for the FE002 cell-seeded Infinity-Lock 3 constructs, the functional biological aspects were documented at the cellular and proteomic levels, which are more informative/relevant (i.e., functionally impactful) than gene expression profiles, for example. In particular, such functional attributes of the cellular active substance (i.e., 3D cellular attachment and proliferation, ECM scaffold fiber coating) may be used as in vitro potency assays for alternative cytotherapeutic formulations (e.g., injectable FE002 cell suspensions in HA-based hydrogels or in autologous human serum-supplemented saline solutions) containing viable FE002 primary progenitor tenocytes [56].

Overall, both the FE002 progenitor cellular active substance and the combined finished product were shown to possess attributes and functions which are in line with the intended use of the bio-enhanced constructs, in view of optimizing musculoskeletal tissue reconstruction processes (Figure 4, Table 1). Specifically, quality- and functionality-related parameters/attributes of the FE002 primary progenitor tenocytes have been analyzed and investigated in light of pre-existing work in cartilage tissue engineering. This angle is especially interesting, as the scientific, clinical, and regulatory dimensions of chondrocyte-based therapy are much more advanced and accepted than those in the scarce current field of clinical tenocyte-based regenerative therapies, providing a tangible comparison point within the musculoskeletal system.

### 4.2. *Applicability of FE002 Primary Progenitor Tenocyte-Bearing Constructs in Allogeneic Cell-Assisted Hand Ligament Regenerative Medicine*

For the sound development of novel cell-based or cell-containing combination products, several regulatory and clinical risks may be mitigated by the use of a material or device which has been previously approved and clinically used successfully (i.e., documented track-record). While several technologies and materials are currently commercialized for tendon and ligament reconstruction, the Neoligaments devices were selected based on the extensive available clinical hindsight and the high versatility in available device designs, enabling eventual widening of the clinical indications for alternative FE002 progenitor cell-seeded constructs (e.g., progenitor cell-assisted rotator cuff repair, Tables S6–S8) [20,24–26,59–68].

In detail, the studied Infinity-Lock 3 system is a CE-marked medical device in the form of an open weave tape with densely woven sections (https://www.neoligaments.com/, accessed on 8 June 2023, Figure 5). This device is a sterile and single-use, non-absorbable, implantable tape made from polyester (i.e., 100% polyethylene terephthalate). Listed clinical indications comprise soft tissue approximation and structural reconstruction in musculoskeletal surgical procedures, such as the reconstruction of damaged or torn ligaments and tendons. The Infinity-Lock system is an adaptation of the Leeds-Keio ligament (LK ligament), which has been tested and validated in porcine and in canine in vivo models (Table S6) [75,76]. The LK synthetic scaffolds were developed several decades ago and were clinically used for ligament and tendon repair surgeries, wherein long-term patient follow-up data are available (Tables S7 and S8) [62–64,66,67].

Importantly, notable studies on the biocompatibility of such devices with human hand tendon tissues (e.g., study of tendon tissue ingrowth) have been considered to constitute the technical foundations for the design of the presented FE002 primary progenitor tenocyte-bearing bio-enhanced graft [60,68]. Therein, healthy human adult extensor tendon tissue was sutured on both ends of 0.5-cm synthetic scaffold segments and then kept in culture for several weeks [60]. Cell migration and proliferation from the tendon tissue onto the scaffold were observed [60]. Overall, the original experimental in vitro data gathered in the present study have demonstrated that FE002 primary progenitor cells and patient primary tenocytes could adhere to the Infinity-Lock 3 scaffold and that the local 3D environment was also suitable for cell proliferation, migration, and ECM protein deposition (Figure 4). Combined with the historical preclinical and clinical data available on the scaffold material itself, a clear demonstration was laid down herein for the applicability of the bio-enhanced graft in the intended clinical uses (Tables S7 and S8).

Of note, retrospective analyses and prospective investigations have highlighted several risks associated with the use of the considered synthetic tapes, such as minimal acute inflammatory tissue reaction, transitory local irritation, allergic reaction and discomfort, or skin breakdown due to prominent knots or fixation devices under the skin (Tables S7 and S8). Such elements were interpreted as being coherent with the process of implanting a biocompatible material in the human body, where the considered material passively and progressively undergoes encasement and colonization by the surrounding native tissues and cellular components [4,6,9]. While the structural and topographical specificities of the implanted device may play a role in the rate of colonization, it is known that suboptimal integration may be characterized by tissue adhesions (i.e., incurring additional morbidity) [14–17,22]. This bottleneck may be averted with the use of a silicone sheath during surgical hand tendon or ligament reconstruction, to limit the occurrence of tissular adhesions. Furthermore, based on the known behaviors of the polyester scaffold itself in vivo, the considered use of biologically-enhanced constructs bears the potential of optimizing colonization by native tissues and bio-integration, through "priming" of the synthetic surfaces with FE002 primary progenitor tenocyte materials [60,75,76]. The objective of such an approach consists in potentially diminishing the rate of tissular adhesions and the need for secondary/corrective surgeries in the clinical setting. Overall, the existing body of knowledge on the Infinity-Lock 3 scaffold, on the FE002 primary progenitor tenocytes, and on the combination thereof enables to confirm and set forward the applicability of the considered progenitor cell-bearing constructs in allogeneic cell-assisted hand ligament regenerative medicine.

### *4.3. Current Translational Development of Cell Therapies for Tendon & Ligament Repair/Regeneration: Alternative Tenocyte-Based Regenerative Medicine Protocols*

While novel CAR-T cell therapies attract much of the attention in the current field of oncology, somatic cell therapy is notably already effectively used at large scales in orthopedics for the treatment of large cartilage defects. First-in-human autologous chondrocyte implantations (ACI) date back to 1994 with the original Brittberg studies and the technique has incrementally evolved over time to optimize the cell delivery methods to the chondral/osteochondral defect site [96]. Long-term studies are now available for ACI and demonstrate the positive clinical outcomes of such regenerative strategies, encouraging the development of similar technologies for the treatment of other musculoskeletal pathologies and affections [97]. Namely, multiple therapeutic cell-based approaches (i.e., autologous and allogeneic, cell-based and cell-free) have been investigated in vivo and at clinical levels for tendon tissue regenerative medicine (Table S9) [2,3,12,13,98,99].

For optimal contextualization of the allogeneic bioengineering solution investigated herein (i.e., cytotherapeutic application of FE002 primary progenitor tenocytes) and comparison to similar protocols in use at the clinical level, the autologous example of the Ortho-ATI (Orthocell, Murdoch, Australia) technology is presented and discussed. Orthocell Ltd., an Australian biotechnology company, transposed the accumulated knowledge around ACI to the development of an autologous tenocyte injection (ATI) strategy. Autologous tenocyte supplementation efficacy has firstly been demonstrated in rabbit models of acute and chronic tendinopathy, in which autologous tenocytes were delivered through grafting of a tenocyte-seeded biological scaffold (i.e., ACI Maix and Restore matrix) or through direct cell injection, respectively, at the site of injury [100,101]. After 8 weeks, a clear improvement in the healing process compared to the no cell treatment groups was observed. Specifically, inflammation and angiogenesis were reduced, collagen I expression was increased, and tendon fiber structure, arrangement, or ultimate load failure were improved [100,101]. The therapeutic tenocytes also accelerated the scaffold absorption by the host and part of the injected cells were still identified at the injured site at the end of the studies. These experimental observations strongly suggested that tenocyte delivery enhanced the intrinsically limited healing process of tendon tissues and could constitute a clinically potent treatment in effective tendinopathy management [100,101].

The first long-term clinical study results were reported for the use of Ortho-ATI in the treatment of chronic resistant lateral epicondylitis (LE) (i.e., clinical trial number ACTRN12607000402448) [43,52]. Therein, 16 patients assessed as refractory to classical non-surgical treatments were enrolled in the study. Patellar tendon biopsies were performed under local anesthesia and the autologous tenocytes (i.e., starting cellular materials) were isolated for expansion. The therapeutic cell lots (i.e., cellular active substance) were validated through the analysis of a panel of CD markers (i.e., CD18, CD34, CD44, CD45, CD90, CD106, CD46, and Stro-1) and the gene expression analysis of specific genes (i.e., ACAN, Col I, Col III, decorin, MAGP2, Mohawk, scleraxis, and TGF-β). As concerns the finished product, 4–10 $\times$ $10^6$ cells were formulated with autologous human serum (aHS) and injected under ultrasound guidance into the tendinopathic site [43,52]. At 4 weeks post-surgery, the patients could resume sport activities. Lasting symptom improvements were recorded after a mean follow-up time of 4.5 years. Therein, the VAS pain, QuickDASH, and grip strength scores improved by 78%, 84%, and 132.6% respectively and no ossification was observed at the elbow injection site [43,52].

The efficacy of Ortho-ATI does not seem limited to LE, as sustained improvements of symptoms have also been recorded in rotator cuff repair (i.e., clinical trial number ACTRN12617000684325) and for gluteal tendinopathy [102]. Based on the currently available data, the ATI therapeutic approach appears to provide a safe and effective way to provide quick and lasting symptom improvements in patients who suffered for several months, did not respond to classical treatments (e.g., PRP, corticosteroids), and eventually would have to go through more invasive surgeries [100–102]. Similarly to ACI, the exact mechanism of action of Ortho-ATI is unknown but most probably impacts multiple aspects of tendinopathy (i.e., cellular integration and ECM synthesis, growth factor supply, inflammation modulation), shifting the balance from a degenerative state to a regenerative state, which is not possible with conventional treatments [100–102].

Considering the promising Ortho-ATI safety and efficacy results, development of the next generation of tenocyte-based cell therapies using an allogeneic clinical grade cell source (e.g., FE002 progenitor cell sources) can tangibly be envisioned [39,100,101]. Allogeneic cell sources (e.g., stem and progenitor cells) have been previously proposed by several authors for musculoskeletal tissue engineering and for the optimal restoration promotion of tendons in particular [103–106]. Specific focus was set on the therapeutic contributions of ECM components, given their strong implications in specific tissular healing processes [107–113]. As concerns the specific use of the FE002 primary progenitor tenocyte source of interest for tendon and ligament regenerative medicine, several formulation approaches and bioengineering concepts have previously been reported (e.g., injectable cellular hydrogel suspension, cell seeding of decellularized equine tendons, use in biofabrication settings) [39,54,56–58]. Generally, FE002 primary progenitor tenocytes have been extensively studied and have demonstrated the potential of becoming a standardized cell source for tendon and ligament disorder treatment [39,71]. Specifically, FE002 primary progenitor tenocytes are stable and pre-terminally differentiated cells, the safety profile shows low risks (i.e., no anchorage-independent cell growth potential, limited lifespan in culture, low telomerase activity), and extensive cryopreserved lots of cellular active substance can be established and validated (Table S1) [39]. Thereafter, FE002 primary progenitor tenocytes were shown to be compatible with hyaluronic acid formulations, remained viable after extrusion through syringes, can be lyophilized, and can be seeded onto biological and synthetic scaffolds (Figure 4) [19,39,54,56–58]. Such approaches have confirmed the high versatility of FE002 primary progenitor tenocytes for novel allogeneic cell-based and cell-containing therapies in a number of clinical indications (i.e., with adapting of the synthetic scaffold nature/shape/size and the surgical protocol) [39,56]. This versatility opens a multitude of options for the development of new allogeneic cell-based therapeutic products tailored to specific musculoskeletal pathologies.

### 4.4. Study Limitations and Future Perspectives

Several limitations have been identified within this study. From a first technical viewpoint, the finished product conditioning and transport medium still needs to be specified and validated, while allowing for conservation of critical quality attributes for the entire finished product validity period. Based on parallel research, the product transport medium may be constituted by a hyaluronan-based hydrogel or an autologous serum-based saline solution with appropriate supplements [54,71]. From a second technical viewpoint, upscaling of the manufacturing protocol to whole Infinity-Lock 3 scaffolds shall be performed, in order to obtain clinically usable constructs of appropriate dimensions, based on the surgical needs and clinical demands (i.e., excess product length manufacture, Figure 5) [114–118]. While the scale of cell seeding and construct incubation may be different using whole Infinity-Lock 3 scaffolds, the extent of process validation studies performed using 1-cm scaffold subunits enables to robustly predict construct behavior in vitro. Specifically, appropriate methodological elements shall be used for the evaluation of the impact of changes in the cytotherapeutic product manufacturing process (e.g., ICH Q5E methodology). From a third technical viewpoint, further development and full validation of the control assays described in the present study shall be performed, specifically as concerns efficacy-related parameters. These aspects are however of prime importance only at later stages of clinical investigational use, according to applicable guidance documents (e.g., Potency Tests for Cellular and Gene Therapy Products) [119].

Future perspectives based on this study consist in the further translational qualification and investigational work around the FE002 primary progenitor tenocytes of cytotherapeutic interest (i.e., primarily in regenerative medicine applications for the hand, e.g., acute sharp force trauma or degenerative pathologies) [120]. Based on the fact that the FE002 primary progenitor tenocyte cellular active substance has been characterized and qualified using multiple safety-related assays and that in vivo cellular implantation has already been performed in a rabbit GLP study, the next steps of the planned translational work comprise a first-in-man clinical trial [39]. As previously mentioned, the present study sets forth important functionality-related parameters for the FE002 primary progenitor tenocytes (e.g., ECM component synthesis and deposition in 3D culture), contributing to the qualification of such primary allogeneic cells for alternative tissue engineering applications [121]. Specifically, diversification of the clinical indications for products containing such FE002 cells comprise the original protocols set forth by the authors for this cell source, namely the use of cellular hydrogel suspensions for intra-tendinous or peritendinous injection treatment of tendinopathies/tendinosis [39,56]. This approach, technically simplified as compared to the tissue engineering protocol using the synthetic Infinity-Lock 3 scaffold, may represent an optimized solution for overall cost management and for widespread clinical applicability, similarly to the well-known autologous ultrasound-guided use of PRP for tendinopathies in sports medicine [47,56].

## 5. Conclusions

The aim of the present study was to establish novel tissue engineering and surgical proofs-of-concept for a bio-enhanced artificial Neoligaments graft bearing cultured viable allogeneic FE002 primary progenitor tenocytes (i.e., clinical grade standardized cellular active substance). In vitro studies confirmed that the progenitor cell-seeded constructs could be obtained using optimized and GMP-transposable processes and were characterized by good quality and functionality-related parameters/attributes. The results of the study have notably shown that FE002 primary progenitor tenocytes were capable of cellular adhesion, proliferation, and homogeneous tendon ECM component synthesis/deposition throughout the Infinity-Lock 3 scaffold, with progressive and structurally-organized biological coating of the synthetic fibers. Ex vivo cadaveric work confirmed that the Infinity-Lock 3 constructs could be clinically applied in two indications of cell-assisted hand surgery (i.e., ligamento-suspension plasty after trapeziectomy and thumb metacarpo-phalangeal ulnar collateral ligamentoplasty). These original data were analyzed and discussed in light of the known behaviors of the synthetic Neoligaments scaffolds following in vivo implantation and of existing clinical practices using cultured autologous tenocytes for bioengineering and cell therapies (e.g., Ortho-ATI). Generally, specific discussion points about the available body of knowledge for the allogeneic FE002 progenitor cellular source and about the retained synthetic scaffold materials enabled the comprehensive assessment and general mitigation of the risks associated with the presented novel tissue engineering solution. Overall, this study enabled to set forth important proofs-of-concept for the translational development of an allogeneic tissue engineering protocol for hand ligament regenerative medicine, in view of further investigative clinical work.

**Supplementary Materials:** The following supporting information can be downloaded at: https://www.mdpi.com/article/10.3390/pharmaceutics15071873/s1, Figure S1A: General study design overview; Figure S1B: Illustrated study design phases; Figure S2: Results of in vitro cellular adhesion assays; Figure S3: Results of β-galactosidase staining assays; Figure S4: Results of Live-Dead assays for primary tenocytes on synthetic Infinity-Lock 3 scaffolds; Figure S5: Results of immunofluorescence assays for FE002 primary progenitor tenocytes on synthetic Infinity-Lock 3 scaffolds; Figure S6: Results of immunofluorescence assays for primary patient tenocytes on synthetic Infinity-Lock 3 scaffolds; Figure S7: Results of MTT-based cytocompatibility assays for primary patient tenocytes on synthetic Infinity-Lock 3 scaffolds; Figure S8: Whole gel imaging for collagen I Western blot analyses; Figure S9: Whole gel imaging for decorin Western blot analyses; Figure S10: Experimental model for the description of functionality-related attributes of FE002 primary progenitor tenocytes on synthetic Infinity-Lock 3 scaffolds; Figure S11: Results of Live-Dead assays for the assessment of the impact of cell-seeded construct processing; Figure S12: Results of immunofluorescence assays for the assessment of the impact of cell-seeded construct processing; Figure S13: Parametric and controlled manufacturing process established for the FE002 primary progenitor tenocyte cellular active substance; Figure S14: Parametric and controlled manufacturing process established for the cell-seeded constructs; Figure S15: Results of Live-Dead assays for the validation of the optimized construct manufacturing protocol; Figure S16: Results of Live-Dead assays for the validation of the optimized construct manufacturing protocol; Figure S17: Results of immunofluorescence assays for the validation of the optimized construct manufacturing protocol; Figure S18: Results immunofluorescence assays for the validation of the optimized construct manufacturing protocol; Table S1: Results of the telomerase activity quantification study; Table S2: Listing of CPP/KPP for cellular active substance manufacture; Table S3: Listing of CPP/KPP for finished product manufacture; Table S4: Listing of CQA/KQA for the cellular active substance; Table S5: Listing of CQA/KQA for the finished product; Table S6: Listing of available preclinical in vivo data on the synthetic constructs; Table S7: Listing of the available in vivo clinical data on the synthetic constructs; Table S8: Listing of post-market clinical follow-up studies performed on the synthetic constructs; Table S9: Summarized listing of human clinical trials using therapeutic cell-based products/therapies for tendon repair and regenerative medicine; Video A: Illustration for damaged UCL distal suture testing; Video B: Illustration for damaged UCL complete suture testing.

**Author Contributions:** Conceptualization, A.J., J.M., L.A.A., W.R. and A.L.; methodology, A.J., J.M., C.P., S.J., M.C., A.T., Z.L., N.H.-B., L.A.A., W.R. and A.L.; software, A.J., J.M., C.P., P.A.-S., N.H.-B., L.A.A., W.R. and A.L.; validation, A.J., J.M., C.P., S.J., M.C., A.T., Z.L., P.A.-S., C.S., N.H.-B., L.A.A., W.R. and A.L.; formal analysis, A.J., J.M., C.P., P.A.-S., C.S., N.H.-B., L.A.A., W.R. and A.L.; investigation, A.J., J.M., C.P., M.C., A.T., Z.L., C.S., L.A.A., W.R. and A.L.; resources, L.A.A., W.R. and A.L.; data curation, A.J., J.M., C.P., N.H.-B., L.A.A., W.R. and A.L.; writing—original draft preparation A.J., J.M., L.A.A. and A.L.; writing—review and editing, A.J., J.M., C.P., S.J., M.C., A.T., Z.L., P.A.-S., C.S., N.H.-B., L.A.A., W.R. and A.L.; visualization, A.J., J.M., M.C., A.T., Z.L., N.H.-B., L.A.A., W.R. and A.L.; supervision, L.A.A., W.R. and A.L.; project administration, L.A.A., W.R. and A.L.; funding acquisition, L.A.A., W.R. and A.L. All authors have read and agreed to the published version of the manuscript.

**Funding:** The S.A.N.T.E and Sandoz Foundations have contributed to fund the Swiss progenitor cell transplantation program during the past fourteen years. This study was in part financed by the Service of Promotion of the Economy and Innovation of the Canton of Vaud (SPEI), in accordance with the Vaud Cantonal Law on Economic Development Support of 12 June 2007 (LADE), reference number LADE 20-472. The funders had no role or involvement in study design, in the collection, analysis and interpretation of data, in the writing of the report, or in the decision to submit the article for publication. This study was not supported by other specific grants or institutional programs.

**Institutional Review Board Statement:** The procurement of the biological starting materials used for the present study was conducted according to the guidelines of the Declaration of Helsinki and was approved by the appropriate Cantonal Ethics Committee [122]. The FE002 primary progenitor tenocyte cell source used in the present study was established from the FE002 organ donation, as approved by the Vaud Cantonal Ethics Committee (University Hospital of Lausanne–CHUV, Ethics Committee Protocol #62/07). The FE002 organ donation was registered under a federal cell transplantation program (i.e., Swiss progenitor cell transplantation program). Obtention and use of patient cellular materials followed the regulations of the Biobank of the CHUV Department of Musculoskeletal Medicine.

**Informed Consent Statement:** Appropriate informed consent was obtained from and confirmed by starting material donors at the time of inclusion in the Swiss progenitor cell transplantation program, following specifically devised protocols and procedures, which were validated by the appropriate health authorities. Informed consent (i.e., formalized in a general informed consent agreement) was obtained from all patients or from their legal representatives at the time of treatment, for unrestricted use of the gathered and anonymized patient data or anonymized biological materials.

**Data Availability Statement:** The data presented in this study are not publicly available due to legal and statutory restrictions. The data presented in this study are available upon written and reasonable request from the corresponding authors.

**Acknowledgments:** We would like to thank the S.A.N.T.E and Sandoz Foundations for their unconditional commitments to the Swiss progenitor cell transplantation program through the years. We would like to thank the Canton of Vaud for their partial economic support of this study. We would like to thank Bahaa Seedhom and Xiros Ltd. for the provision of the Neoligaments devices and surgical materials used for the study. We would like to thank the Proteomics Core Facility and Technology Platform at the Ecole Polytechnique Fédérale de Lausanne for their provided support. We would like to thank the Pharmaceutical Technology group at the Institute of Pharmaceutical Sciences of Western Switzerland and the University of Geneva for the provided support in sterilization protocol establishment. We would like to thank the Orthopedics and Traumatology Service at the Lausanne University Hospital for the shared time and close collaboration. We would like to thank the Musculoskeletal Research Unit at the University of Zurich for the provision of control cell lines, for the shared time, and for the historic collaborations. Artwork templates were partly created with www.biorender.com, accessed on 18 May 2023.

**Conflicts of Interest:** Authors A.J., C.P. and A.L. were employed by LAM Biotechnologies SA during the course of the study. The remaining authors declare no conflict of interest.

## Abbreviations

| | |
|---|---|
| ACL | anterior cruciate ligament |
| ADRC | adipose-derived regenerative cells |
| APL | abductor pollicis longus |
| ASC | adipose-derived stem cells |
| BCA | bicinchoninic acid |
| BM-MSC | bone marrow-derived mesenchymal stem cells |
| BSA | bovine serum albumin |
| CAM | chorioallantoic membrane model |
| cATMP | combined advanced therapy medicinal product |
| CE | European conformity certification |
| CHUV | centre hospitalier universitaire vaudois |
| CPP | critical process parameter |
| CQA | critical quality attribute |
| CT | cycle threshold |
| DMEM | Dulbecco's modified Eagle medium |
| DMSO | dimethyl sulfoxide |
| DNA | deoxyribonucleic acid |
| DTT | dithiothreitol |
| ECL | electrochemiluminescence |
| ECM | extracellular matrix |
| EDTA | ethylenediaminetetraacetic acid |
| ELISA | enzyme-linked immunosorbent assay |
| EPB | extensor pollicis brevis |
| EU | European Union |
| EU | endotoxin unit |
| FACS | fluorescence-activated cell sorting |
| FASP | filter-aided sample preparation |
| FBS | fetal bovine serum |
| FC | fold change |
| FCR | flexor carpi radialis |
| FDR | false discovery rate |
| FE002 | clinical grade primary progenitor cell sources |
| GLP | good laboratory practices |
| GMP | good manufacturing practices |
| HA | hyaluronic acid |
| HRP | horseradish peroxidase |
| IPC | in-process control |
| kDa | kiloDaltons |
| kGy | kiloGray |
| KPP | key process parameter |
| KQA | key quality attribute |
| LC-MS/MS | liquid chromatography tandem mass spectrometry |
| LE | lateral epicondylitis |
| MCB | master cell bank |
| MD | medical device |
| MoA | mechanism of action |
| MOPS | 3-(N-Morpholino)propanesulfonic acid |
| MRI | magnetic resonance imaging |
| MSC | mesenchymal stem cell |
| MTT | 3-(4,5-dimethylthiazol-2-yl)-2,5-diphenyltetrazolium bromide |
| NA | not applicable |
| NAT | nucleic acid amplification technique |
| OD | optical density |

| | |
|---|---|
| PAF | paraformaldehyde |
| PBS | phosphate-buffered saline |
| PCB | parental cell bank |
| PDGF-BB | platelet-derived growth factor-BB |
| Ph. Eur. | European Pharmacopoeia |
| PMSF | phenylmethanesulfonyl fluoride |
| PPC | post-process control |
| PRP | platelet-rich plasma |
| PTRCT | partial-thickness rotator cuff tears |
| QA | quality assurance |
| QC | quality control |
| qPCR | quantitative polymerase chain reaction |
| RH | relative humidity |
| RIPA | radio-immunoprecipitation assay |
| SDS | sodium dodecyl sulfate |
| TrSt | standardized transplant |
| UCL | ulnar collateral ligament |
| UK | United Kingdom |
| USA | United States of America |
| UVEC | umbilical vein endothelial cell |
| Vs | vs. |
| WCB | working cell bank |

## References


1. Clayton, R.A.; Court-Brown, C.M. The epidemiology of musculoskeletal tendinous and ligamentous injuries. *Injury* **2008**, *39*, 1338–1344. [CrossRef] [PubMed]
2. Freedman, B.R.; Mooney, D.J.; Weber, E. Advances toward transformative therapies for tendon diseases. *Sci. Transl. Med.* **2022**, *14*, eabl8814. [CrossRef] [PubMed]
3. Bianchi, E.; Ruggeri, M.; Rossi, S.; Vigani, B.; Miele, D.; Bonferoni, M.C.; Sandri, G.; Ferrari, F. Innovative strategies in tendon tissue engineering. *Pharmaceutics* **2021**, *13*, 89. [CrossRef] [PubMed]
4. Chen, J.; Mo, Q.; Sheng, R.; Zhu, A.; Ling, C.; Luo, Y.; Zhang, A.; Chen, Z.; Yao, Q.; Cai, Z.; et al. The application of human periodontal ligament stem cells and biomimetic silk scaffold for in situ tendon regeneration. *Stem Cell Res. Ther.* **2021**, *12*, 596. [CrossRef]
5. Steinmann, S.; Pfeifer, C.G.; Brochhausen, C.; Docheva, D. Spectrum of tendon pathologies: Triggers, trails and end-state. *Int. J. Mol. Sci.* **2020**, *21*, 844. [CrossRef]
6. Sharma, P.; Maffulli, N. Tendon injury and tendinopathy: Healing and repair. *J. Bone Jt. Surg. Am.* **2005**, *87*, 187–202. [CrossRef]
7. Hopkins, C.; Fu, S.C.; Chua, E.; Hu, X.; Rolf, C.; Mattila, V.M.; Qin, L.; Yung, P.S.; Chan, K.M. Critical review on the socio-economic impact of tendinopathy. *Asia Pac. J. Sport. Med. Arthrosc. Rehabil. Technol.* **2016**, *4*, 9–20. [CrossRef]
8. Van der Vlist, A.C.; Winters, M.; Weir, A.; Ardern, C.L.; Welton, N.J.; Caldwell, D.M.; Verhaar, J.A.; de Vos, R.J. Which treatment is most effective for patients with Achilles tendinopathy? A living systematic review with network meta-analysis of 29 randomised controlled trials. *Br. J. Sport. Med.* **2021**, *55*, 249–256. [CrossRef]
9. Brebels, J.; Mignon, A. Polymer-based constructs for flexor tendon repair: A review. *Polymers* **2022**, *14*, 867. [CrossRef] [PubMed]
10. Abate, M.; Schiavone, C.; Salini, V. The use of hyaluronic acid after tendon surgery and in tendinopathies. *BioMed. Res. Int.* **2014**, *2014*, 783632. [CrossRef]
11. Romero, A.; Barrachina, L.; Ranera, B.; Remacha, A.R.; Moreno, B.; de Blas, I.; Sanz, A.; Vasquez, F.J.; Vitoria, A.; Junquera, C.; et al. Comparison of autologous bone marrow and adipose tissue derived mesenchymal stem cells, and platelet-rich plasma, for treating surgically induced lesions of the equine superficial digital flexor tendon. *Vet. J.* **2017**, *224*, 76–84. [CrossRef] [PubMed]
12. Mirghaderi, S.P.; Valizadeh, Z.; Shadman, K.; Lafosse, T.; Oryadi-Zanjani, L.; Yekaninejad, M.S.; Nabian, M.H. Cell therapy efficacy and safety in treating tendon disorders: A systemic review of clinical studies. *J. Exp. Orthop.* **2022**, *9*, 85. [CrossRef] [PubMed]
13. Ho, J.O.; Sawadkar, P.; Mudera, V. A review on the use of cell therapy in the treatment of tendon disease and injuries. *J. Tissue Eng.* **2014**, *5*, 2041731414549678. [CrossRef]
14. Amadio, P.C. Gliding resistance and modifications of gliding surface of tendon: Clinical perspectives. *Hand Clin.* **2013**, *29*, 159–166. [CrossRef]
15. Nichols, A.E.C.; Best, K.T.; Loiselle, A.E. The cellular basis of fibrotic tendon healing: Challenges and opportunities. *Transl. Res.* **2019**, *209*, 156–168. [CrossRef]
16. Galatz, L.M.; Gerstenfeld, L.; Heber-Katz, E.; Rodeo, S.A. Tendon regeneration and scar formation: The concept of scarless healing. *J. Orthop. Res.* **2015**, *33*, 823–831. [CrossRef]

17. Ratcliffe, A.; Butler, D.L.; Dyment, N.A.; Cagle, P.J., Jr.; Proctor, C.S.; Ratcliffe, S.S.; Flatow, E.L. Scaffolds for tendon and ligament repair and regeneration. *Ann. Biomed. Eng.* **2015**, *43*, 819–831. [CrossRef]
18. Wong, J.K.; Cerovac, S.; Ferguson, M.W.; McGrouther, D.A. The cellular effect of a single interrupted suture on tendon. *J. Hand Surg.* **2006**, *31*, 358–367. [CrossRef]
19. Aeberhard, P.A.; Grognuz, A.; Peneveyre, C.; McCallin, S.; Hirt-Burri, N.; Antons, J.; Pioletti, D.; Raffoul, W.; Applegate, L.A. Efficient decellularization of equine tendon with preserved biomechanical properties and cytocompatibility for human tendon surgery indications. *Artif. Organs* **2020**, *44*, E161–E171. [CrossRef] [PubMed]
20. Sahoo, S. Biologic- and synthetic-based scaffolds for tendon regeneration. In *Tendon Regeneration–Understanding Tissue Physiology and Development to Engineer Functional Substitutes*; Gomes, M.E., Reis, R.L., Rodrigues, M.T., Eds.; Academic Press: Cambridge, MA, USA, 2015; pp. 243–255. [CrossRef]
21. Pridgen, B.C.; Woon, C.Y.; Kim, M.; Thorfinn, J.; Lindsey, D.; Pham, H.; Chang, J. Flexor tendon tissue engineering: Acellularization of human flexor tendons with preservation of biomechanical properties and biocompatibility. *Tissue Eng. Part C Methods* **2011**, *17*, 819–828. [CrossRef]
22. Lovati, A.B.; Bottagisio, M.; Moretti, M. Decellularized and engineered tendons as biological substitutes: A critical review. *Stem Cells Int.* **2016**, *2016*, 7276150. [CrossRef]
23. Chong, A.K.; Riboh, J.; Smith, R.L.; Lindsey, D.P.; Pham, H.M.; Chang, J. Flexor tendon tissue engineering: Acellularized and reseeded tendon constructs. *Plast. Reconstr. Surg.* **2009**, *123*, 1759–1766. [CrossRef]
24. Longo, U.G.; Lamberti, A.; Petrillo, S.; Maffulli, N.; Denaro, V. Scaffolds in tendon tissue engineering. *Stem Cells Int.* **2012**, *2012*, 517165. [CrossRef] [PubMed]
25. Vasiliadis, A.V.; Katakalos, K. The role of scaffolds in tendon tissue engineering. *J. Funct. Biomater.* **2020**, *11*, 78. [CrossRef]
26. Mao, Z.; Fan, B.; Wang, X.; Huang, X.; Guan, J.; Sun, Z.; Xu, B.; Yang, M.; Chen, Z.; Jiang, D.; et al. A systematic review of tissue engineering scaffold in tendon bone healing in vivo. *Front. Bioeng. Biotechnol.* **2021**, *9*, 621483. [CrossRef]
27. Lui, H.; Vaquette, C.; Bindra, R. Tissue engineering in hand surgery: A technology update. *J. Hand Surg.* **2017**, *42*, 727–735. [CrossRef]
28. Kloczko, E.; Nikkhah, D.; Yildirimer, L. Scaffolds for hand tissue engineering: The importance of surface topography. *J. Hand Surg.* **2015**, *40*, 973–985. [CrossRef] [PubMed]
29. Zhang, Q.; Yang, Y.; Yildirimer, L.; Xu, T.; Zhao, X. Advanced technology-driven therapeutic interventions for prevention of tendon adhesion: Design, intrinsic and extrinsic factor considerations. *Acta Biomater.* **2021**, *124*, 15–32. [CrossRef] [PubMed]
30. Hasslund, S.; Jacobson, J.A.; Dadali, T.; Basile, P.; Ulrich-Vinther, M.; Søballe, K.; Schwarz, E.M.; O'Keefe, R.J.; Mitten, D.J.; Awad, H.A. Adhesions in a murine flexor tendon graft model: Autograft versus allograft reconstruction. *J. Orthop. Res.* **2008**, *26*, 824–833. [CrossRef] [PubMed]
31. Liu, C.F.; Aschbacher-Smith, L.; Barthelery, N.J.; Dyment, N.; Butler, D.; Wylie, C. What we should know before using tissue engineering techniques to repair injured tendons: A developmental biology perspective. *Tissue Eng. Part B Rev.* **2011**, *17*, 165–176. [CrossRef]
32. Kaux, J.F.; Samson, A.; Crielaard, J.M. Hyaluronic acid and tendon lesions. *Muscles Ligaments Tendons J.* **2016**, *5*, 264–269. [CrossRef] [PubMed]
33. Looney, A.M.; Leider, J.D.; Horn, A.R.; Bodendorfer, B.M. Bioaugmentation in the surgical treatment of anterior cruciate ligament injuries: A review of current concepts and emerging techniques. *SAGE Open Med.* **2020**, *8*, 2050312120921057. [CrossRef] [PubMed]
34. Barber, F.A.; Herbert, M.A.; Coons, D.A. Tendon augmentation grafts: Biomechanical failure loads and failure patterns. *Arthroscopy* **2006**, *22*, 534–538. [CrossRef] [PubMed]
35. Woon, C.Y.; Farnebo, S.; Schmitt, T.; Kraus, A.; Megerle, K.; Pham, H.; Yan, X.; Gambhir, S.S.; Chang, J. Human flexor tendon tissue engineering: Revitalization of biostatic allograft scaffolds. *Tissue Eng. Part A* **2012**, *18*, 2406–2417. [CrossRef]
36. Laurencin, C.T.; Freeman, J.W. Ligament tissue engineering: An evolutionary materials science approach. *Biomaterials* **2005**, *26*, 7530–7536. [CrossRef]
37. Seo, Y.K.; Yoon, H.H.; Song, K.Y.; Kwon, S.Y.; Lee, H.S.; Park, Y.S.; Park, J.K. Increase in cell migration and angiogenesis in a composite silk scaffold for tissue-engineered ligaments. *J. Orthop. Res.* **2009**, *27*, 495–503. [CrossRef]
38. Costa-Almeida, R.; Calejo, I.; Gomes, M.E. Mesenchymal stem cells empowering tendon regenerative therapies. *Int. J. Mol. Sci.* **2019**, *20*, 3002. [CrossRef]
39. Laurent, A.; Abdel-Sayed, P.; Grognuz, A.; Scaletta, C.; Hirt-Burri, N.; Michetti, M.; de Buys Roessingh, A.S.; Raffoul, W.; Kronen, P.; Nuss, K.; et al. Industrial development of standardized fetal progenitor cell therapy for tendon regenerative medicine: Preliminary safety in xenogeneic transplantation. *Biomedicines* **2021**, *9*, 380. [CrossRef]
40. Meier Bürgisser, G.; Evrova, O.; Calcagni, M.; Scalera, C.; Giovanoli, P.; Buschmann, J. Impact of PDGF-BB on cellular distribution and extracellular matrix in the healing rabbit Achilles tendon three weeks post-operation. *FEBS Open Bio* **2020**, *10*, 327–337. [CrossRef]
41. Zhang, Z.; Li, Y.; Zhang, T.; Shi, M.; Song, X.; Yang, S.; Liu, H.; Zhang, M.; Cui, Q.; Li, Z. Hepatocyte growth factor-induced tendon stem cell conditioned medium promotes healing of injured Achilles tendon. *Front. Cell Dev. Biol.* **2021**, *9*, 654084. [CrossRef]

42. Andriolo, L.; Altamura, S.A.; Reale, D.; Candrian, C.; Zaffagnini, S.; Filardo, G. Nonsurgical treatments of patellar tendinopathy: Multiple injections of platelet-rich plasma are a suitable option: A systematic review and meta-analysis. *Am. J. Sport. Med.* **2019**, *47*, 1001–1018. [CrossRef]
43. Wang, A.; Mackie, K.; Breidahl, W.; Wang, T.; Zheng, M.H. Evidence for the durability of autologous tenocyte injection for treatment of chronic resistant lateral epicondylitis: Mean 4.5-year clinical follow-up. *Am. J. Sport. Med.* **2015**, *43*, 1775–1783. [CrossRef]
44. Van den Boom, N.A.C.; Winters, M.; Haisma, H.J.; Moen, M.H. Efficacy of stem cell therapy for tendon disorders: A systematic review. *Orthop. J. Sport. Med.* **2020**, *8*, 2325967120915857. [CrossRef] [PubMed]
45. Kryger, G.S.; Chong, A.K.; Costa, M.; Pham, H.; Bates, S.J.; Chang, J. A comparison of tenocytes and mesenchymal stem cells for use in flexor tendon tissue engineering. *J. Hand Surg. Am.* **2007**, *32*, 597–605. [CrossRef] [PubMed]
46. Migliorini, F.; Tingart, M.; Maffulli, N. Progress with stem cell therapies for tendon tissue regeneration. *Exp. Opin. Biol. Ther.* **2020**, *20*, 1373–1379. [CrossRef] [PubMed]
47. Sebbagh, P.; Hirt-Burri, N.; Scaletta, C.; Abdel-Sayed, P.; Raffoul, W.; Gremeaux, V.; Laurent, A.; Applegate, L.A.; Gremion, G. Process optimization and efficacy assessment of standardized PRP for tendinopathies in sports medicine: Retrospective study of clinical files and GMP manufacturing records in a Swiss university hospital. *Bioengineering* **2023**, *10*, 409. [CrossRef] [PubMed]
48. Sato, D.; Takahara, M.; Narita, A.; Yamakawa, J.; Hashimoto, J.; Ishikawa, H.; Ogino, T. Effect of platelet-rich plasma with fibrin matrix on healing of intrasynovial flexor tendons. *J. Hand Surg. Am.* **2012**, *37*, 1356–1363. [CrossRef]
49. Jo, C.H.; Chai, J.W.; Jeong, E.C.; Oh, S.; Kim, P.S.; Yoon, J.Y.; Yoon, K.S. Intratendinous injection of autologous adipose tissue-derived mesenchymal stem cells for the treatment of rotator cuff disease: A first-in-human trial. *Stem Cells* **2018**, *36*, 1441–1450. [CrossRef]
50. Hurd, J.L.; Facile, T.R.; Weiss, J.; Hayes, M.; Hayes, M.; Furia, J.P.; Maffulli, N.; Winnier, G.E.; Alt, C.; Schmitz, C.; et al. Safety and efficacy of treating symptomatic, partial-thickness rotator cuff tears with fresh, uncultured, unmodified, autologous adipose-derived regenerative cells (UA-ADRCs) isolated at the point of care: A prospective, randomized, controlled first-in-human pilot study. *J. Orthop. Surg. Res.* **2020**, *15*, 122. [CrossRef]
51. Chun, S.W.; Kim, W.; Lee, S.Y.; Lim, C.Y.; Kim, K.; Kim, J.G.; Park, C.H.; Hong, S.H.; Yoo, H.J.; Chung, S.G. A randomized controlled trial of stem cell injection for tendon tear. *Sci. Rep.* **2022**, *12*, 818. [CrossRef]
52. Wang, A.; Breidahl, W.; Mackie, K.E.; Lin, Z.; Qin, A.; Chen, J.; Zheng, M.H. Autologous tenocyte injection for the treatment of severe, chronic resistant lateral epicondylitis: A pilot study. *Am. J. Sport. Med.* **2013**, *41*, 2925–2932. [CrossRef] [PubMed]
53. Gaspar, D.; Spanoudes, K.; Holladay, C.; Pandit, A.; Zeugolis, D. Progress in cell-based therapies for tendon repair. *Adv. Drug Del. Rev.* **2015**, *84*, 240–256. [CrossRef]
54. Liu, H.; Chansoria, P.; Delrot, P.; Angelidakis, E.; Rizzo, R.; Rütsche, D.; Applegate, L.A.; Loterie, D.; Zenobi-Wong, M. Filamented light (flight) biofabrication of highly aligned tissue-engineered constructs. *Adv. Mater.* **2022**, *34*, 2204301. [CrossRef]
55. Jeannerat, A.; Peneveyre, C.; Armand, F.; Chiappe, D.; Hamelin, R.; Scaletta, C.; Hirt-Burri, N.; de Buys Roessingh, A.; Raffoul, W.; Applegate, L.A.; et al. Hypoxic incubation conditions for optimized manufacture of tenocyte-based active pharmaceutical ingredients of homologous standardized transplant products in tendon regenerative medicine. *Cells* **2021**, *10*, 2872. [CrossRef]
56. Grognuz, A.; Scaletta, C.; Farron, A.; Pioletti, D.P.; Raffoul, W.; Applegate, L.A. Stability enhancement using hyaluronic acid gels for delivery of human fetal progenitor tenocytes. *Cell Med.* **2016**, *8*, 87–97. [CrossRef] [PubMed]
57. Laurent, A.; Porcello, A.; Fernandez, P.G.; Jeannerat, A.; Peneveyre, C.; Abdel-Sayed, P.; Scaletta, C.; Hirt-Burri, N.; Michetti, M.; de Buys Roessingh, A.; et al. Combination of hyaluronan and lyophilized progenitor cell derivatives: Stabilization of functional hydrogel products for therapeutic management of tendinous tissue disorders. *Pharmaceutics* **2021**, *13*, 2196. [CrossRef] [PubMed]
58. Laurent, A.; Porcello, A.; Jeannerat, A.; Peneveyre, C.; Coeur, A.; Abdel-Sayed, P.; Scaletta, C.; Michetti, M.; de Buys Roessingh, A.; Jordan, O.; et al. Lyophilized progenitor tenocyte extracts: Sterilizable cytotherapeutic derivatives with antioxidant properties and hyaluronan hydrogel functionalization effects. *Antioxidants* **2023**, *12*, 163. [CrossRef] [PubMed]
59. Fujikawa, K.; Ohtani, T.; Matsumoto, H.; Seedhom, B.B. Reconstruction of the extensor apparatus of the knee with the Leeds-Keio ligament. *J. Bone Jt. Surg. Br.* **1994**, *76*, 200–203. [CrossRef]
60. Abdullah, S.; Mohtar, F.; Abdul Shukor, N.; Sapuan, J. In vitro evaluation of human hand tendon ingrowth into a synthetic scaffold. *J. Hand Surg. (Asian-Pac. Vol.)* **2017**, *22*, 429–434. [CrossRef]
61. Fujikawa, K.; Iseki, F.; Seedhom, B.B. Arthroscopy after anterior cruciate reconstruction with the Leeds-Keio ligament. *J. Bone Jt. Surg. Br.* **1989**, *71*, 566–570. [CrossRef]
62. Zaffagnini, S.; Marcheggiani Muccioli, G.M.; Chatrath, V.; Bondi, A.; De Pasquale, V.; Martini, D.; Bacchelli, B.; Marcacci, M. Histological and ultrastructural evaluation of Leeds-Keio ligament 20 years after implant: A case report. *Knee Surg. Sport. Traumatol. Arthrosc.* **2008**, *16*, 1026–1029. [CrossRef] [PubMed]
63. Marcacci, M.; Zaffagnini, S.; Visani, A.; Iacono, F.; Neri, M.P.; Petitto, A. Arthroscopic reconstruction of the anterior cruciate ligament with Leeds-Keio ligament in non-professional athletes. Results after a minimum 5 years' follow-up. *Knee Surg. Sport. Traumatol. Arthrosc.* **1996**, *4*, 9–13. [CrossRef] [PubMed]
64. Schroven, I.T.; Geens, S.; Beckers, L.; Lagrange, W.; Fabry, G. Experience with the Leeds-Keio artificial ligament for anterior cruciate ligament reconstruction. *Knee Surg. Sport. Traumatol. Arthrosc.* **1994**, *2*, 214–218. [CrossRef]
65. Fukuta, S.; Kuge, A.; Nakamura, M. Use of the Leeds-Keio prosthetic ligament for repair of patellar tendon rupture after total knee arthroplasty. *Knee* **2003**, *10*, 127–130. [CrossRef] [PubMed]

66. Ghalayini, S.R.; Helm, A.T.; Bonshahi, A.Y.; Lavender, A.; Johnson, D.S.; Smith, R.B. Arthroscopic anterior cruciate ligament surgery: Results of autogenous patellar tendon graft versus the Leeds-Keio synthetic graft five year follow-up of a prospective randomised controlled trial. *Knee* **2010**, *17*, 334–339. [CrossRef] [PubMed]
67. Jones, A.P.; Sidhom, S.; Sefton, G. Long-term clinical review (10–20 years) after reconstruction of the anterior cruciate ligament using the Leeds-Keio synthetic ligament. *J. Long-Term Eff. Med. Implant.* **2007**, *17*, 59–69. [CrossRef] [PubMed]
68. Abdullah, S.; Gill Narin Singh, P.S.; Zi Fan, E.S.; Ahmad, A.A.; Mohd Haflah, N.H.; Sapuan, J. Long-term follow-up of synthetic ligament (Orthotape) usage in reconstructive surgery of the hand. *J. Hand Surg. Glob. Online* **2021**, *3*, 195–203. [CrossRef]
69. Sato, N.; Taniguchi, T.; Goda, Y.; Kosaka, H.; Higashino, K.; Sakai, T.; Katoh, S.; Yasui, N.; Sairyo, K.; Taniguchi, H. Proteomic analysis of human tendon and ligament: Solubilization and analysis of insoluble extracellular matrix in connective tissues. *J. Proteome Res.* **2016**, *15*, 4709–4721. [CrossRef]
70. Rowland, J.R.; Tsukazaki, S.; Kikuchi, T.; Fujikawa, K.; Kearney, J.; Lomas, R.; Wood, E.; Seedhom, B.B. Radiofrequency-generated glow discharge treatment: Potential benefits for polyester ligaments. *J. Orthop. Sci.* **2003**, *8*, 198–206. [CrossRef]
71. Grognuz, A.; Scaletta, C.; Farron, A.; Raffoul, W.; Applegate, L.A. Human fetal progenitor tenocytes for regenerative medicine. *Cell Transplant.* **2016**, *25*, 463–479. [CrossRef]
72. Laurent, A.; Rey, M.; Scaletta, C.; Abdel-Sayed, P.; Michetti, M.; Flahaut, M.; Raffoul, W.; de Buys Roessingh, A.; Hirt-Burri, N.; Applegate, L.A. Retrospectives on three decades of safe clinical experience with allogeneic dermal progenitor fibroblasts: High Versatility in topical cytotherapeutic care. *Pharmaceutics* **2023**, *15*, 184. [CrossRef] [PubMed]
73. Hiyama, E.; Hiyama, K. Telomere and telomerase in stem cells. *Br. J. Cancer* **2007**, *96*, 1020–1024. [CrossRef]
74. Evans, C.H. The vicissitudes of gene therapy. *Bone Jt. Res.* **2019**, *8*, 469–471. [CrossRef]
75. Otani, T. Development of ligament-bone junction in anterior cruciate ligament reconstruction with the scaffold type polyester artificial ligament (Leeds-Keio) in the dog. *Nihon Seikeigeka Gakkai Zasshi* **1992**, *66*, 264–278.
76. Kawakubo, M. An experimental study on tissue induction in anterior cruciate ligament reconstruction with the scaffold-type polyester artificial ligament (Leeds-Keio). *Nihon Seikeigeka Gakkai Zasshi* **1992**, *66*, 1016–1030. [PubMed]
77. Taye, N.; Karoulias, S.Z.; Hubmacher, D. The "other" 15–40%: The role of non-collagenous extracellular matrix proteins and minor collagens in tendon. *J. Orthop. Res.* **2020**, *38*, 23–35. [CrossRef]
78. Chen, X.; Song, X.H.; Yin, Z.; Zou, X.H.; Wang, L.L.; Hu, H.; Cao, T.; Zheng, M.; Ouyang, H.W. Stepwise differentiation of human embryonic stem cells promotes tendon regeneration by secreting fetal tendon matrix and differentiation factors. *Stem Cells* **2009**, *27*, 1276–1287. [CrossRef] [PubMed]
79. Chen, H.S.; Su, Y.T.; Chan, T.M.; Su, Y.J.; Syu, W.S.; Harn, H.J.; Lin, S.Z.; Chiu, S.C. Human adipose-derived stem cells accelerate the restoration of tensile strength of tendon and alleviate the progression of rotator cuff injury in a rat model. *Cell Transplant.* **2015**, *24*, 509–520. [CrossRef] [PubMed]
80. Xu, W.; Wang, Y.; Liu, E.; Sun, Y.; Luo, Z.; Xu, Z.; Liu, W.; Zhong, L.; Lv, Y.; Wang, A.; et al. Human iPSC-derived neural crest stem cells promote tendon repair in a rat patellar tendon window defect model. *Tissue Eng. Part A* **2013**, *19*, 2439–2451. [CrossRef]
81. Chong, A.K.; Ang, A.D.; Goh, J.C.; Hui, J.H.; Lim, A.Y.; Lee, E.H.; Lim, B.H. Bone marrow-derived mesenchymal stem cells influence early tendon-healing in a rabbit Achilles tendon model. *J. Bone Jt. Surg. Am.* **2007**, *89*, 74–81. [CrossRef]
82. Watts, A.E.; Yeager, A.E.; Kopyov, O.V.; Nixon, A.J. Fetal derived embryonic-like stem cells improve healing in a large animalflexor tendonitis model. *Stem Cell Res.* **2011**, *2*, 4. [CrossRef]
83. Ellera Gomes, J.L.; da Silva, R.C.; Silla, L.M.; Abreu, M.R.; Pellanda, R. Conventional rotator cuff repair complemented by the aid of mononuclear autologous stem cells. *Knee Surg. Sport. Traumatol. Arthrosc.* **2012**, *20*, 373–377. [CrossRef] [PubMed]
84. Song, I.; Rim, J.; Lee, J.; Jang, I.; Jung, B.; Kim, K.; Lee, S. Therapeutic potential of human fetal mesenchymal stem cells in musculoskeletal disorders: A narrative review. *Int. J. Mol. Sci.* **2022**, *23*, 1439. [CrossRef] [PubMed]
85. Durgam, S.S.; Stewart, A.A.; Sivaguru, M.; Wagoner Johnson, A.J.; Stewart, M.C. Tendon-derived progenitor cells improve healing of collagenase-induced flexor tendinitis. *J. Orthop. Res.* **2016**, *34*, 2162–2171. [CrossRef] [PubMed]
86. Chen, E.; Yang, L.; Ye, C.; Zhang, W.; Ran, J.; Xue, D.; Wang, Z.; Pan, Z.; Hu, Q. An asymmetric chitosan scaffold for tendon tissue engineering: In vitro and in vivo evaluation with rat tendon stem/progenitor cells. *Acta Biomater.* **2018**, *73*, 377–387. [CrossRef]
87. Oshita, T.; Tobita, M.; Tajima, S.; Mizuno, H. Adipose-derived stem cells improve collagenase-induced tendinopathy in a rat model. *Am. J. Sport. Med.* **2016**, *44*, 1983–1989. [CrossRef]
88. Deng, D.; Wang, W.; Wang, B.; Zhang, P.; Zhou, G.; Zhang, W.J.; Cao, Y.; Liu, W. Repair of Achilles tendon defect with autologous ASCs engineered tendon in a rabbit model. *Biomaterials* **2014**, *35*, 8801–8809. [CrossRef]
89. Hoffmann, A.; Pelled, G.; Turgeman, G.; Eberle, P.; Zilberman, Y.; Shinar, H.; Keinan-Adamsky, K.; Winkel, A.; Shahab, S.; Navon, G.; et al. Neotendon formation induced by manipulation of the Smad8 signalling pathway in mesenchymal stem cells. *J. Clin. Investig.* **2006**, *116*, 940–952. [CrossRef]
90. Alberton, P.; Popov, C.; Prägert, M.; Kohler, J.; Shukunami, C.; Schieker, M.; Docheva, D. Conversion of human bone marrow-derived mesenchymal stem cells into tendon progenitor cells by ectopic expression of scleraxis. *Stem Cells Dev.* **2012**, *21*, 846–858. [CrossRef]
91. Zhang, M.; Liu, H.; Shi, M.; Zhang, T.; Lu, W.; Yang, S.; Cui, Q.; Li, Z. Potential mechanisms of the impact of hepatocyte growth factor gene-modified tendon stem cells on tendon healing. *Front. Cell Dev. Biol.* **2021**, *9*, 659389. [CrossRef]
92. Gulotta, L.V.; Kovacevic, D.; Packer, J.D.; Deng, X.H.; Rodeo, S.A. Bone marrow-derived mesenchymal stem cells transduced with scleraxis improve rotator cuff healing in a rat model. *Am. J. Sport. Med.* **2011**, *39*, 1282–1289. [CrossRef] [PubMed]

93. Papalamprou, A.; Yu, V.; Chen, A.; Stefanovic, T.; Kaneda, G.; Salehi, K.; Castaneda, C.M.; Gertych, A.; Glaeser, J.D.; Sheyn, D. Directing iPSC differentiation into iTenocytes using combined scleraxis overexpression and cyclic loading. *J. Orthop. Res.* **2023**, *41*, 1148–1161. [CrossRef] [PubMed]
94. Tsutsumi, H.; Kurimoto, R.; Nakamichi, R.; Chiba, T.; Matsushima, T.; Fujii, Y.; Sanada, R.; Kato, T.; Shishido, K.; Sakamaki, Y.; et al. Generation of a tendon-like tissue from human iPS cells. *J. Tissue Eng.* **2022**, *13*, 20417314221074018. [CrossRef]
95. Ni, M.; Sun, W.; Li, Y.; Ding, L.; Lin, W.; Peng, H.; Zheng, Q.; Sun, J.; Li, J.; Liu, H.; et al. Sox11 modified tendon-derived stem cells promote the repair of osteonecrosis of femoral head. *Cell Transplant.* **2021**, *30*, 9636897211053870. [CrossRef] [PubMed]
96. Brittberg, M. Cell carriers as the next generation of cell therapy for cartilage repair: A review of the matrix-induced autologous chondrocyte implantation procedure. *Am. J. Sport. Med.* **2010**, *38*, 1259–1271. [CrossRef]
97. Brittberg, M. Autologous chondrocyte implantation--technique and long-term follow-up. *Injury* **2008**, *39*, S40–S49. [CrossRef]
98. Lu, V.; Tennyson, M.; Zhang, J.; Khan, W. Mesenchymal stem cell-derived extracellular vesicles in tendon and ligament repair-A systematic review of in vivo studies. *Cells* **2021**, *10*, 2553. [CrossRef]
99. Wellings, E.P.; Huang, T.C.; Li, J.; Peterson, T.E.; Hooke, A.W.; Rosenbaum, A.; Zhao, C.D.; Behfar, A.; Moran, S.L.; Houdek, M.T. Intrinsic tendon regeneration after application of purified exosome product: An in vivo study. *Orthop. J. Sport. Med.* **2021**, *9*, 23259671211062929. [CrossRef] [PubMed]
100. Chen, J.; Yu, Q.; Wu, B.; Lin, Z.; Pavlos, N.J.; Xu, J.; Ouyang, H.; Wang, A.; Zheng, M.H. Autologous tenocyte therapy for experimental Achilles tendinopathy in a rabbit model. *Tissue Eng. Part A* **2011**, *17*, 2037–2048. [CrossRef]
101. Chen, J.M.; Willers, C.; Xu, J.; Wang, A.; Zheng, M.H. Autologous tenocyte therapy using porcine-derived bioscaffolds for massive rotator cuff defect in rabbits. *Tissue Eng.* **2007**, *13*, 1479–1491. [CrossRef]
102. Bucher, T.A.; Ebert, J.R.; Smith, A.; Breidahl, W.; Fallon, M.; Wang, T.; Zheng, M.H.; Janes, G.C. Autologous tenocyte injection for the treatment of chronic recalcitrant gluteal tendinopathy: A prospective pilot study. *Orthop. J. Sport. Med.* **2017**, *5*, 2325967116688866. [CrossRef]
103. Steiner, M.M.; Calandruccio, J.H. Biologic approaches to problems of the hand and wrist. *Orthop. Clin. N. Am.* **2017**, *48*, 343–349. [CrossRef]
104. Gonçalves, A.I.; Gershovich, P.M.; Rodrigues, M.T.; Reis, R.L.; Gomes, M.E. Human adipose tissue-derived tenomodulin positive subpopulation of stem cells: A promising source of tendon progenitor cells. *J. Tissue Eng. Regen. Med.* **2018**, *12*, 762–774. [CrossRef] [PubMed]
105. Shen, W.; Chen, J.; Yin, Z.; Chen, X.; Liu, H.; Heng, B.C.; Chen, W.; Ouyang, H.W. Allogenous tendon stem/progenitor cells in silk scaffold for functional shoulder repair. *Cell Transplant.* **2012**, *21*, 943–958. [CrossRef]
106. Khodabukus, A.; Guyer, T.; Moore, A.C.; Stevens, M.M.; Guldberg, R.E.; Bursac, N. Translating musculoskeletal bioengineering into tissue regeneration therapies. *Sci. Transl. Med.* **2022**, *14*, eabn9074. [CrossRef]
107. Dahlgren, L.A.; Mohammed, H.O.; Nixon, A.J. Temporal expression of growth factors and matrix molecules in healing tendon lesions. *J. Orhtop. Res.* **2005**, *23*, 84–92. [CrossRef]
108. Ribitsch, I.; Bileck, A.; Aldoshin, A.D.; Kańduła, M.M.; Mayer, R.L.; Egerbacher, M.; Gabner, S.; Auer, U.; Gültekin, S.; Huber, J.; et al. Molecular mechanisms of fetal tendon regeneration versus adult fibrous repair. *Int. J. Mol. Sci.* **2021**, *22*, 5619. [CrossRef]
109. Schneider, M.; Angele, P.; Järvinen, T.A.H.; Docheva, D. Rescue plan for Achilles: Therapeutics steering the fate and functions of stem cells in tendon wound healing. *Adv. Drug Delivery Rev.* **2018**, *129*, 352–375. [CrossRef] [PubMed]
110. Costa-Almeida, R.; Calejo, I.; Reis, R.L.; Gomes, M.E. Crosstalk between adipose stem cells and tendon cells reveals a temporal regulation of tenogenesis by matrix deposition and remodeling. *J. Cell. Physiol.* **2018**, *233*, 5383–5395. [CrossRef]
111. Badylak, S.F.; Freytes, D.O.; Gilbert, T.W. Extracellular matrix as a biological scaffold material: Structure and function. *Acta Biomaterialia* **2009**, *5*, 1–13. [CrossRef] [PubMed]
112. Beredjiklian, P.K. Biologic aspects of flexor tendon laceration and repair. *J. Bone Jt. Surg.* **2003**, *85*, 539–550. [CrossRef]
113. Singh, R.; Rymer, B.; Theobald, P.; Thomas, P.B. A review of current concepts in flexor tendon repair: Physiology, biomechanics, surgical technique and rehabilitation. *Orthop. Rev.* **2015**, *7*, 6125. [CrossRef]
114. Carpenter, J.E.; Hankenson, K.D. Animal models of tendon and ligament injuries for tissue engineering applications. *Biomaterials* **2004**, *25*, 1715–1722. [CrossRef]
115. Derwin, K.A.; Baker, A.R.; Spragg, R.K.; Leigh, D.R.; Iannotti, J.P. Commercial extracellular matrix scaffolds for rotator cuff tendon repair. Biomechanical, biochemical, and cellular properties. *J. Bone Jt. Surg.* **2006**, *88*, 2665–2672. [CrossRef]
116. Zhang, A.Y.; Bates, S.J.; Morrow, E.; Pham, H.; Pham, B.; Chang, J. Tissue-engineered intrasynovial tendons: Optimization of acellularization and seeding. *J. Rehabil. Res. Dev.* **2009**, *46*, 489–498. [CrossRef]
117. Lomas, A.J.; Ryan, C.N.; Sorushanova, A.; Shologu, N.; Sideri, A.I.; Tsioli, V.; Fthenakis, G.C.; Tzora, A.; Skoufos, I.; Quinlan, L.R.; et al. The past, present and future in scaffold-based tendon treatments. *Adv. Drug Deliv. Rev.* **2015**, *84*, 257–277. [CrossRef]
118. Chen, X.; Qi, Y.Y.; Wang, L.L.; Yin, Z.; Yin, G.L.; Zou, X.H.; Ouyang, H.W. Ligament regeneration using a knitted silk scaffold combined with collagen matrix. *Biomaterials* **2008**, *29*, 3683–3692. [CrossRef] [PubMed]
119. US Food and Drug Administration. *Guidance for Industry; Potency Tests for Cellular and Gene Therapy Products*; FDA: Silver Spring, MA, USA, 2011.
120. Durdzińska, A.T.; Arnaud, P.B.; Durand, S. Osteoarticular surgery of the hand in rheumatoid patients. *Rev. Med. Suisse* **2023**, *19*, 526–529. [CrossRef]

121. Blache, U.; Stevens, M.M.; Gentleman, E. Harnessing the secreted extracellular matrix to engineer tissues. *Nat. Biomed. Eng.* **2020**, *4*, 357–363. [CrossRef]
122. World Medical Association. World Medical Association Declaration of Helsinki: Ethical principles for medical research involving human subjects. *JAMA* **2013**, *310*, 2191–2194. [CrossRef] [PubMed]

*pharmaceutics*

*Article*

# Autologous and Allogeneic Cytotherapies for Large Knee (Osteo)Chondral Defects: Manufacturing Process Benchmarking and Parallel Functional Qualification

**Virginie Philippe [1,2,*,†], Annick Jeannerat [3,†], Cédric Peneveyre [3], Sandra Jaccoud [2,4], Corinne Scaletta [2], Nathalie Hirt-Burri [2], Philippe Abdel-Sayed [2,5], Wassim Raffoul [2], Salim Darwiche [6,7], Lee Ann Applegate [2,7,8], Robin Martin [1,‡] and Alexis Laurent [2,3,*,‡]**

1 Orthopedics and Traumatology Service, Lausanne University Hospital, University of Lausanne, CH-1011 Lausanne, Switzerland; robin.martin@chuv.ch
2 Regenerative Therapy Unit, Plastic, Reconstructive and Hand Surgery Service, Lausanne University Hospital, University of Lausanne, CH-1066 Epalinges, Switzerland; sandra.jaccoud@chuv.ch (S.J.); corinne.scaletta@chuv.ch (C.S.); nathalie.burri@chuv.ch (N.H.-B.); philippe.abdel-sayed@chuv.ch (P.A.-S.); wassim.raffoul@chuv.ch (W.R.); lee.laurent-applegate@chuv.ch (L.A.A.)
3 Preclinical Research Department, LAM Biotechnologies SA, CH-1066 Epalinges, Switzerland; annick.jeannerat@lambiotechnologies.com (A.J.); cedric.peneveyre@lambiotechnologies.com (C.P.)
4 Laboratory of Biomechanical Orthopedics, Federal Polytechnic School of Lausanne, CH-1015 Lausanne, Switzerland
5 STI School of Engineering, Federal Polytechnic School of Lausanne, CH-1015 Lausanne, Switzerland
6 Musculoskeletal Research Unit, Vetsuisse Faculty, University of Zurich, CH-8057 Zurich, Switzerland; sdarwiche@vetclinics.uzh.ch
7 Center for Applied Biotechnology and Molecular Medicine, University of Zurich, CH-8057 Zurich, Switzerland
8 Oxford OSCAR Suzhou Center, Oxford University, Suzhou 215123, China
* Correspondence: virginie.philippe@chuv.ch (V.P.); alexis.laurent@lambiotechnologies.com (A.L.); Tel.: +41-21-314-90-18 (V.P.); +41-21-546-42-00 (A.L.)
† These authors contributed equally to this work.
‡ These authors also contributed equally to this work.

**Abstract:** Cytotherapies are often necessary for the management of symptomatic large knee (osteo)-chondral defects. While autologous chondrocyte implantation (ACI) has been clinically used for 30 years, allogeneic cells (clinical-grade FE002 primary chondroprogenitors) have been investigated in translational settings (Swiss progenitor cell transplantation program). The aim of this study was to comparatively assess autologous and allogeneic approaches (quality, safety, functional attributes) to cell-based knee chondrotherapies developed for clinical use. Protocol benchmarking from a manufacturing process and control viewpoint enabled us to highlight the respective advantages and risks. Safety data (telomerase and soft agarose colony formation assays, high passage cell senescence) and risk analyses were reported for the allogeneic FE002 cellular active substance in preparation for an autologous to allogeneic clinical protocol transposition. Validation results on autologous bioengineered grafts (autologous chondrocyte-bearing Chondro-Gide scaffolds) confirmed significant chondrogenic induction (*COL2* and *ACAN* upregulation, extracellular matrix synthesis) after 2 weeks of co-culture. Allogeneic grafts (bearing FE002 primary chondroprogenitors) displayed comparable endpoint quality and functionality attributes. Parameters of translational relevance (transport medium, finished product suturability) were validated for the allogeneic protocol. Notably, the process-based benchmarking of both approaches highlighted the key advantages of allogeneic FE002 cell-bearing grafts (reduced cellular variability, enhanced process standardization, rationalized logistical and clinical pathways). Overall, this study built on our robust knowledge and local experience with ACI (long-term safety and efficacy), setting an appropriate standard for further clinical investigations into allogeneic progenitor cell-based orthopedic protocols.

**Keywords:** allogeneic cytotherapies; autologous chondrocyte implantation; cartilage defect; chondrogenesis; cell therapy; FE002 primary chondroprogenitors; manufacturing process; standardized transplant product; tissue engineering; translational research

## 1. Introduction

Patients presenting symptomatic large knee cartilage lesions often report pain, swelling, joint locking, stiffness, and clicking [1–4]. The resulting functional impairments often negatively impact daily life activities, and untreated cartilage lesions predispose for osteoarthritis (OA) [4–6]. Therefore, early treatment for the restoration of cartilage structure and function could lead to measurable benefits for patient quality of life and tangibly limit the progression of OA [4,6]. However, articular cartilage is characterized by poor self-healing potential due to low vascularity and a limited supply of adjacent cells able to migrate to the lesion and mediate a healing response [2,3,6]. Therefore, various therapeutic approaches have been developed for the treatment of moderate knee chondropathies, such as microfracture (MFx) or osteochondral autografts and allografts, yet their use and efficacy are limited by the lesion type, size, and grade [7–14]. Importantly, the onset of severe OA often leads to the need to replace the arthritic surface with a synthetic prosthesis. While this approach is the current standard in older sedentary patients, it is less desirable for active and young patients [4,6].

From a specific cytotherapeutic viewpoint, Brittberg et al. have reported autologous chondrocyte implantation (ACI) clinical protocols for articular cartilage defect treatment since 1994 [3,7,8,15–18]. Applications of cultured autologous chondrocytes aim to promote the restauration of hyaline cartilage, providing the structural and biomechanical properties required to sustain normal joint load-bearing and function [1,2,7,11]. Despite documented inhomogeneity in cell therapy manufacturing processes and surgical approaches, the accumulated evidence points toward a beneficial effect of ACI over MFx in the medium and long term [5,9,16,18–26]. Since the initial reports on ACI, thousands of patients have been successfully treated, and the technique has evolved to further improve clinical outcomes [8,14,27–31]. Specifically, third-generation ACI involves the use of a synthetic scaffold/matrix for autologous graft bioengineering before surgical implantation [11,12,21,24,26,31–37]. This approach involves less invasive surgical procedures, and modern synthetic scaffolds are less fragile than the periosteal flaps used in previous ACI generations [2,8,38–40]. In addition to improved therapeutic cell localization, the 3D scaffold-based co-culture step induces internal re-differentiation and the expression of specific chondrogenic genes such as *COL2* and *ACAN* [31,41–47].

Whilst ACI has been clinically investigated for three decades and yielded significant beneficial results, the technique is scarcely implanted, mainly due to limited good manufacturing practice (GMP)-compliant production capabilities [4,48]. Therefore, building on our in-house translational experience regarding second-generation ACI (i.e., NCT04296487 clinical trial), a local multi-centric clinical study was approved for third-generation ACI (i.e., NCT05651997 clinical trial) [8,11,12,26,35,48]. Specifically, the studied autologous chondral graft is indicated for large ICRS grade III or IV localized and symptomatic knee cartilage lesions [4,48]. Parallelly to this autologous approach, multifaceted translational work was carried out under the Swiss progenitor cell transplantation program for the eventual cytotherapeutic use of allogeneic primary chondroprogenitors (i.e., FE002 clinical-grade cells) in human orthopedics [49–54]. Given that both tissue engineering approaches share technical, clinical, and regulatory similarities, both options are currently being locally investigated [48,50].

Generally, various therapeutic cell sources (e.g., mesenchymal stem cells, infant polydactyly chondrocytes, genetically engineered cells) were considered up to the clinical investigation and post-market follow-up (FU) stages of cartilage regenerative medicine [10,11,33,55–64]. Importantly, FE002 primary chondroprogenitors have been established as a standardized clinical-grade cell source and preclinically qualified for tissue engineering purposes [49–53].

Ten years of multicentric translational research and their good safety profile have validated the robustness and versatility of FE002 progenitor cells for industrial cytotherapeutic formulation in cartilage tissue engineering [50–53]. Specifically, clinical-grade FE002 cell source establishment and upscaled cell manufacturing optimization have validated their adequation with standard industrial biotechnology and biobanking workflows [50]. Importantly, the technical aspects of manufacturing and clinical safety risk analyses regarding FE002 primary chondroprogenitors were based on the international clinical uses of alternative FE002 progenitor cell sources [65]. Overall, several advantages were outlined regarding the considered cytotherapeutic use of FE002 primary chondroprogenitors over autologous chondrocytes, such as reduced operative burdens and optimized serial bioengineered graft manufacturing possibilities [50].

Therefore, the objective of this study was to comparatively assess the autologous and allogeneic approaches to large knee (osteo)-chondral defect cytotherapeutic management that have been locally developed for clinical application. The translational significance of this work lies in the use of a regulatorily validated autologous somatic cell therapy protocol as the baseline for benchmarking with a novel allogeneic approach valorizing a clinical-grade allogeneic FE002 progenitor cell source. Our specific areas of experimental focus included the comparative translational qualification and validation of combined cytotherapeutic product quality, safety, and functional attributes. The benchmarking of both protocols for chondral graft preparation from a manufacturing process and control viewpoint enabled us to discuss the respective opportunities, advantages, and risks of each approach. Overall, this study set forth the robust research and local clinical experience reported with respect to ACI for large knee (osteo)-chondral defects. By extension, this work also enabled the authors to establish an appropriate continuum for further local clinical investigations into cell-based orthopedic protocols, with a specific focus on autologous to allogeneic approach transposition.

## 2. Materials and Methods

### 2.1. Reagents and Consumables Used for the Study

The reagents and consumables were as follows: purified water (Bichsel, Unterseen, Switzerland); DMEM cell culture medium, L-glutamine, TrypLE, Opti-MEM, penicillin-streptomycin, dexamethasone, TRIzol, BCA assay kits, NuPAGE Bis-Tris 4–12% protein gels, MOPS buffer, loading buffer, DTT, gel migration buffer antioxidant, page ruler protein ladder, MTT, β-mercaptoethanol, PMSF, microAmp fast 96-well reaction plates, optical adhesive covers, and 96-well PCR plates (Thermo Fisher Scientific, Waltham, MA, USA); C-Chip Neubauer hemocytometers (NanoEntek, Seoul, Republic of Korea); KAPA SYBR Fast (Roche, Basel, Switzerland); PrimeScript RT reagent kits (Takara Bio, San Jose, CA, USA); X-gal powder (Chemie Brunschwig, Basel, Switzerland); HAM's F12 nutrient mix and papain (Sigma Aldrich, Buchs, Switzerland); Millipore Stericup, Trypan Blue, FBS, VitCp, sodium acetate, EDTA, low-melting point agarose, and cysteine HCl (Merck, Darmstadt, Germany); HPL (Sexton Biotechnologies, Indianapolis, IN, USA); human insulin (Novo Nordisk, Bagsværd, Danemark); ascorbic acid (Streuli Pharma, Uznach, Switzerland); ITS 100× (PAN-Biotech, Aidenbach, Germany); cell culture vessels, assay tubes, and plastic assay surfaces (Greiner BioOne, Frickenhausen, Germany; Corning, Corning, NY, USA; TPP, Trasadingen, Switzerland); TGF-β1 and TGF-β3 (PeproTech, London, UK); Chondro-Gide membranes (Geistlich Pharma, Wolhusen, Switzerland); Hyalograft membranes (Anika Therapeutics, Bedford, MA, USA); Blyscan-sulfated glycosaminoglycan assay kits (BioColor, Carrickfergus, UK); telomerase activity quantification qPCR assay kits (ScienCell, Carlsbad, CA, USA); Monosyn 6/0 suture kits (B. Braun, Melsungen, Germany).

### 2.2. Instruments and Equipment Used for the Study

Component weighing was performed using a laboratory scale (Ohaus, Parsippany, NJ, USA). Sample centrifugation was performed using a Rotina 420R centrifuge (Hettich, Tuttlingen, Germany) or on a Sorvall Legend Micro 21R microcentrifuge (Thermo Fisher Scientific, Waltham, MA, USA). Colorimetric and luminescence measurements were taken using a Varioskan LUX multimode plate reader (Thermo Fisher Scientific, Waltham, MA, USA). Telomerase activity and chondrogenic gene expression quantification assays were run on a StepOne Real-time PCR System instrument (Thermo Fisher Scientific, Waltham, MA, USA). Spectrophotometric analyses were performed using a NanoDrop instrument (Thermo Fisher Scientific, Waltham, MA, USA). Immunohistochemistry imaging was performed using an inverted IX81 fluorescence microscope (Olympus, Tokyo, Japan).

### *2.3. Ethical Compliance of the Study and Regulatory Approval of Investigative Cytotherapeutic Protocols*

This study was performed using autologous biological materials (patient primary articular chondrocytes) gathered in the context of an authorized clinical trial (www.ClinicalTrials.gov, accessed on 4 August 2023, identifier NCT04296487, "Introduction of ACI for Cartilage Repair", Lausanne, Switzerland) and/or included in the Biobank of the Department of Musculoskeletal Medicine in the Lausanne University Hospital [48]. Appropriate data security protocols were followed during the study. The described biological materials were used within the registration process of a second clinical trial (NCT05651997, "Study Comparing Two Methods for the Treatment of Large Chondral and Osteochondral Defects of the Knee", Lausanne and Fribourg, Switzerland). The second clinical trial was approved by the local cantonal ethics committee (Vaud Cantonal Ethics Committee, CER-VD authorization N°2020-01707). The corresponding clinical trial was registered following federal authorization by Swissmedic (authorization N°2021TpP2004).

The allogeneic FE002 primary chondroprogenitor cell source used in the study (the clinical-grade FE002 progenitor cell source) was established from a registered organ donation, as approved by the Vaud Cantonal Ethics Committee (Ethics Committee Protocol N°62/07). The FE002 organ donation was registered under a federal cell transplantation program (the Swiss progenitor cell transplantation program) [50]. Full material traceability was ensured during the study.

### *2.4. Autologous Primary Chondrocyte Sourcing and Chondrogenic Cellular Active Substance Lot Manufacturing*

The clinical-grade autologous primary chondrocytes (human articular chondrocytes [HAC] from orthopedic patients) used for the study consisted of banked human diploid cells. Cell type establishment was performed following cartilage biopsy procurement by the Orthopedics and Traumatology Service of the Lausanne University Hospital (Lausanne, Switzerland). The cryopreserved HACs were obtained from the biobank of the Department of Musculoskeletal Medicine in the Lausanne University Hospital. Patient-specific primary cell type establishment was performed in-house as described previously [48]. The HACs were manufactured using serial in vitro cellular expansions and were used in the present study at passage levels 3–4.

Briefly, the harvested healthy cartilage biopsies were rinsed, manually fragmented, and enzymatically treated (using pronase/collagenase) for HAC isolation. Following sample filtration on a cell sieve, the cell suspensions were expanded in vitro using human platelet lysate (HPL)-enriched culture medium (DMEM–HAM's F12 base). After 1–2 cell passage procedures, the expanded HACs were formulated for cryopreservation and stored until further use [48]. The described processes were approved by the relevant health authorities in the framework of a clinical trial (NCT04296487).

### *2.5. Allogeneic FE002 Primary Chondroprogenitor Sourcing and Chondrogenic Cellular Active Substance Lot Manufacturing*

The FE002 primary chondroprogenitor cell source used for the study consisted of banked primary human diploid cells from a clinical-grade source, as previously described [50]. The considered FE002 primary progenitor cells were procured and produced under the Swiss progenitor cell transplantation program and were made available as cryopreserved stocks. The FE002 primary chondroprogenitors were manufactured using a serial in vitro cellular expansion workflow and were used in the study at in vitro passages 6–7.

Briefly, the cryopreserved cell vials were used as cellular seeding materials for in vitro monolayer expansions. Following thawing, the cells were cultured in fetal bovine serum (FBS)-enriched or HPL-enriched cell culture medium (DMEM base). Following the in vitro monolayer expansion phase, the expanded cells were formulated for cryopreservation and stored until further use [50].

### 2.6. FE002 Primary Chondroprogenitor Cellular Active Substance Characterization Assays

Extensive characterization and qualification work was already reported for the considered clinical-grade FE002 primary chondroprogenitors [49–53]. Specifically, the cellular active substance quality-related attributes and technical specifications for industrial scale cell bank manufacture had already been published [50]. Additionally, several in vivo studies have been performed on bioengineered product prototypes bearing viable allogeneic FE002 primary chondroprogenitors, confirming their safety and functionality in the retained setups [49–53]. Therefore, primarily based on a gap analysis of the safety characterization of FE002 primary chondroprogenitors, several in vitro assays were conducted for this study to further confirm their applicability in a translational setting.

#### 2.6.1. Allogeneic FE002 Cellular Active Substance Characterization: Cell Expansion Medium Selection

The previously reported work on FE002 primary chondroprogenitors was performed using FBS-supplemented cell proliferation medium [50]. In order to investigate whether alternative cell proliferation media could be used while maintaining cellular quality attributes, comparative proliferation assays were performed. Firstly, three different cell proliferation media (10% FBS in DMEM; 5% HPL in DMEM; Brittberg medium) and two different cell culture surfaces were used to assess the robustness of FE002 primary chondroprogenitors in culture. The Brittberg medium was composed of DMEM–HAM's F12 (1:1) with 2 mM L-glutamine and 25 μg/mL ascorbic acid. Culture vessel incubation was performed in humidified incubators under 5% $CO_2$ at 37 °C, and the cell proliferation medium was exchanged twice weekly. Operator assessments were performed regularly and recorded. Secondly, quantitative proliferation assays were performed using various HPL concentrations with a 10% FBS control, and the corresponding growth curves were recorded.

#### 2.6.2. Allogeneic FE002 Cellular Active Substance Characterization: Multiplex Proteomic Analyses

Soluble protein quantification was performed for the cellular materials of interest using specific multiplex analyses (Eve Technologies, Calgary, AB, Canada). The analyses (Discovery Assays) comprised the human angiogenesis array and growth factor 17-plex array, the human cytokine/chemokine 65-plex panel, the human-soluble cytokine receptor 14-plex array, the human MMP (matrix metalloproteinases) and TIMP (tissue inhibitors of metalloproteinases) panel for cell cultures, the cytokine TGF-β (transforming growth factor-β) 3-plex array, and the HFNFS-04 array. Briefly, the samples were prepared using bulk FE002 primary chondroprogenitor lysate with $10^7$ cell equivalents/mL. The samples were centrifuged at 13,000 rpm at 4 °C for 5 min. The resulting supernatants were frozen and shipped on dry ice for proteomic analyses. Simultaneously, the total protein contents of the samples were determined using colorimetric BCA assay kits and following the manufacturer's instructions.

#### 2.6.3. Allogeneic FE002 Cellular Active Substance Qualification: β-Galactosidase Staining for In Vitro Senescence Assessment

An in vitro β-galactosidase assay (i.e., cellular senescence marker) was performed to confirm that FE002 primary chondroprogenitors did not yet reach senescence in culture at a passage level superior to that used in the allogeneic chondral grafts (i.e., passages 7–8). Briefly, FE002 primary chondroprogenitors were seeded in T25 cell culture flasks at $1.5 \times 10^3$ cells/cm$^2$ and expanded until they reached 70% confluency. Culture vessel incubation was performed in humidified incubators under 5% $CO_2$ at 37 °C, and the cell proliferation medium was exchanged twice weekly. The cells were then fixed for 5 min in 10 mL of fixation solution containing 1.85% formaldehyde with 0.2% glutaraldehyde. The cells were then rinsed twice using PBS. The cells were stained overnight at 37 °C with a SA-β-gal staining solution consisting of 0.1% X-gal, 5 mM potassium ferrocyanide, 5 mM potassium ferricyanide, 150 mM NaCl, and 2 mM $MgCl_2$ in a 40 mM citric acid/sodium phosphate solution at pH 6.0. The cells were washed twice with PBS and once with DMSO to remove the staining solution. The presence of β-galactosidase-positive (i.e., blue staining) cells was observed microscopically using 40× and 100× magnification. Random field acquisition was performed using the same microscopy setup, and the obtained images were used for β-galactosidase-positive cell operator enumeration.

#### 2.6.4. Allogeneic FE002 Cellular Active Substance Qualification: Telomerase Activity Quantification for In Vitro Tumorigenicity Assessment

An in vitro telomerase assay was performed using a qPCR telomerase activity quantification kit to confirm the non-tumorigenic potential of FE002 primary chondroprogenitors. Telomerase activity quantification was performed using frozen cellular dry pellets. HeLa and HCT-116 cancerous cell lines were used as positive controls. For sample preparation, cell lysis was performed using 20 μL of lysis buffer (supplemented with PMSF and β-mercaptoethanol) per $10^6$ cells before a 30 min incubation phase on ice. The samples were centrifuged at 12,000× *g* at 4 °C for 20 min. The supernatants were transferred to new Eppendorf tubes. For telomerase activity detection, 0.5 μL of sample, 4 μL of 5× telomerase reaction buffer, and 15.5 μL of nuclease-free water were mixed and incubated at 37 °C for 3 h. The reaction was quenched by heating the samples at 85 °C for 10 min. The samples were centrifuged at 1500× *g* for 10 s and stored on ice. The qPCR reactions were prepared in triplicate by mixing 1 μL of the prepared sample, 2 μL of primers, 10 μL of TaqGreen qPCR master mix, and 7 μL of nuclease-free water. The qPCR plates were sealed and centrifuged at 1500× *g* at ambient temperature for 15 s. The qPCR run conditions included an initial denaturation step of 10 min at 95 °C and 36 amplification cycles (i.e., denaturation over 20 s at 95 °C, annealing for over 20 s at 52 °C, and extension for over 45 s at 72 °C). Samples with a cycle threshold (Ct) > 33 were assessed as negative. The relative telomerase activity quantification between two samples was based on the $2^{-\Delta Ct}$ calculation method.

#### 2.6.5. Allogeneic FE002 Cellular Active Substance Qualification: Soft Agarose Colony Formation Assay for In Vitro Semi-Quantitative Tumorigenicity Assessment

A standard soft agarose cell colony formation assay (cell transformation assay) was used to assess the potential of FE002 primary chondroprogenitors to proliferate in non-adherent settings. The assays were performed in 24-well microplates. The solid agarose layer (i.e., the bottom layer) was composed of 0.6% agarose in PBS- and FBS-supplemented growth medium with 1% penicillin-streptomycin. The soft agarose layer (i.e., the top layer) was composed of 0.4% agarose and contained the investigated cellular materials (i.e., 125 viable cells/well to $10^4$ viable cells/well). Both agarose layers were sequentially prepared and of equal volumes. The tested cellular samples were FE002 primary chondroprogenitors that had been freshly harvested from confluent cultures. Positive control samples contained HeLa cancerous cells freshly harvested from confluent cultures. FBS-supplemented growth medium with 1% penicillin-streptomycin was added on top of the soft agarose layer, and the assay plates were incubated at 37 °C under 5% $CO_2$ in a humidified incubator for 21 days. The plates were regularly microscopically assessed, and representative imaging was performed to comparatively assess the formation of non-adherent cell colonies.

### 2.7. *Cytotherapeutic Finished Product Manufacturing Process: Chondrogenic Induction of Cell-Bearing Chondro-Gide Constructs*

Autologous and allogeneic cellular active substance lots were used to seed Chondro-Gide scaffolds, which were incubated under chemical chondrogenic induction (i.e., two weeks of incubation). Technical specificities characterized each protocol (e.g., cellular active substance, chondrogenic induction medium composition). Overall, most of the parameters and technical specifications of the autologous and allogeneic protocols were similar, and any specific variations or differences were analyzed according to quality, functional attributes, and risk viewpoints. While maximal finished product dimensions correspond to 20 $cm^2$ (i.e., 4 cm × 5 cm Chondro-Gide), smaller finished product units were experimentally investigated for sparing material use.

#### 2.7.1. Autologous Chondrocyte-Bearing Graft Manufacturing Process

Autologous chondrocytes were expanded in vitro before scaffold seeding. Chondro-Gide subunits with 1 cm × 1 cm dimensions were placed rough side up in 12-well plates and soaked with HPL for 1 h. Then, the seeding cell suspension (i.e., autologous cellular active substance in cell proliferation medium, passages 3–4, final cellular concentration of $2 \times 10^6$ cells/$cm^2$ scaffold) was homogeneously dispensed on the scaffold. The plates were incubated overnight at 37 °C under 5% $CO_2$ in a humidified incubator. Residual seeding cell suspension was used for cell recovery controls. Then, volumes of 1 mL of autologous chondrogenic medium (i.e., DMEM–HAM's F12 [1:1]; HPL 10%; L-glutamine; ascorbic acid 0.025 mg/mL; TGF-β1 10 ng/mL; ITS 1×; dexamethasone $10^{-7}$ M) were dispensed in each well, and the plates were incubated again. The cell-seeded scaffolds were maintained under chondrogenic induction for 16 ± 4 days, and medium exchanges were performed twice weekly. The constructs were finally rinsed thrice via immersion in warm PBS and were made available for further in vitro studies. The described processes were approved by the relevant health authorities in the framework of a clinical trial (i.e., NCT05651997).

#### 2.7.2. Allogeneic FE002 Chondroprogenitor-Bearing Graft Manufacturing Process

Cryopreserved FE002 primary chondroprogenitors were thawed and directly used for scaffold seeding. Chondro-Gide subunits (0.5–1 cm × 1 cm dimensions) were placed rough side up in 12-well plates, and the seeding cell suspension (i.e., allogeneic cellular active substance in cell proliferation medium, passage 6, final cellular concentration of $2 \times 10^6$ cells/$cm^2$ scaffold) was homogeneously dispensed on the scaffold. The plates were incubated overnight at 37 °C under 5% $CO_2$ in a humidified incubator. Residual seeding cell suspension was used for cell recovery controls. The cell-seeded constructs were covered with 1 mL of allogeneic chondrogenic medium (i.e., high-glucose DMEM; 2 mM L-glutamine; ITS 1×; 10 nM dexamethasone; 10 ng/mL TGF-β3; 82 µg/mL VitCp). The cell-seeded scaffolds were maintained under chondrogenic induction for 15–18 days, and medium exchanges were performed thrice weekly. Macroscopic evaluation of the constructs was regularly performed over the course of the chondrogenic incubation phase. The constructs were finally rinsed thrice via immersion in warm PBS and were made available for further in vitro studies. To investigate the impact of scaffold size on the manufacturing process and endpoint functional attributes of the allogeneic finished product, 5 $cm^2$ Chondro-Gide subunits were subsequently used for process validation.

### 2.8. *Cytotherapeutic Finished Product Controls: Functional Validation*

To comparatively assess the quality- and functionality-related attributes of the finished products (i.e., the autologous and allogeneic grafts), several in-process controls (IPC) and post-process controls (PPC) were performed. Specifically, cellular distribution throughout the constructs and cellular metabolic activity maintenance were assessed. Specific functionality parameters such as chondrogenic gene induction in 3D and ECM synthesis/deposition throughout the constructs were also assessed.

#### 2.8.1. MTT Staining for Assessing Metabolic Activity and Cell Distribution throughout the Constructs

An MTT assay was used to assess the endpoint cellular metabolic activity and cellular distribution throughout the Chondro-Gide scaffolds after incubation. Specifically, the MTT assay was used to confirm the adherence of the cells to the scaffold, the maintenance of cellular metabolic activity within the scaffold, and the quality of cellular colonization of the scaffold (i.e., the homogeneous repartition of the cells on the available surfaces). For endpoint analysis, the constructs were incubated at 37 °C for 2 h in a 5 mg/mL MTT solution. Following the rinsing of the constructs, photographic imaging was performed.

#### 2.8.2. Evaluation of Chondrogenic Gene Induction in the Constructs via RT-PCR

At various timepoints of the in vitro chondrogenic induction phase, the constructs were harvested and frozen at −80 °C for subsequent RNA extraction and gene expression analysis. The constructs were then mechanically disrupted in liquid nitrogen. The resulting powder was transferred to Eppendorf tubes containing TRIzol, and RNA extraction was performed according to the manufacturer's protocol. RNA purity and concentration were quantified via spectrophotometry. Reverse transcription into cDNA was performed using 1 μg of RNA in a final volume of 20 μL using a PrimeScript RT reagent kit according to the manufacturer's protocol. The reverse transcription cycle conditions were as follows: 37 °C for 15 min and 85 °C for 5 s. A real-time polymerase chain reaction (RT-PCR) was then performed in 96-well microplates. The reaction was performed using 1 μL of cDNA for a final volume of 20 μL using the KAPA SYBR Fast according to the manufacturer's protocol. Fluorescence was acquired using the following cycling conditions: 95 °C for 3 min (i.e., enzyme activation) and 40 amplification cycles (i.e., 95 °C for 3 s and annealing extension at 60 °C for 30 s). Each sample was run in triplicate, and the relative expression level for each gene was normalized to GAPDH. Gene expression levels (for *Sox9*, *COL2*, and *ACAN*) were quantified using the $2^{-\Delta\Delta Ct}$ calculation method, as described elsewhere [66].

#### 2.8.3. DMMB Quantification for Assessment of ECM Synthesis and Deposition throughout the Constructs

The quantification of total glycosaminoglycans (GAG) in the cell-seeded constructs was performed using a DMMB kit according to the manufacturer's protocol. Briefly, the constructs were harvested, washed once with PBS, weighed, and stored at −80 °C until further use. For the analysis, the samples were cut into small fragments with a scalpel. The fragments were transferred into Eppendorf tubes, and 1 mL of papain digestion buffer was added to each sample. Incubation was performed overnight at 65 °C for complete sample digestion, and the tubes were centrifuged at 10,000 rpm for 10 min. The supernatants were transferred into new Eppendorf tubes. Samples and analytical standard were diluted and mixed with 1 mL of dye reagent before incubation for 30 min at ambient temperature under gentle mechanical agitation. The samples were then centrifuged at 12,000 rpm for 10 min and carefully inverted to discard all the supernatant without disturbing the GAG pellet. Volumes of 0.5 mL of dissociation reagent were added on top of the pellets, and the samples were incubated for 10 min at ambient temperature with regular vortexing. Following the complete dissociation of the dye from the GAG pellet, the samples were centrifuged for 5 min at 12,000 rpm. Finally, volumes of 100 μL of standard or sample were transferred into 96-well microtitration plates, and the absorbance was determined at a wavelength of 656 nm. The relative GAG contents were determined with reference to the net weight of the constructs following harvest.

#### 2.8.4. Staining and Immunohistology for Specific ECM Component Visualization in the Constructs

At various timepoints of the in vitro chondrogenic induction phase, the constructs were harvested and fixed overnight at 4 °C in a 4% formalin solution, rinsed thrice with PBS, and transferred in 70% EtOH at 4 °C until inclusion in paraffin. After methyl methacrylate inclusion, thin 5-μm sections were cut and placed onto microscope slides, deparaffinized, and stained for over 30 min for specific ECM component visualization. The direct staining types were hematoxylin and eosin (H&E) and Alcian Blue (AB). Thereafter, the prepared immunohistology slides were processed using antibodies against specific ECM components, namely aggrecan (ACAN; Invitrogen primary antibody, N°AHP0022) and collagen I (COL1; Abcam antibody, N°ab138492). Following final revelation, the slides were microscopically assessed and imaged.

### *2.9. Translational Qualification of the Allogeneic Cytotherapeutic Finished Products*

In order to further qualify the allogeneic cytotherapeutic finished products from a translational viewpoint, several assays were performed to validate the product validity period and its physical applicability for surgical suturing.

#### 2.9.1. Qualification of Allogeneic Finished Product Transport Medium and Product Validity Period Validation

Following manufacture and before surgical implantation, the finished product must be harvested, conditioned, and transported from the production suite to the clinical center. The transport medium for the autologous finished product was specified as normal saline with 20% autologous human serum (AHS) for a validity period of 6 h post-manufacture. For the allogeneic finished product, several synthetic conditioning and transport media were assessed to avoid the use of AHS and the related blood draw/blood product processing steps. Allogeneic finished product stability was experimentally investigated at ambient temperature over a time-period of 6 h using a diversified readout panel (i.e., grading of quality and functionality attributes). Specifically, 3 distinct conditioning and transport media were evaluated. The allogeneic finished products were produced over a period of 15 days, as previously described. Following harvest and rinsing, the constructs were transferred into transport tubes containing either (i) normal saline, NaCl 0.9%, (ii) PBS with 0.25% sodium hyaluronate, molecular weight range 1.0–1.25 MDa, or (iii) Opti-MEM medium without phenol red. The control samples were maintained under incubation in chondrogenic medium, while the other samples were submitted to a standardized transport protocol of 45 min over 12 km, followed by static storage (i.e., total transport and storage time-period of 6 h; all phases performed at controlled ambient temperature). All samples were finally harvested and controlled via MTT staining, total GAG quantification, and immunohistology.

#### 2.9.2. Validation of Allogeneic Finished Product Implantability via Suture Testing

The Chondro-Gide scaffold (with or without cells) can be implanted using fibrin glue and/or sutures depending on the retained clinical protocol. To verify that the allogeneic finished product possessed the appropriate structural/physical attributes for suture-based surgical implantation in the knee (i.e., the maintenance of physical integrity upon transport, handling, and suturing), an endpoint suture test was performed. After a manufacturing period of 15 days, the finished product samples were submitted to the standardized transport and storage protocol. Then, a standard knot was tied in each sample using a Monosyn 6/0 suture kit, and a gentle mechanical challenge was applied to the finished products (i.e., simulation of finished product handling and surgical knot tightening). An endpoint MTT assay was performed before and after suturing, and imaging was performed.

### *2.10. Statistical Analysis and Data Presentation*

To statistically compare the average values from the two datasets, a paired Student's $t$-test was applied. The normality of data distribution was appropriately validated prior to the application of parametric tests. A $p$-value $< 0.05$ was used to determine statistical significance. Discrete data are presented using histograms and box-and-whisker plots, while continuous data are presented using broken-line graphs. Calculations and data presentation were carried out using Microsoft Excel, Microsoft PowerPoint (Microsoft Corporation, Redmond, WA, USA), and GraphPad Prism version 8.0.2 (GraphPad Software, San Diego, CA, USA).

## 3. Results

### *3.1. FE002 Primary Chondroprogenitors Possess Quality and Safety Attributes Compatible with Clinical Tissue Engineering*

Within existing clinical ACI applications, the use of HPL as a cell proliferation medium supplement has been implemented successfully following functional validation against the historically used FBS [66]. Therefore, our experimental results initially confirmed that 5% HPL could technically be used as an alternative to 10% FBS for the monolayer expansion of FE002 primary chondroprogenitors (Figures S1 and S2). However, based on the existing body of research on clinical-grade FE002 primary chondroprogenitors, the substitution of FBS by HPL has not yet been undertaken (mainly for stability reasons), and all further data presented herein were gathered with FBS-cultured cells.

From a quality point of view, the proteomic characterization of the allogeneic FE002 cellular active substance yielded some insights into the potential molecular contributions underlaying the intended therapeutic effects of the cells (Table S1). Specifically, cell therapies are postulated to partly act by means of paracrine effects, a concept which directed the analyses toward the soluble fraction of FE002 primary chondroprogenitor lysates. These were found to mainly contain (in relatively high abundance) MMPs/TIMPs, growth factors, and cytokines (Table S1). Notably, MMP-2, MMP-13, TIMP-1, and TIMP-2 were identified in concentrations > 30 ng/mg of total proteins (Table S1). MMPs/TIMPs are conjointly involved in the processes of ECM regulation, which is of high functional relevance in chondral defects [67]. The growth factor FGF-2 is known to stimulate chondrocyte or mesenchymal stem cell proliferation and plays a positive role in cartilage healing [67]. The growth factor HGF has been shown to induce in vitro rodent chondrocyte proliferation and ECM synthesis [68]. Another identified protein, sgp130, is a negative regulator of IL-6, with the latter being involved in cartilage degradation (Table S1). Similarly, sTNFRI and IL-1Ra are negative inhibitors of TNF and IL-1 signaling (i.e., they are proinflammatory, negatively impacting cartilage), respectively. Overall, FE002 primary chondroprogenitors were found to contain potentially useful proteinic components for orthopedic cytotherapeutic applications (Table S1).

From an efficacy point of view, it was firstly confirmed that FE002 primary chondroprogenitors could not yet reach senescence at passage levels equal or superior to that of the cellular active substance lots (i.e., the maintenance of physiological activity at passages 7–8, Figure S3). Furthermore, from a preliminary safety viewpoint, the small amounts of isolated senescent cells (i.e., 1.5–3.0% of total cells) that were recorded confirmed that FE002 primary chondroprogenitors are not immortal and therefore present low potential for uncontrolled and indefinite proliferation (Figure S3). Secondly, specific in vitro safety characterization of the allogeneic cellular active substance was performed to complement and support existing in vivo safety data. In the soft agarose assay, significant non-adherent colonies of HeLa cells were rapidly observed, and they continued to grow over the 21-day incubation phase (Figure S4). Conversely, no anchorage-independent cellular proliferation or tumoral growth-like activity was recorded for the FE002 progenitor cell group (Figure S4). In the telomerase activity assay, the FE002 cells (i.e., clinically usable passage levels) were found to possess low telomerase activities (i.e., at the lower limit of detection of the test) that were comparable in value to those of seven patient primary HAC cell types (i.e., previously safely clinically used for ACI, Figure S5). Conversely, both positive controls (i.e., HeLa and HCT-116 cancerous cells) were found to possess high telomerase activity (as expected), thereby confirming the validity of the experimental setup (Figure S5). Overall, no safety-related concerns were evidenced in vitro for the FE002 primary chondroprogenitors (congruent with and complementary to existing safety data, including a large animal GLP study), further confirming their applicability in subsequent translational applications.

### 3.2. FE002 Primary Chondroprogenitors Possess Quality and Functionality Attributes Compatible with the Controlled GMP Manufacturing of Chondrogenic Cellular Active Substances

Based on the existing research on clinical-grade primary HAC cell type establishment and GMP manufacturing, the stability of the FE002 primary chondroprogenitors was firstly assessed following 3 years of cryostorage. Following parallel in vitro initiation with primary HACs, it was confirmed that the FE002 cells possessed appropriate key and critical quality attributes (e.g., adherence, morphology, proliferation) in recovery cultures after storage (Figure S6). Based on this validation of the cryopreservation phase, a parametrically defined and controlled manufacturing process was devised for the chondrogenic cellular active substances (designed to be applicable to both autologous HACs and allogeneic FE002 primary chondroprogenitors, Figure 1).

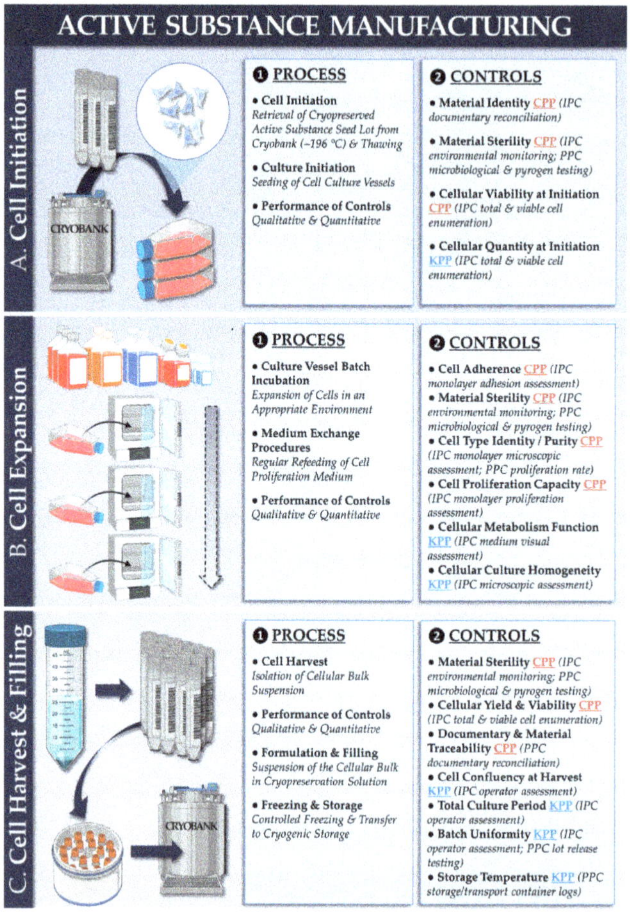


**Figure 1.** Schematic presentation of the manufacturing and control processes for the autologous or allogeneic chondrogenic cellular active substances. The process describes a primary cell amplification and cryopreservation cycle, starting with master cell bank (MCB) or working cell bank (WCB) vials of HACs or FE002 primary chondroprogenitors. (**A**) Cellular seeding material initiation from cryopreservation with rapid thawing and culture vessel seeding. (**B**) In vitro cellular expansion in monolayers for cellular active substance lot manufacture. (**C**) Cellular bulk harvest and cellular active substance lot processing for cryopreservation. CPP, critical process parameter; HAC, human articular chondrocytes; IPC, in-process control; KPP, key process parameter; MCB, master cell bank; PPC, post-process control; WCB, working cell bank.

The corresponding quality attributes (i.e., active substance) are presented in Table S2. From a technical standpoint, the most significant difference between the autologous and allogeneic workflows is the possibility to serially manufacture extensive allogeneic cell lots, contrasting with patient-specific autologous HAC manufacturing campaigns. Regarding finished product manufacturing, a second parametrically defined and controlled manufacturing process was devised (designed to be applicable to autologous and allogeneic protocols) based on the approved autologous protocol (Figure 2).

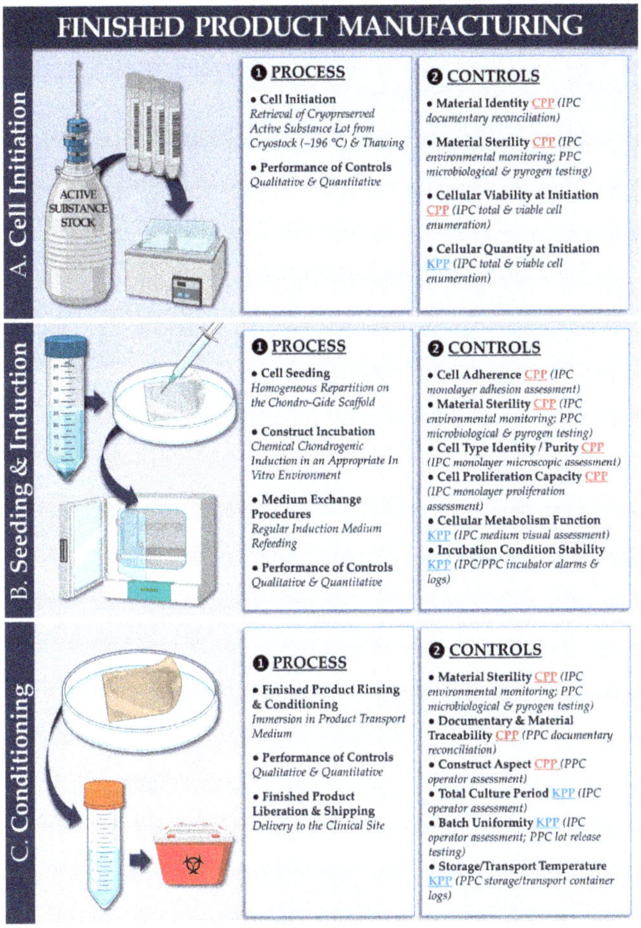


**Figure 2.** Schematic presentation of the manufacturing and control processes for the allogeneic finished cytotherapeutic product (i.e., Chondro-Gide scaffolds bearing FE002 primary chondroprogenitors). The process describes cellular active substance lot initiation, scaffold seeding and chondrogenic induction, and finished product conditioning for transport. (**A**) Cellular active substance initiation from cryopreservation with rapid thawing. It is important to note that, in the autologous protocol, an additional in vitro HAC monolayer expansion phase is carried out at this point. (**B**) Seeding of the cellular active substance on the Chondro-Gide scaffold and incubation of the constructs under chemical chondrogenic induction. (**C**) Endpoint harvest of the finished cytotherapeutic product lot and conditioning for transport to the clinical site. CPP, critical process parameter; HAC, human articular chondrocytes; IPC, in-process control; KPP, key process parameter; PPC, post-process control.

The corresponding quality attributes (i.e., finished products) are presented in Table S3. Illustrative experimental records from the autologous and allogeneic finished product manufacturing campaigns are presented in Figure S7a,b (i.e., upscaling studies using 5 cm$^2$ Chondro-Gide subunits), respectively. For simplified manufacturing process benchmarking (i.e., autologous versus allogeneic protocol), a list of the production process parameters (i.e., cellular active substance and finished product manufacturing) is presented in Table 1.

**Table 1.** Parametric benchmarking of the manufacturing processes for the autologous and the allogeneic protocols. Manufacturing process technical benchmarking may highlight the specific points that require additional data and specific risk analyses for the allogeneic protocol based on a gap analysis and using the approved autologous protocol as a baseline. AHS, autologous human serum; DMEM, Dulbecco's modified Eagle medium; ECM, extracellular matrix; FBS, fetal bovine serum; HAC, human articular chondrocytes; HPL, human platelet lysate; NA, non-applicable.

| Parameter/Specification | | Autologous Protocol | Allogeneic Protocol | Purpose/Targets | Resource Requirements [1] (Allogeneic vs. Autologous) |
|---|---|---|---|---|---|
| Regulatory Status of the Protocol for Clinical Investigational Use | | Approved [2] (Swissmedic) | Pending Submission | NA | Increased |
| 1. Cellular Active Substance | Cellular Active Substance Proliferation Medium | DMEM–Ham's F12; L-glutamine; HPL 10% | DMEM; L-glutamine; FBS 10% | Obtention of $\geq 40 \times 10^6$ cells for a cellular active substance lot | Decreased |
| | Cellular Active Substance Lot Cryopreservation | Yes; Liquid nitrogen | Yes; liquid nitrogen | Maintenance of appropriate biological functionalities | Conserved |
| | Cellular Active Substance Lot Processing for Scaffold Seeding | HACs expanded once in 2D before scaffold seeding | FE002 primary chondroprogenitors directly seeded after initiation | Use of cellular active substance materials with optimal quality and functionality attributes | Decreased |
| 2. Finished Cytotherapeutic Product | Matrix/Scaffold | Chondro-Gide $\leq 20$ cm$^2$ | Chondro-Gide $\leq 20$ cm$^2$ | Use of cyto-/bio-compatible scaffold of appropriate dimensions with appropriate functionalities | Conserved |
| | Cell Seeding Density on the Scaffold | $[2 \pm 0.5] \times 10^6$ cells/cm$^2$ | $[2 \pm 0.5] \times 10^6$ cells/cm$^2$ | Obtention of homogeneous scaffold cell seeding | Conserved |
| | Chondrogenic Induction Medium Composition | DMEM–Ham's F12; HPL 10%; L-glutamine; ascorbic acid 0.025 mg/mL; TGF-β1 10 ng/mL; Insulin 10 µg/mL; dexamethasone 100 nM | DMEM; L-glutamine; ITS; TGF-β3 10 ng/mL; VitCp 82 µg/mL; dexamethasone 10 nM | Induction of chondrogenic genes and ECM deposition by viable cells | Conserved |
| | Chondrogenic Induction Time-Period | $16 \pm 4$ days | $14 \pm 2$ days | Induction of chondrogenic genes and ECM deposition by viable cells | Decreased |
| | Transport Medium Composition | NaCl 0.9%; AHS 20% | NaCl 0.9% | Maintenance of appropriate physical and biological functionalities | Decreased |
| | Finished Product Validity Period | 6 h after end of manufacture | 6 h after end of manufacture | Maintenance of appropriate physical and biological functionalities | Conserved |

[1] Combination of global financial, regulatory, material, and scientific resources. [2] NCT05651997 clinical trial, Lausanne and Fribourg, Switzerland.

An illustrated workflow describing the temporal constraints and the risks associated with the autologous and/or the allogeneic protocol is presented in Figure S8. Generally, the two processes were considered to be technically overlapping. The main differences in the allogeneic process were the use of FBS instead of HPL for cell expansions, the direct use of cryopreserved cellular active substance for Chondro-Gide seeding, and the tailoring of the chondrogenic induction medium for optimal ECM deposition (Table 1).

### 3.3. FE002 Primary Chondroprogenitors Possess Functional Attributes Comparable to Those of Clinical-grade HACs within Chondrogenically Induced Chondro-Gide Constructs

To maximize the therapeutic potential of the intervention, the presence of viable and functional cells at the time of construct implantation in the knee is required. Endpoint MTT assays were performed on the autologous and allogeneic finished products, initially confirming that the cells homogeneously colonized the Chondro-Gide scaffolds and retained significant metabolic activity (Figure S7(aE,bF2)). Furthermore, the cells colonized one of the two scaffold layers (i.e., rough side), as expected (Figure S7b).

Regarding specific chondrogenic function in the constructs, the cultured cells must be able to readopt a chondrogenic phenotype after monolayer expansion (i.e., where transient de-differentiation occurs). The results of finished product functional characterization at the gene expression level showed that, during the in vitro 3D chondrogenic induction phase, specific genes of interest were induced in HACs and in FE002 primary chondroprogenitors (Figure 3).

Specifically, previous internal research showed that HAC chondrogenic genes (*COL2*, *ACAN*, *Sox9*) were induced following the chemical induction of 3D cell pellets [66]. In the present study, our results showed that similar functions could be obtained upon placing HACs within two types of implantable sheet scaffolds, with highly significant chondrogenic gene induction taking place at the 16-day timepoint (Figure 3A). As the Chondro-Gide scaffold was already clinically implemented for the second-generation ACI protocol (i.e., NCT04296487) and retained for the MACT protocol (i.e., NCT05651997), it was used for the functional qualification of the FE002 primary chondroprogenitors as well (Figure 3B). Notably, regarding the allogeneic cell group, *Sox9* expression was constitutively high and was not significantly ($p$-value = 0.296) induced following the construct incubation phase (Figure 3(B3)). However, extremely potent *COL2* and *ACAN* induction were recorded in the FE002 groups, with endpoint values over 10× higher than those of the autologous HAC-based constructs (Figure 3(B1,B2)). Overall, it was shown that the autologous and allogeneic cells were capable of re-expressing specific chondrogenic genes following appropriate chemical induction in 3D, with quantitative advantages favoring the allogeneic FE002 cells (Figure 3). Additionally, it was shown that a two-week chondrogenic induction period resulted in the exponential induction of *COL2* and *ACAN* genes and that, from a functional standpoint, a two-week chondrogenic induction period is preferrable over a 7-day induction period (Figure 3).

To validate the functional advantages generated by the chondrogenic induction phase and measured via gene expression analysis, finished product functional characterization was performed at the protein level, focusing on ECM components. A DMMB assay for total GAG quantification was employed in various experimental setups (Figure 4).

In the allogeneic FE002 cell group, a time-course of GAG deposition in the Chondro-Gide scaffold showed a significant ($p$-value < 0.05) increase between the 7-day and 14-day timepoints but no further rise at the 21-day timepoint (Figure 4A). Such results were congruent with the data gathered at the gene expression level and validated the chondrogenic induction phase duration of approximatively two weeks (Figure 3). Then, the DMMB assay was used to assess the interpatient variability in endpoint total GAG contents within the autologous finished product (Figure 4B). Furthermore, mean endpoint total GAG contents were compared between the autologous and allogeneic groups, wherein the FE002 cells were found to deposit much more ECM throughout the constructs than the HACs (Figure 4C).

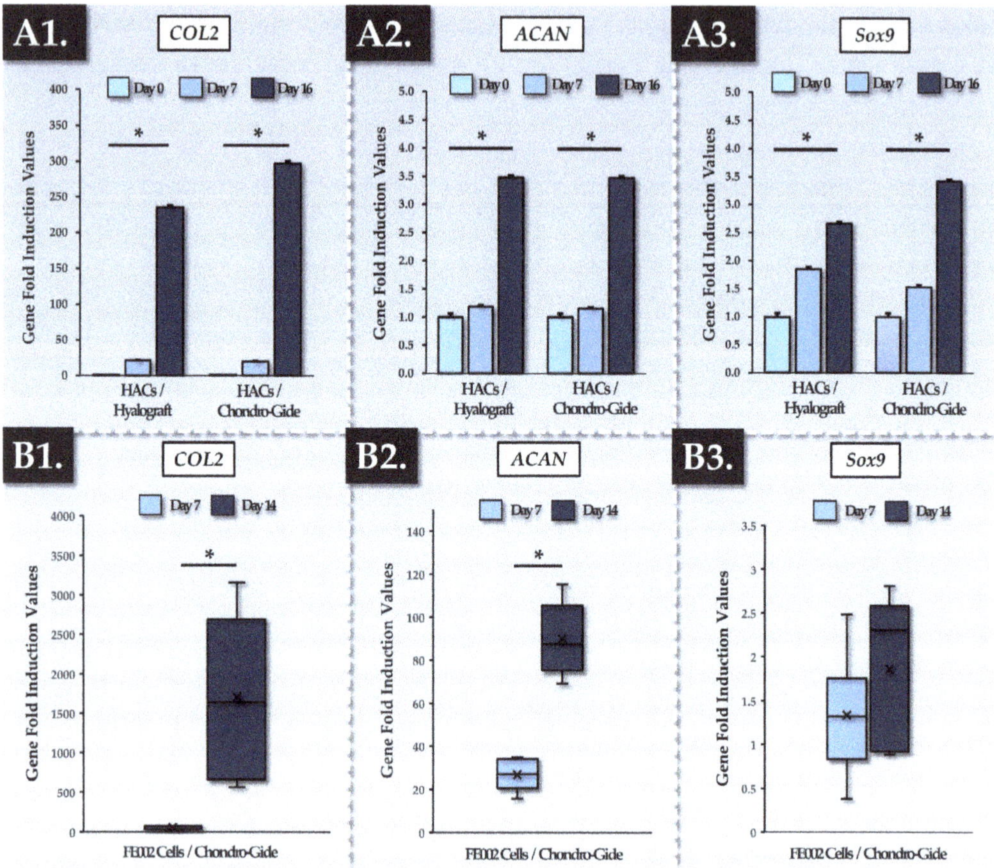


**Figure 3.** Functional characterization of the autologous and allogeneic finished products, as assessed according to their evolutive chondrogenic gene expression levels during construct incubation. (**A1–A3**) Relative chondrogenic gene (i.e., *COL2*, *ACAN*, *Sox9*) fold induction values at various timepoints of autologous finished product incubation (assessed for Hyalograft and Chondro-Gide scaffolds, respectively). Both scaffolds were assessed as being functionally equivalent, and endpoint chondrogenic gene expression was highly significantly increased compared to the baseline in all groups ($p$-values < 0.01). (**B1–B3**) Relative chondrogenic gene (i.e., *COL2*, *ACAN*, *Sox9*) fold induction values at various timepoints of allogeneic finished product incubation (assessed for Chondro-Gide scaffolds). Endpoint chondrogenic gene expression was highly significantly increased for *COL2* ($p$-value < 0.01) and *ACAN* ($p$-value < 0.0001). Furthermore, endpoint chondrogenic gene expression was significantly higher in value for *COL2* and *ACAN* ($p$-values < 0.01) compared to the respective endpoint induction levels of the same genes in the autologous finished products (i.e., the Chondro-Gide groups). Experimental replicates ($n \geq 3$) and repetitions were used for the assays. Statistically significant differences are marked by an asterisk (i.e., "*"). ACAN, aggrecan; COL, collagen.

For a qualitatively enhanced investigation of the ECM deposition activities in the Chondro-Gide constructs by HACs and FE002 primary chondroprogenitors, several histology assays were performed. Firstly, endpoint cellular localization and ECM organization were visualized in the autologous constructs, showing appropriate structural and composition attributes (Figure 5).

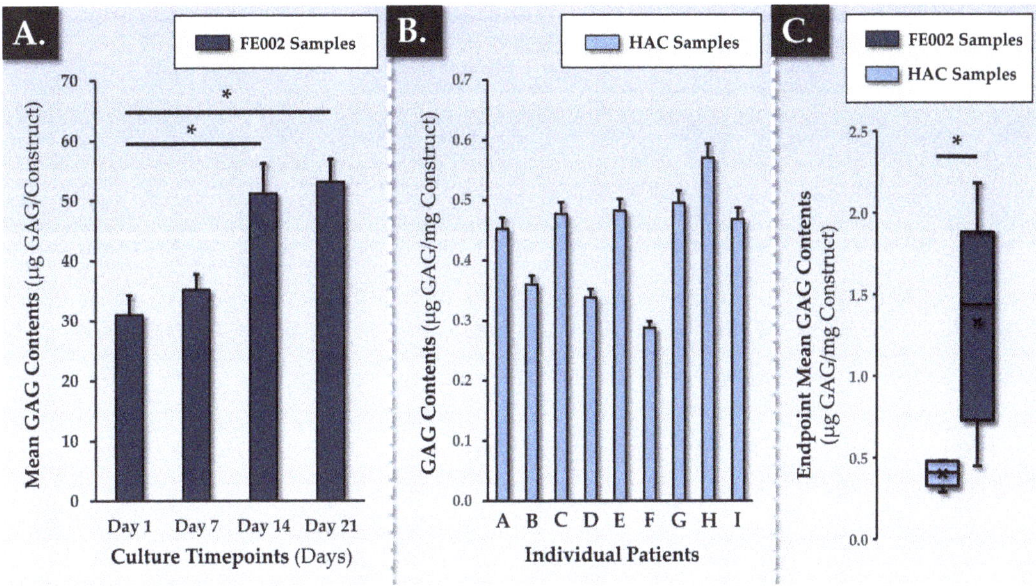


**Figure 4.** Functional characterization of the autologous and allogeneic finished products, as assessed via total GAG quantification within the constructs. (**A**) Increase in GAG contents over time within constructs bearing allogeneic FE002 primary chondroprogenitors. Experimental replicates ($n \geq 6$) and repetitions were used for the assay. Statistically significant differences ($p$-values < 0.05) are marked by an asterisk (i.e., "*"). (**B**) Interpatient variability in terms of endpoint GAG contents within freshly harvested autologous constructs. Experimental replicates ($n \geq 3$) from nine different donors were used for the assay. (**C**) Comparison of endpoint GAG contents between constructs bearing HACs (i.e., 16 days of induction) and constructs bearing FE002 primary chondroprogenitors (i.e., 14 days of induction). Experimental replicates ($n \geq 6$) and repetitions were used for the assay. Statistically significant differences ($p$-value < 0.05) are marked by an asterisk (i.e., "*"). GAG, glycosaminoglycan; HAC, human articular chondrocytes.

As expected, cellular presence and ECM deposition were concentrated within one layer of the scaffold (the rough side; Figure 5). Furthermore, cellular morphology was observed to be rounded, and the cells were embedded in the lacunae (Figure 5(A3,B3)). Regarding the allogeneic grafts, progressive ECM deposition was observed in a time-course immunohistology setup (Figure 6). Therein, the experimental results were congruent with the gene expression and GAG quantification readouts, showing a strong increase in ECM deposition between the 7-day and the 14-day timepoints (Figure 6). Furthermore, no significant increase in ECM content was evidenced at the 21-day timepoint, and the homogeneity in the aggrecan deposition was lower than that at the 14-day timepoint (Figure 6).

Subjecting the allogeneic grafts to multiparametric endpoint histological evaluation enabled us to confirm that appropriate structural and qualitative attributes were obtained and were comparable to those of the autologous grafts following two weeks of chondrogenic induction (Figures 5 and 7).

The various control parameters, methods, and acceptance criteria used for the parallel functional qualification of the autologous and allogeneic constructs are presented in Table 2, along with the corresponding experimental assessments.

A summary of the various relevant finished product attributes (classified by control parameter type) is presented in Table 3.

**Table 2.** Control parameters for the autologous and allogeneic finished products (i.e., in-process indirect assessments and endpoint direct assessments). AB, Alcian Blue; ACAN, aggrecan; C, conforming; COL 2, collagen II; DMMB, dimethylmethylene blue; ECM, extracellular matrix; GAG, glycosaminoglycan; h, hours; HE, hematoxylin and eosin; MTT, 3-(4,5-dimethylthiazol-2-yl)-2,5-diphenyltetrazolium bromide; NC, non-conforming; PBS, phosphate-buffered saline; RT-PCR, real-time polymerase chain reaction.

| Control/Assessment Type | Control Parameters | Control Methods | Targets/Acceptance Criteria | Autologous Protocol Assessment | | Allogeneic Protocol Assessment | |
|---|---|---|---|---|---|---|---|
| | | | | C | NC | C | NC |
| 1. Endpoint Direct Assessment [1] of Finished Product Lot | Chondrogenic Gene Induction in 3D | RT-PCR | Induction of *COL2* and *ACAN* | ✓ | - | ✓ | - |
| | Cartilage GAG Presence (Total) in 3D | DMMB | Cartilage GAG presence ≥ 0.25 µg/mg | ✓ | - | ✓ | - |
| | Cartilage ECM Presence (Histology) in 3D | HE | Presence of staining | ✓ | - | ✓ | - |
| | | ACAN | Presence of staining | ✓ | - | ✓ | - |
| | | AB | Presence of staining | ✓ | - | ✓ | - |
| | Cellular Viability in 3D | MTT | Presence of MTT signal | ✓ | - | ✓ | - |
| | Homogeneity of Cell Presence Across the Construct | MTT signal homogeneity; Histology | Homogeneous staining of the whole surface of the construct | ✓ | - | ✓ | - |
| | Cells and Synthetized ECM Localized in 1 Layer of the Construct | MTT; Histology | Presence of cells and ECM in one layer of the construct (absent from the other layer) | ✓ | - | ✓ | - |
| | Cells Localized in Lacunae | Histology | Presence of cells in the lacunae | ✓ | - | ✓ | - |
| | Cellular Morphology | Histology | Rounded cellular morphology | ✓ | - | ✓ | - |
| | Homogeneous ECM Presence Across the Construct | Histology | Homogeneous presence of ECM across the construct | ✓ | - | ✓ | - |
| | Significant ECM Deposition Within the Construct | Histology | Significant ECM deposition in one layer of the construct | ✓ | - | ✓ | - |
| 2. In-Process Indirect Assessment [2] of Finished Product Lot | Cell Viability in Monolayer Control Cultures | Cell enumeration; Operator assessment | Cellular viability ≥ 75% before control plate seeding; limited amounts of floating dead cells; induction medium consumption | ✓ | - | ✓ | - |
| | Cellular Adhesion in Monolayer Control Cultures | Operator assessment | Presence of ≥60% adherent cells 24 h after seeding; absence of significant cellular detachment | ✓ | - | ✓ | - |

**Table 2.** *Cont.*

| Control/Assessment Type | Control Parameters | Control Methods | Targets/Acceptance Criteria | Autologous Protocol Assessment | | Allogeneic Protocol Assessment | |
|---|---|---|---|---|---|---|---|
| | | | | C | NC | C | NC |
| 2. In-Process Indirect Assessment [2] of Finished Product Lot | Cellular Proliferation in Monolayer Control Cultures | Operator assessment | Appropriate proliferative cellular morphology adoption, proliferation rate, and proliferation homogeneity in monolayer | ✓ | - | ✓ | - |
| | Cellular Population Purity in Monolayer Control Cultures | Operator assessment | Absence of observable cell sub-population presence | ✓ | - | ✓ | - |

[1] Destructive control process performed directly on the finished product, requires dedicated replicate production.
[2] Non-destructive control process performed on cell recovery control cultures or on manufacturing process retention samples.

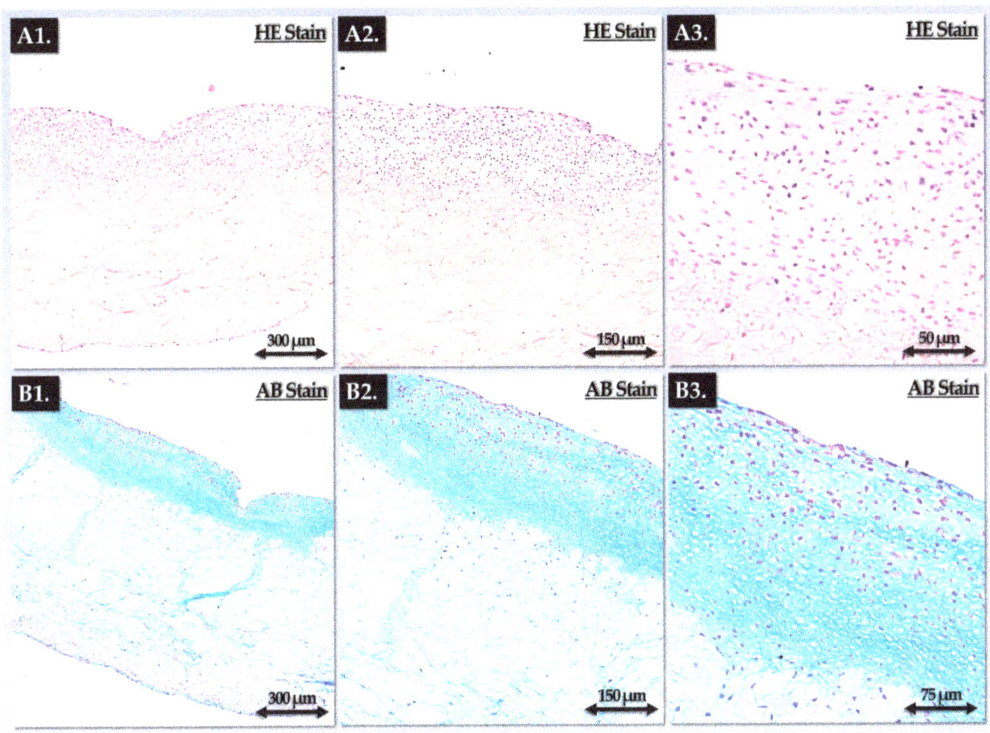


**Figure 5.** Endpoint functional characterization of the autologous finished product (as assessed by immunohistology for constructs bearing HACs). (**A1–A3**) Sections of a construct following HE staining. (**B1–B3**) Sections of a construct following AB staining. The results showed the zone-specific localization of the HACs (i.e., rounded cells within lacunae) and the deposited ECM (i.e., one defined construct zone), as expected. AB, Alcian Blue; ECM, extracellular matrix; HAC, human articular chondrocytes; HE, hematoxylin and eosin.

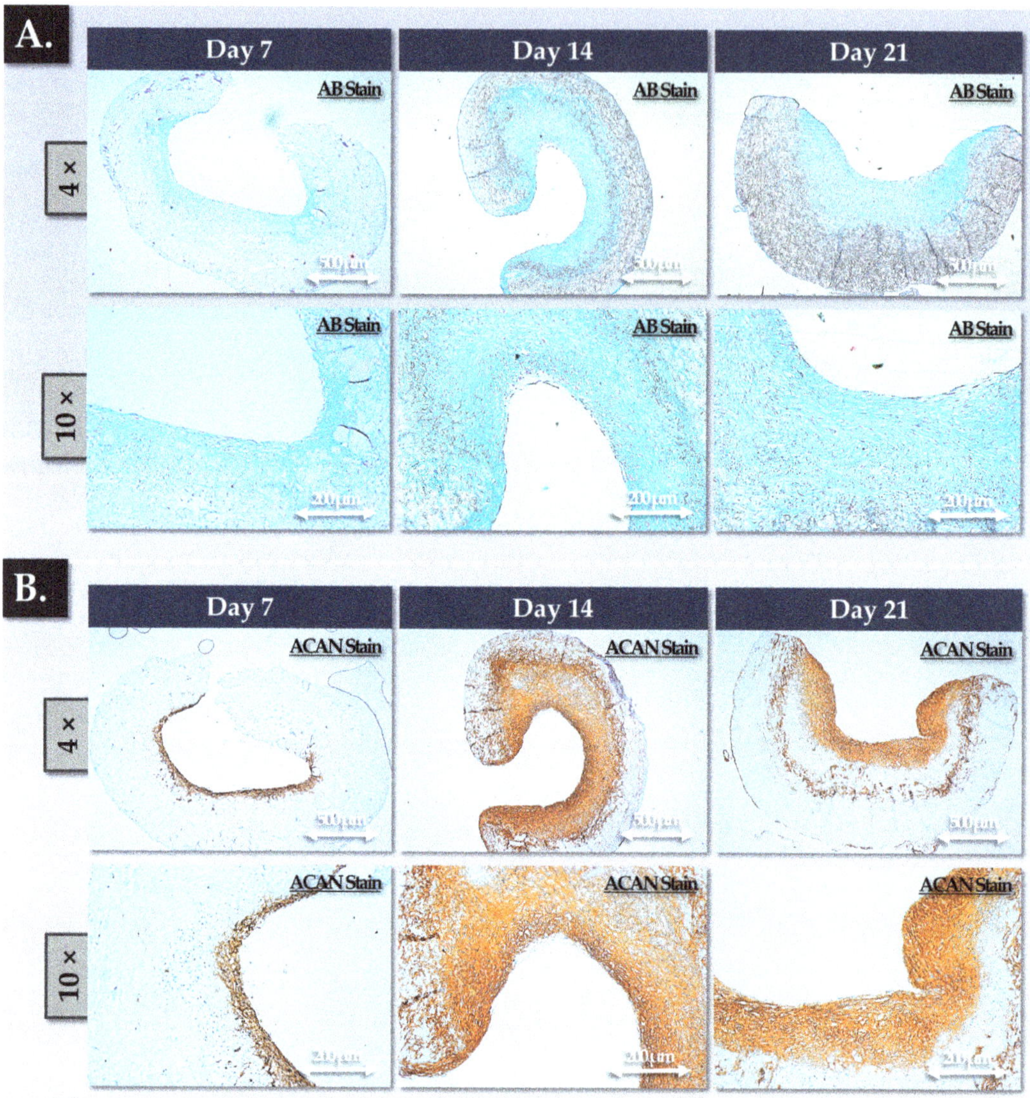


**Figure 6.** Functional characterization (time-course) of the allogeneic finished product, as assessed via immunohistology for constructs bearing FE002 primary chondroprogenitors. (**A**) Construct sections at various timepoints of the incubation phase following AB staining. (**B**) Construct sections at various timepoints of the incubation phase following ACAN staining. Overall, the results showed that significant ECM deposition occurred between days 7 and 14 of the construct incubation phase. AB, Alcian blue; ACAN, aggrecan; ECM, extracellular matrix.

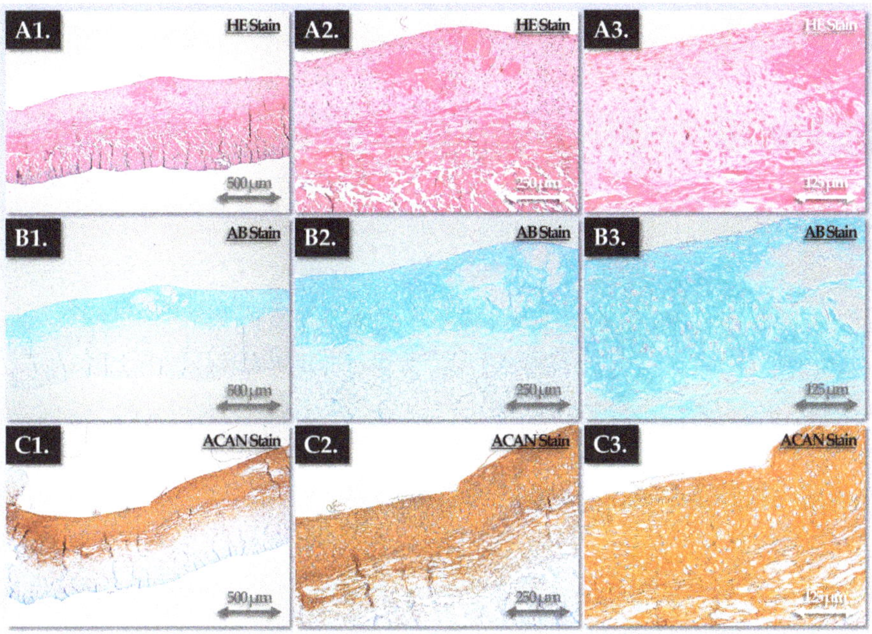


**Figure 7.** Endpoint characterization of the allogeneic finished products (as assessed via immunohistology for constructs bearing FE002 primary chondroprogenitors). In addition to significant ECM deposition in one layer of the constructs, the cells were observed to be rounded and localized in the lacunae, as expected. (**A1–A3**) Hematoxylin and eosin staining. (**B1–B3**) Alcian Blue staining. (**C1–C3**) Aggrecan staining. AB, Alcian Blue; ACAN, aggrecan; ECM, extracellular matrix; HE, hematoxylin and eosin.

**Table 3.** Autologous and allogeneic finished product attributes used for the parametric description and multi-phasic control of the in vitro manufacturing process. CQA, critical quality attribute; ECM, extracellular matrix; IPC, in-process control; PPC, post-process control.

| Parameter Type | Control Parameters | IPC [1] | PPC [2] | Process Development /Validation [3] | Release Criterion |
|---|---|---|---|---|---|
| 1. Quality | Cell viability (monolayer recovery) | ✓ | - | ✓ | ✓ |
| | Cell viability (3D) | - | ✓ | ✓ | ✓ |
| | Cell proliferation rate (monolayer recovery) | ✓ | - | ✓ | ✓ |
| | Endpoint cell yield (monolayer recovery) | ✓ | - | ✓ | - |
| | Cell morphology (3D) | - | ✓ | ✓ | - |
| | Localization of cells in the lacunae | - | ✓ | ✓ | - |
| 2. Purity | Microscopic cell morphology assessment (monolayer recovery) | ✓ | - | ✓ | ✓ |
| | Cell proliferation rate (monolayer recovery) | ✓ | - | ✓ | ✓ |
| 3. Efficacy | Cell viability (3D) | - | ✓ | ✓ | ✓ |
| | Chondrogenic gene induction (3D) | - | ✓ | ✓ | - |
| | Cartilage-specific ECM synthesis and deposition in 3D | - | ✓ | ✓ | - |
| | Macroscopic change in construct color and rigidity | ✓ | ✓ | ✓ | ✓ |

**Table 3.** *Cont.*

| Parameter Type | Control Parameters | IPC [1] | PPC [2] | Process Development /Validation [3] | Release Criterion |
|---|---|---|---|---|---|
| 4. Safety | In vitro and in vivo tumorigenicity assessment; telomerase activity quantification; cell type senescence assessment; karyotyping; literature review | - | - | ✓ | - |
| | Microbiological safety (manufacturing system) | ✓ | ✓ | ✓ | ✓ |
| | Microbiological safety (raw/starting materials, retention samples) | ✓ | ✓ | ✓ | ✓ |
| | Microbiological safety (finished product lot) | - | ✓ | ✓ | ✓ |
| 5. Stability | Finished product CQA maintenance after storage | - | ✓ | ✓ | - |
| | Finished product CQA maintenance after transport | - | ✓ | ✓ | - |

[1] Performed on cell recovery control cultures or on manufacturing process retention samples. [2] Performed on the finished product or on manufacturing process retention samples. [3] These activities are characterized by the enhanced scope and granularity of their technical validation compared to the routine finished product release criteria.

Specifically, each control parameter subtype was identified with respect to its use in the finished product manufacturing process itself (i.e., IPC vs. PPC), in its development/validation, and in its implementation (i.e., release criterion, Table 3). Overall, the gathered experimental data confirmed that the produced allogeneic grafts were qualitatively non-inferior or functionally superior to the autologous grafts, with the latter being approved for clinical investigational use (i.e., NCT05651997). Multi-parametric functional data confirmed and validated that a two-week chondrogenic induction period was most appropriate for the considered finished products (Figures 3–7). Furthermore, no differences were observed between the 1 $cm^2$ and 5 $cm^2$ allogeneic constructs in terms of endpoint functional attributes, confirming that the described manufacturing protocol is readily upscalable (Figure S7).

### *3.4. Allogeneic Finished Products Possess an Appropriate Pharmaceutical Form and Stability Attributes for Clinical Orthopedic Bioengineering*

In order to confirm that the allogeneic finished products maintained appropriate quality and functionality attributes at least up until surgical implantation in the knee, specific validation studies were performed. Firstly, it was confirmed that ambient temperature storage and transport for a total time-period of 6 h did not significantly impact cellular colonization and viability nor the total GAG contents of the constructs (Figure 8).

Similar results were obtained for the three types of tested transport media (Figure 8). At the end of the manufacturing phase and following transport/storage, the constructs were evaluated via macroscopic assessment, cell viability assessment, total GAG quantification, and histology for three different transport media (Table 4).

While the GAG contents were found to be 25% lower on average in the NaCl group compared to the control group, no statistically significant difference was found ($p$-value = 0.370, Figure 8C). Macroscopically, no inexplicable or unusual changes in construct physical attributes were noted after harvest (Figure 8A). Structurally, no significant modifications were evidenced between the groups via our histological analyses (Table 4). Secondly, it was shown that the constructs could be handled and sutured using standard surgical threads (Figure S9). Specifically, it was shown that construct handling, suturing, and gentle mechanical challenging did not result in the disturbance of the biological materials present on the samples (Figure 8B, top row). Overall, it was experimentally confirmed that the retained manufacturing process and technical specifications enable the production of clinically usable allogeneic grafts of appropriate quality for orthopedic implantation.

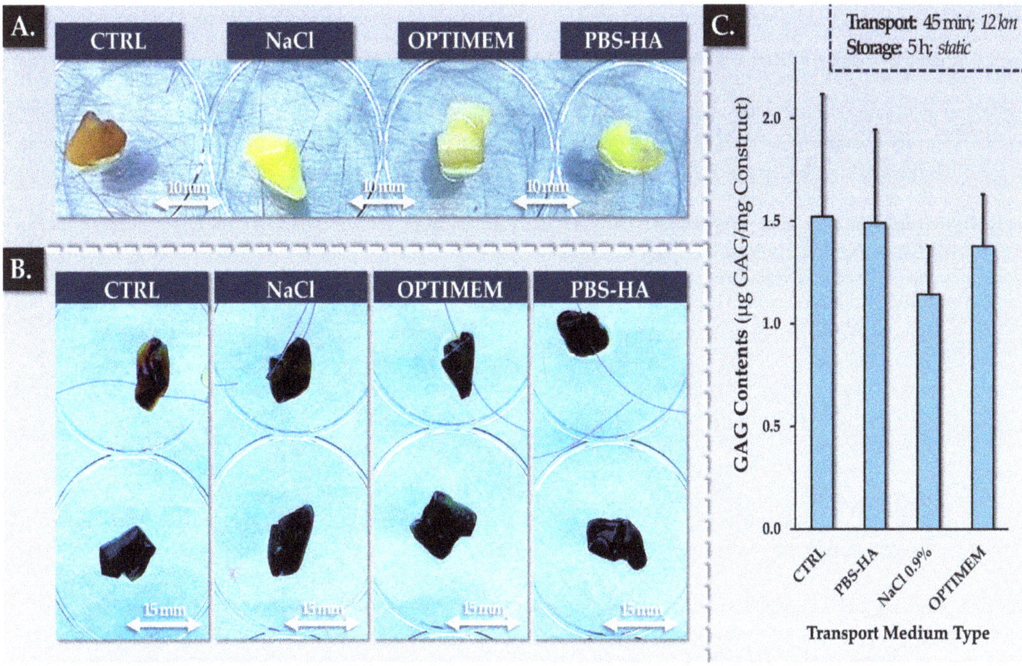


**Figure 8.** Validation results for allogeneic finished product transport medium and construct suturability. (**A**) Freshly harvested finished products before conditioning for transport/storage. Experimental replicates (n = 3) were used for the assay. (**B**) MTT-stained finished products after the application of the standardized transport protocol. Constructs presented in the top row were additionally submitted to the suture test before MTT staining. Experimental replicates (n = 3) were used for the assay. (**C**) Impact of the transport protocol on the total GAG contents of the constructs. Experimental replicates (n = 6) were used for the assay. CTRL, control; HA, hyaluronic acid; PBS, phosphate-buffered saline.

**Table 4.** Parametric grading table of allogeneic finished products after 6 h of transport and storage. AB, Alcian Blue; ACAN, aggrecan; DMMB, dimethylmethylene blue; GAG, glycosaminoglycan; HA, hyaluronic acid; HE, hematoxylin and eosin; MTT, 3-(4,5-dimethylthiazol-2-yl)-2,5-diphenyltetrazolium bromide; NaCl, sodium chloride; PBS, phosphate-buffered saline.

| Parameter | Controls | Targets/Acceptance Criteria | Endpoint Construct Grading [1] | | |
|---|---|---|---|---|---|
| | | | NaCl | OPTIMEM | HA-PBS |
| Cellular Viability | MTT | Presence of viable cells on the constructs | +++ | +++ | +++ |
| Cellular Repartition | MTT/HE | Homogeneous viable cell repartition on one side of the scaffold | +++ | +++ | +++ |
| Construct Morphology | Operator Assessment | Specific macroscopic change in construct color and rigidity | +++ | +++ | +++ |
| GAG Content | DMMB | Maintenance of total GAG contents | ++ | +++ | +++ |
| Aggrecan Presence | Histology | Maintenance of positive ACAN staining on one side of the construct | +++ | +++ | +++ |
| Alcian Blue Staining | Histology | Maintenance of positive AB staining on one side of the construct | +++ | +++ | +++ |

[1] Semi-quantitative grading was performed using the abbreviated nomenclature presented hereafter. (++) = satisfactory; (+++) = optimal.

## 4. Discussion

### *4.1. Progressive Translational Development of Cell Therapies for Cartilage Repair/Regeneration: Extensive Manufacturing Experience and Long-Term Clinical Research on ACI*

Cartilage-oriented regenerative strategies are currently far from being fully satisfactory, and the search for effective disease-modifying interventions is ongoing [69–71]. In order to meet increasing clinical needs, important translational efforts are being allocated toward the optimization of existing ACI protocols or the creation of novel approaches [11,12,72–76]. Several generations of ACI have been clinically investigated and shown to yield positive impacts for treated patients [1–3,11–15]. Importantly, extensive, long-term, and large-scale clinical human data are available for ACI [15,22,29,30]. In one study, first-generation ACI involved the arthrotomic implantation of expanded HACs under a periosteal flap [7,14]. The aim of this study was to durably restore tissular structures and functions following lesion debridement and the creation of an optimal local environment for the cell-based product. Good clinical outcomes were obtained, yet a major cause of failure was the development of periosteal hypertrophy, requiring new surgical interventions [8,13,14]. Additionally, the surgery requires an open-joint procedure and the harvest of a periosteal flap, which is fragile and can tear during suturing.

In second-generation ACI, the periosteal flap was replaced by an artificial membrane (e.g., Chondro-Gide) [8,14]. This substitution improved outcomes, as the procedure was less invasive (no periosteal tissue harvest); less surgical complications were observed, and a reduction in hypertrophy development was recorded [2,8,11]. However, the procedure still required open surgery, which brings risks of complication. Furthermore, a risk of injected cell leakage or inhomogeneous repartition on the lesion surface exists. McCarthy et al. directly compared the clinical and histological outcomes between first- and second-generation ACI [38]. Patients implanted with Chondro-Gide membranes demonstrated a higher cellular morphology score (i.e., ICRS II score), a better surface morphology for treated medial femoral condyle defects, and a higher proportion of hyaline cartilage formation (i.e., OsScore) [38]. These results demonstrated that the use of Chondro-Gide membranes resulted in a better quality of tissular repair [38].

Overall, considering the available clinical data on the various generations of ACI led us to conclude that the interventions are generally safe and effective and that the successive technical updates in therapy/product manufacturing protocols have been clinically beneficial [14–17,77–80]. Specifically, it was shown in multiple settings and by various clinical groups that the use of the Chondro-Gide membrane was of high therapeutic utility in a variety of treatment strategies. The comprehensive consideration of the elements presented hereabove enabled the local implementation of the NCT05651997 clinical trial, which was based on the robust global track records of the Chondro-Gide membrane and third-generation ACI.

### *4.2. Safety, Quality, and Efficacy Attributes: FE002 Primary Chondroprogenitors Are Compatible with Modern Clinical Regenerative Medicine Requirements*

Since the establishment of the cell source in 2009 under the Swiss progenitor cell transplantation program, FE002 primary chondroprogenitors have been exploited as clinical-grade cytotherapeutic materials [49,50]. Specifically, extensive technical work has validated the applicability of such cells in industrial-scale manufacturing workflows for transposition to GMP manufacturing [50]. Furthermore, previous preclinical research has shown the versatility and high potential of FE002 primary chondroprogenitors as promising contenders in cell-based orthopedic regenerative medicine [50–54,81]. Some of the advantages of using such an allogeneic cellular active substance for cartilage bioengineering involve the off-the-freezer availability of standardized biologicals, rationalized manufacturing workflows, and drastically reduced operative burdens [50].

However, major concerns regarding the development of novel cell-based protocols for human cytotherapeutic use are linked to biological material safety, especially in allogeneic contexts. Notably, FE002 primary chondroprogenitors have been implanted in vivo in a variety of xenogeneic settings (including a caprine GLP study of knee cartilage defects) [50–52]. Furthermore, the original experimental results presented in this study have served to complement and enhance the available body of knowledge on the safety attributes of FE002 primary chondroprogenitors (finite in vitro lifespan, low telomerase activity, no anchorage-independent cell growth). From a mechanistic viewpoint, the identification of the main soluble constituents of the FE002 allogeneic biological materials (e.g., growth factors, cytokines) has provided some insight into the possible biochemical cues at play in the paracrine modulation of pathological environments (Table S1).

From a translational viewpoint, our combined cell manufacturing and clinical cytotherapeutic experiences enabled us to tangibly set forward the established protocols and processes (i.e., autologous and allogeneic, Figures 1 and 2). Regarding local GMP manufacturing and the clinical administration of HAC-based preparations, more than 67 patients have been treated to date (NCT04296487 clinical trial) [48]. Regarding GMP manufacturing and the clinical use of primary progenitor cells (e.g., FE002 primary dermal progenitor fibroblasts), more than 300 patients have been treated to date [65]. Overall, the appropriate consolidation of the locally available resources and research should enable the timely transposition of orthopedic protocols from an autologous to an allogeneic setting using FE002 primary chondroprogenitors.

### *4.3. FE002 Primary Chondroprogenitors Are Functionally Comparable to Clinical-grade HACs in Chondro-Gide Constructs*

The functional characterization of FE002 primary chondroprogenitors has previously been reported by multiple research groups and in a variety of product prototypes [50–52,81]. The specific methodological advantage of the present study lied within the use of a regulatorily approved autologous approach and clinical-grade HAC materials as a baseline for manufacturing process benchmarking and parallel functional qualification. Therein, it was shown that FE002 primary chondroprogenitors equaled or outperformed patient primary HAC cell types in terms of function in the retained Chondro-Gide construct (Figures 3 and 4). Specifically, it was shown that finished products with appropriate quality and functionality attributes could be obtained using both protocols, notwithstanding the specific technical adaptations (Tables 1, S2 and S3). The simultaneous consideration of both approaches enabled us to devise optimized manufacturing processes and related controls, which were validated as being applicable to the HAC-based and the FE002 primary chondroprogenitor-based protocols (Figures 1 and 2, Table 2). While direct comparison between the two approaches was not possible (due to specific process adaptations), parallel functional qualification indicated that both finished product types conformed to the specified requirements (Table 2).

To strengthen the rationale of using Chondro-Gide scaffolds for therapeutic cell chondrogenic induction, an alternative autologous approach (i.e., N-TEC, engineered nasal cartilage) has been discussed [32,57,82]. Nasal chondrocyte-based tissue-engineered cartilage has been extensively studied at preclinical and clinical levels, garnering a robust scientific, technical, and clinical track record [32,57,73]. Specifically, chondrocytes isolated from nasal septa were cultured and chondrogenically induced on Chondro-Gide scaffolds for up to two weeks [32,73]. Favorable therapeutic effects have been shown for orthopedic patients following osteoarthritic knee cartilage defect management using the N-TEC protocol [32]. Notably, the methodological elements of the N-TEC protocol and its iterative technical updates were closely considered for devising the autologous and allogeneic workflows presented herein [66,73]. Therein, manufacturing technical specificities and stepwise control implementation from the N-TEC approach were considered as bases for the validation of both reported protocols (autologous and allogeneic) using the Chondro-Gide scaffold [73].

A notable technical divergence in this study between the presented approaches (autologous vs. allogeneic) was the use of HPL for the autologous protocol and the use of FBS in the allogeneic protocol (Table 1). While the implementation of HPL as a cell proliferation medium supplement may easily be justified from a risk reduction viewpoint, the long-term functional impact on expanded chondrogenic cells remains under investigation. Specifically, several studies have shown the functional equivalence of FBS and HPL for the in vitro manufacturing of chondrogenic cells [66,83–89]. Furthermore, the upscaling of cell manufacturing for ACI has technically excluded the use of AHS as a culture supplement due to limited available quantities [72,74]. Therefore, specific concerns have been voiced over the impact of HPL supplementation on the in vitro chondrogenic potential of the cellular active substance; however, the available reports are not all congruent, and the overall impact on the therapeutic efficacy of the intervention remains unknown [74]. Overall, while several new cell proliferation medium supplements are available and conform to the modern standards of animal material-free workflows, FBS remains the gold standard due to its proven manufacturing and clinical track record [84–87]. These elements were considered to justify the maintenance of FBS for the industrial manufacturing of FE002 primary chondroprogenitors, despite the evident technical applicability of HPL (Figures S1 and S2) [50].

### *4.4. Autologous versus Allogeneic Approaches to Large (Osteo)-Chondral Defects of the Knee: Comparative Burden Analysis for Clinical Pathway Rationalization*

A main advantage of adopting an allogeneic cell-based approach to manage large knee (osteo)-chondral defects is the reduction in operative burdens and donor-site morbidity [50,90]. Specifically, allogeneic workflows normally require only one orthopedic intervention at the time of matured graft implantation in the joint (Figure S8). Furthermore, it was validated that AHS was not necessary in the finished product transport medium for the FE002 cell-based allogeneic constructs, removing the need for autologous blood draw (Figure 8, Table 4). Such process simplifications may be interpreted positively in the case of the presented allogeneic protocol and from multiple standpoints (clinical pathways, technical risks, resource allocation).

Regarding the clinical pathway rationalization with the use of the allogeneic protocol, numerous logistical advantages may be yielded by the off-the-freezer availability of the FE002 cellular active substance (Figures 1 and S8) [50]. Specifically, the operative program may be devised around a single orthopedic intervention for graft implantation, and manufacturing activities may be retro-planned accordingly, without the time constraints linked to autologous biopsy processing (Figure S8) [48]. Therefore, the serial manufacturing of FE002 allogeneic cellular active substance lots allow for significant potential organizational gains at the institutional level.

Regarding the technical risk reduction in the allogeneic approach, the amount of process steps and the number of repetitions of said steps is determinant. Indeed, the autologous protocol requires primary patient HAC cell type establishment, HAC expansion, and finished product formulation steps to be performed for each new patient (Figure S8) [48]. Conversely, the exploitation of a standardized allogeneic cell source such as FE002 primary chondroprogenitors does not require renewed cell type establishment, and the same cellular active substance lot may be used quasi-universally for different patients [50]. Therein, standard FE002 cellular active substance manufacturing batches may potentially serve for the serial preparation of >20 allogeneic grafts (40 mm $\times$ 50 mm). Thus, all technical means that result in a reduction in manufacturing steps or repetitions may provide tangible reductions in biosafety-related risks or manufacturing failure-related risks (Figure S8). Importantly, the high inter-patient variability, which impacts autologous cellular active substance manufacturing activities, may be avoided in the allogeneic approach, which enhances process standardization [48]. At the finished product level, the original data presented in the present study showed the superior performance of the FE002 cells in terms of GAG synthesis but also showed higher variability compared to the HAC-based constructs (Figure 4C). Such results were explained by the different scale of chondrogenic gene expression under induction (i.e., >ten-fold higher expression in allogeneic constructs) and were not interpreted negatively due to the fact that only minimal requirements are specified within functional controls (Figure 3, Table 2).

Regarding the comparative analysis of resource allocation for the autologous and allogeneic approaches, the technical and clinical simplifications described hereabove lead to overall cost rationalization within the allogeneic approach (Table 1). Specifically, the sparing use of manufacturing resources may be achieved via serial cell batch production instead of patient-specific production (Figure S8). Furthermore, less surgeon-related and operating room-related resources are needed, as the autologous biopsy harvest procedure is abolished in the allogeneic protocol (Figure S8). Importantly, as the specific case of second-generation ACI is reimbursed as a lump sum by universal healthcare coverage in Switzerland, any means that can lower the overall cost of the cell-based orthopedic intervention may potentially demonstrably lead to higher specific public healthcare efficiency, provided that therapeutic outcomes are at least equivalent [48].

However, the various advantages presented hereabove in favor of the implementation of allogeneic cell-based protocols are counterbalanced by the time- and resource-consuming process of obtaining the ad hoc regulatory approvals [50,91–99]. Specifically, extensive risk-based approaches to the transition from autologous to allogeneic investigational medicinal products (IMP) must be followed, along with appropriate (i.e., specific and general) risk analyses (for product quality, purity, efficacy, safety, and stability; see Tables S4–S7) [48]. The tangible consideration of FE002 allogeneic cellular active substance substitution into an existing technical and clinical workflow (autologous to allogeneic transposition) is highly advisable compared to de novo process development and implementation.

### 4.5. Identified Study Limitations and Future Clinical Research Directions

The main technical limitations of the presented study were related to the use of specific manufacturing processes for the autologous and allogeneic materials, which did not enable a strict comparison of both approaches. Importantly, both manufacturing processes were developed and optimized, respectively, around HACs and FE002 primary chondroprogenitors to maximize cellular active substance and finished product quality and functionality attributes [48–50,66,100,101]. Therefore, we chose to parallelly qualify the two types of finished products using the respective technical specifications of both protocols (i.e., those regulatorily approved for the autologous protocol and those used for the industrial manufacturing of the allogeneic grafts). This was preferred to using an identical manufacturing process for the autologous and allogeneic cells, which would have enabled the strict functional benchmarking of the materials. This option was not favored, as the relevance of appropriate functional attribute development is generally higher than that of process technical specificities (all risks being equal and mitigated). By extension, the strict quantitative benchmarking of both approaches is probably of low translational relevance as, for such similarly behaving biologicals (i.e., in terms of endpoint functional attributes), it is unclear if superior in vitro performance would correspond to differential therapeutic benefits for the patients [102–105].

Regarding the scale of the presented work (i.e., Chondro-Gide membrane sub-units), further validation studies are warranted in order to generate constructs of appropriate dimensions for the management of large knee (osteo)-chondral defects (>10 cm$^2$). When working with qualified scaffold lots, high robustness in finished product manufacturing processes was recorded, and our experimental results regarding manufacturing protocol upscaling confirmed endpoint functional equivalence at two different size scales (1 cm$^2$ vs. 5 cm$^2$). Therefore, the use of full 20 cm$^2$ Chondro-Gide membranes would require the adaptation of incubation vessels and contact–process consumables for ease of processing in GMP manufacturing environments.

As previously mentioned, a large body of scientific and technical research regarding the clinical-grade allogeneic FE002 primary chondroprogenitor cell source is currently available. Notably, the in vitro and in vivo safety of the FE002 cells has been studied and validated by several research groups [50–54]. Based on the presented technical data and the current clinical developments of autologous and allogeneic cell-based solutions for knee chondral lesion management, a pilot clinical trial is being devised around the therapeutic FE002 progenitor cell source. Therein, two cytotherapeutic formulation options may tangibly be considered, namely the bioengineered graft presented herein (i.e., chondrogenically induced cells on Chondro-Gide scaffolds) and an injectable FE002 cell suspension to be used in a setup similar to second-generation ACI [48,50]. Therein, injectable FE002 primary chondroprogenitor suspensions may be simply obtained for additionally rationalized manufacturing and clinical workflows.

## 5. Conclusions

The aim of the present study was to perform manufacturing process benchmarking and parallel functional qualification for matrix-associated autologous and allogeneic approaches to large knee (osteo)-chondral defect cytotherapeutic management. Our experimental results confirmed that both types of bioengineered constructs could be manufactured using overlapping and optimized GMP-transposable processes. Specifically, the obtained constructs were characterized by comparable quality- and functionality-related attributes (e.g., *COL2* and *ACAN* induction, GAG deposition, Chondro-Gide scaffold maturation), where quantitative results were relatively superior in the allogeneic sample groups. Based on the existing evidence on the use of HAC/Chondro-Gide combinations, this study confirmed that allogeneic FE002 primary chondroprogenitors were compatible with the Chondro-Gide scaffold and that they could form a functionally sound (i.e., 3D chondrogenic gene induction, ECM deposition) finished product. Additionally, complementary in vitro safety data enabled us to further characterize FE002 primary chondroprogenitors from a preclinical safety viewpoint. The presented data were specifically considered for establishing the rationale around an autologous to allogeneic cell-based orthopedic protocol transposition. These undertakings were based on a gap analysis between the autologous and allogeneic protocols, on the reported functional comparability at the finished product level, and on risk analyses for the use of FE002 primary allogeneic biologicals. Considering the specific discussion points about the available body of research on the current cell-based approaches to large knee (osteo)-chondral defect management enabled us to highlight their respective opportunities, advantages, and risks. Overall, building on the available clinical research on ACI, the present study could enable the establishment of an appropriate standard for the further clinical investigation of FE002 allogeneic cell-based orthopedic protocols.

**Supplementary Materials:** The following supporting information can be downloaded at https://www.mdpi.com/article/10.3390/pharmaceutics15092333/s1: Figure S1: Comparative cellular proliferation assays; Figure S2: Comparative cellular proliferation curves; Figure S3: Cellular senescence detection assays; Figure S4: Soft agarose colony formation assay; Figure S5: Comparative telomerase activity quantification assay; Figure S6: Cellular active substance stability studies; Figure S7: Finished cytotherapeutic product manufacturing steps; Figure S8: Comparative technical and clinical workflow for the autologous and allogeneic protocols; Figure S9: Finished product suture tests; Table S1: Proteomic characterization results of FE002 allogeneic cellular materials; Table S2: Established cryopreserved cellular active substance quality attributes; Table S3: Established finished product quality attributes; Table S4: Risk analysis matrix for human FE002 primary chondroprogenitor cell type establishment; Table S5: Risk analysis matrix for human FE002 primary chondroprogenitor cell banking; Table S6: Specific risk analysis matrix established for the assessment of the microbiological safety of FE002 primary chondroprogenitors; Table S7: General risk analysis matrix established for the finished products.

**Author Contributions:** Conceptualization, V.P., A.J., L.A.A., R.M. and A.L.; methodology, V.P., A.J., C.P., S.J., C.S., N.H.-B., S.D., L.A.A., R.M. and A.L.; software, V.P., A.J., C.P., and A.L.; validation, V.P., A.J., C.P., S.J., C.S., N.H.-B., P.A.-S., W.R., S.D., L.A.A., R.M. and A.L.; formal analysis, V.P., A.J., C.P., N.H.-B., S.D., L.A.A. and A.L.; investigation, V.P., A.J., C.P., S.J., C.S., N.H.-B., S.D., R.M. and A.L.; resources, L.A.A., R.M. and A.L.; data curation, V.P., A.J., C.P., S.J., C.S., S.D., L.A.A. and A.L.; writing—original draft preparation, V.P., A.J., N.H.-B., L.A.A. and A.L.; writing—review and editing, V.P., A.J., C.P., S.J., C.S., N.H.-B., P.A.-S., W.R., S.D., L.A.A., R.M. and A.L.; visualization, V.P., A.J., C.P., N.H.-B., S.D. and A.L.; supervision, V.P., A.J., S.D., L.A.A., R.M. and A.L.; project administration, V.P., L.A.A., R.M. and A.L.; funding acquisition, V.P., L.A.A., R.M. and A.L. All authors have read and agreed to the published version of the manuscript.

**Funding:** The S.A.N.T.E and Sandoz Foundations have contributed to funding the Swiss progenitor cell transplantation program during the past fourteen years, reference numbers 27846-06 and 27866-06, respectively. This research received general funding from the Lausanne Orthopedics Research Foundation (LORF), reference number LORF31018-Chondro. This study was partly financed by the Service of Promotion of the Economy and Innovation of the Canton of Vaud (SPEI), in accordance with the Vaud Cantonal Law on Economic Development Support of 12 June 2007 (LADE), reference number LADE 20-472. The funders had no role or involvement in design of the study; in the collection, analysis, and interpretation of data; in the writing of the report; or in the decision to submit the article for publication. This study was not supported by other specific grants or institutional programs.

**Institutional Review Board Statement:** The biological starting materials used for the present study were procured according to the guidelines of the Declaration of Helsinki and the ICH-GCP, and their procurement was approved by the appropriate Cantonal Ethics Committee [106]. The clinical-grade FE002 primary chondroprogenitor cell source used in the present study was established from the FE002 organ donation, as approved by the Vaud Cantonal Ethics Committee (University Hospital of Lausanne–CHUV, Ethics Committee Protocol N°62/07). The FE002 organ donation was registered under a federal cell transplantation program (Swiss progenitor cell transplantation program). This study was performed using materials and information gathered in the context of two authorized clinical trials (www.ClinicalTrials.gov, accessed on 4 August 2023, identifiers: NCT04296487 and NCT05651997) in Switzerland [107].

**Informed Consent Statement:** Appropriate informed consent was obtained from and confirmed by starting material donors at the time of inclusion in the Swiss progenitor cell transplantation program following specifically devised protocols and procedures that were validated by the appropriate health authorities. Informed consent (formalized in a general informed consent agreement) was obtained from all patients or from their legal representatives at the time of treatment for the unrestricted use of the gathered and anonymized patient data or anonymized biological materials (i.e., donors for primary cell types included in institutional biobanks).

**Data Availability Statement:** The data presented in this study are available from the corresponding authors upon written and reasonable request.

**Acknowledgments:** We would like to thank the S.A.N.T.E and Sandoz Foundations for their unconditional commitment to the Swiss progenitor cell transplantation program through the years. We would like to thank the Lausanne Orthopedics Research Foundation (LORF) for their continued support and commitment. We would like to thank the Canton of Vaud for their continued support and commitment. We would like to thank Aymone Lenisa and Mara Heinold for their technical contributions. Artwork templates were partly created using www.biorender.com, accessed on 20 July 2023.

**Conflicts of Interest:** Authors A.J., C.P. and A.L. were employed by LAM Biotechnologies SA (Epalinges, Switzerland) during the production of this work. The remaining authors declare no conflicts of interest.

## References

1. Niemeyer, P.; Hanus, M.; Belickas, J.; László, T.; Gudas, R.; Fiodorovas, M.; Cebatorius, A.; Pastucha, M.; Hoza, P.; Magos, K.; et al. Treatment of large cartilage defects in the knee by hydrogel-based autologous chondrocyte implantation: Two-year results of a prospective, multicenter, single-arm phase III trial. *Cartilage* **2022**, *13*, 19476035221085146. [CrossRef]
2. Makris, E.A.; Gomoll, A.H.; Malizos, K.N.; Hu, J.C.; Athanasiou, K.A. Repair and tissue engineering techniques for articular cartilage. *Nat. Rev. Rheumatol.* **2015**, *11*, 21–34. [CrossRef]
3. Brittberg, M.; Gomoll, A.H.; Canseco, J.A.; Far, J.; Lind, M.; Hui, J. Cartilage repair in the degenerative ageing knee. *Acta Orthop.* **2016**, *87*, 26–38. [CrossRef]
4. Martin, R.; Laurent, A.; Applegate, L.A.; Philippe, V. Grands défects chondraux et ostéochondraux du genou: Traitement par greffe chondrocytaire autologue. *Rev. Med. Suisse* **2022**, *18*, 2384–2390. [CrossRef]
5. Saris, D.B.; Vanlauwe, J.; Victor, J.; Almqvist, K.F.; Verdonk, R.; Bellemans, J.; Luyten, F.P.; TIG/ACT/01/2000&EXT Study Group. Treatment of symptomatic cartilage defects of the knee: Characterized chondrocyte implantation results in better clinical outcome at 36 months in a randomized trial compared to microfracture. *Am. J. Sports Med.* **2009**, *37*, 10S–19S. [CrossRef]
6. Heidari, B. Knee osteoarthritis prevalence, risk factors, pathogenesis and features: Part I. *Casp. J. Int. Med.* **2011**, *2*, 205–212.
7. Brittberg, M.; Lindahl, A.; Nilsson, A.; Ohlsson, C.; Isaksson, O.; Peterson, L. Treatment of deep cartilage defects in the knee with autologous chondrocyte transplantation. *N. Engl. J. Med.* **1994**, *331*, 889–895. [CrossRef] [PubMed]
8. Brittberg, M. Cell carriers as the next generation of cell therapy for cartilage repair: A review of the matrix-induced autologous chondrocyte implantation procedure. *Am. J. Sports Med.* **2010**, *38*, 1259–1271. [CrossRef] [PubMed]

9. Hoburg, A.; Niemeyer, P.; Laute, V.; Zinser, W.; Becher, C.; Kolombe, T.; Fay, J.; Pietsch, S.; Kuźma, T.; Widuchowski, W.; et al. Sustained superiority in KOOS subscores after matrix-associated chondrocyte implantation using spheroids compared to microfracture. *Knee Surg. Sports Traumatol. Arthrosc.* **2023**, *31*, 2482–2493. [CrossRef] [PubMed]
10. Urlic, I.; Ivkovic, A. Cell sources for cartilage repair-Biological and clinical perspective. *Cells* **2021**, *10*, 2496. [CrossRef] [PubMed]
11. Kon, E.; Roffi, A.; Filardo, G.; Tesei, G.; Marcacci, M. Scaffold-based cartilage treatments: With or without cells? A systematic review of preclinical and clinical evidence. *Arthroscopy* **2015**, *31*, 767–775. [CrossRef] [PubMed]
12. Binder, H.; Hoffman, L.; Zak, L.; Tiefenboeck, T.; Aldrian, S.; Albrecht, C. Clinical evaluation after matrix-associated autologous chondrocyte transplantation: A comparison of four different graft types. *Bone Joint Res.* **2021**, *10*, 370–379. [CrossRef] [PubMed]
13. Kili, S.; Mills, S.; Levine, D.W. Tissue-engineered cartilage products: Clinical experience. In *Principles of Tissue Engineering: Fourth Edition*; Elsevier: Amsterdam, The Netherlands, 2013. [CrossRef]
14. Davies, R.L.; Kuiper, N.J. Regenerative medicine: A review of the evolution of autologous chondrocyte implantation (ACI) therapy. *Bioengineering* **2019**, *6*, 22. [CrossRef] [PubMed]
15. Peterson, L.; Vasiliadis, H.S.; Brittberg, M.; Lindahl, A. Autologous chondrocyte implantation: A long-term follow-up. *Am. J. Sports Med.* **2010**, *38*, 1117–1124. [CrossRef]
16. Brittberg, M.; Recker, D.; Ilgenfritz, J.; Saris, D.B.F.; SUMMIT Extension Study Group. Matrix-applied characterized autologous cultured chondrocytes versus microfracture: Five-year follow-up of a prospective randomized trial. *Am. J. Sports Med.* **2018**, *46*, 1343–1351. [CrossRef]
17. Peterson, L.; Minas, T.; Brittberg, M.; Nilsson, A.; Sjögren-Jansson, E.; Lindahl, A. Two- to 9-year outcome after autologous chondrocyte transplantation of the knee. *Clin. Orthop. Rel. Res.* **2000**, *374*, 212–234. [CrossRef]
18. Kon, E.; Filardo, G.; Brittberg, M.; Busacca, M.; Condello, V.; Engebretsen, L.; Marlovits, S.; Niemeyer, P.; Platzer, P.; Posthumus, M.; et al. A multilayer biomaterial for osteochondral regeneration shows superiority vs microfractures for the treatment of osteochondral lesions in a multicentre randomized trial at 2 years. *Knee Surg. Sports Traumatol. Arthrosc.* **2018**, *26*, 2704–2715. [CrossRef]
19. Oussedik, S.; Tsitskaris, K.; Parker, D. Treatment of articular cartilage lesions of the knee by microfracture or autologous chondrocyte implantation: A systematic review. *Arthroscopy* **2015**, *31*, 732–744. [CrossRef]
20. Saris, D.; Price, A.; Widuchowski, W.; Bertrand-Marchand, M.; Caron, J.; Drogset, J.O.; Emans, P.; Podskubka, A.; Tsuchida, A.; Kili, S.; et al. Matrix-applied characterized autologous cultured chondrocytes versus microfracture: Two-year follow-up of a prospective randomized trial. *Am. J. Sports Med.* **2014**, *42*, 1384–1394. [CrossRef]
21. Gille, J.; Kunow, J.; Boisch, L.; Behrens, P.; Bos, I.; Hoffmann, C.; Köller, W.; Russlies, M.; Kurz, B. Cell-laden and cell-free matrix-induced chondrogenesis versus microfracture for the treatment of articular cartilage defects: A histological and biomechanical study in sheep. *Cartilage* **2010**, *1*, 29–42. [CrossRef]
22. Ibarra, C.; Villalobos, E.; Madrazo-Ibarra, A.; Velasquillo, C.; Martinez-Lopez, V.; Izaguirre, A.; Olivos-Meza, A.; Cortes-Gonzalez, S.; Perez-Jimenez, F.J.; Vargas-Ramirez, A.; et al. Arthroscopic matrix-assisted autologous chondrocyte transplantation versus microfracture: A 6-year follow-up of a prospective randomized trial. *Am. J. Sports Med.* **2021**, *49*, 2165–2176. [CrossRef] [PubMed]
23. Basad, E.; Ishaque, B.; Bachmann, G.; Stürz, H.; Steinmeyer, J. Matrix-induced autologous chondrocyte implantation versus microfracture in the treatment of cartilage defects of the knee: A 2-year randomised study. *Knee Surg. Sports Traumatol. Arthrosc.* **2010**, *18*, 519–527. [CrossRef] [PubMed]
24. Crawford, D.C.; DeBerardino, T.M.; Williams, R.J., 3rd. NeoCart, an autologous cartilage tissue implant, compared with microfracture for treatment of distal femoral cartilage lesions: An FDA phase-II prospective, randomized clinical trial after two years. *J. Bone Joint Surg.* **2012**, *94*, 979–989. [CrossRef] [PubMed]
25. Van Assche, D.; Staes, F.; Van Caspel, D.; Vanlauwe, J.; Bellemans, J.; Saris, D.B.; Luyten, F.P. Autologous chondrocyte implantation versus microfracture for knee cartilage injury: A prospective randomized trial, with 2-year follow-up. *Knee Surg. Sports Traumatol. Arthrosc.* **2010**, *18*, 486–495. [CrossRef]
26. Petri, M.; Broese, M.; Simon, A.; Liodakis, E.; Ettinger, M.; Guenther, D.; Zeichen, J.; Krettek, C.; Jagodzinski, M.; Haasper, C. CaReS (MACT) versus microfracture in treating symptomatic patellofemoral cartilage defects: A retrospective matched-pair analysis. *J. Orthop. Sci.* **2013**, *18*, 38–44. [CrossRef]
27. Cortese, F.; McNicholas, M.; Janes, G.; Gillogly, S.; Abelow, S.P.; Gigante, A.; Coletti, N. Arthroscopic delivery of matrix-induced autologous chondrocyte implant: International experience and technique recommendations. *Cartilage* **2012**, *3*, 156–164. [CrossRef]
28. Abelow, S.P.; Guillen, P.; Ramos, T. Arthroscopic technique for matrix-induced autologous chondrocyte implantation for the treatment of large chondral defects in the knee and ankle. *Oper. Tech. Orthop.* **2006**, *16*, 257–261. [CrossRef]
29. Bentley, G.; Biant, L.C.; Vijayan, S.; Macmull, S.; Skinner, J.A.; Carrington, R.W. Minimum ten-year results of a prospective randomised study of autologous chondrocyte implantation versus mosaicplasty for symptomatic articular cartilage lesions of the knee. *J. Bone Joint Surg.* **2012**, *94*, 504–509. [CrossRef]
30. Biant, L.C.; Bentley, G.; Vijayan, S.; Skinner, J.A.; Carrington, R.W. Long-term results of autologous chondrocyte implantation in the knee for chronic chondral and osteochondral defects. *Am. J. Sports Med.* **2014**, *42*, 2178–2183. [CrossRef]
31. Huang, B.J.; Hu, J.C.; Athanasiou, K.A. Cell-based tissue engineering strategies used in the clinical repair of articular cartilage. *Biomaterials* **2016**, *98*, 1–22. [CrossRef]

32. Mumme, M.; Barbero, A.; Miot, S.; Wixmerten, A.; Feliciano, S.; Wolf, F.; Asnaghi, A.M.; Baumhoer, D.; Bieri, O.; Kretzcchmar, M.; et al. Nasal chondrocyte-based engineered autologous cartilage tissue for repair of articular cartilage defects: An observational first-in-human trial. *Lancet* **2016**, *388*, 1985–1994. [CrossRef]
33. Vinardell, T.; Sheehy, E.J.; Buckley, C.T.; Kelly, D.J. A comparison of the functionality and in vivo phenotypic stability of cartilaginous tissues engineered from different stem cell sources. *Tissue Eng. Part A* **2012**, *18*, 1161–1170. [CrossRef]
34. Almqvist, K.F.; Dhollander, A.A.; Verdonk, P.C.; Forsyth, R.; Verdonk, R.; Verbruggen, G. Treatment of cartilage defects in the knee using alginate beads containing human mature allogenic chondrocytes. *Am. J. Sports Med.* **2009**, *37*, 1920–1929. [CrossRef]
35. Zak, L.; Albrecht, C.; Wondrasch, B.; Widhalm, H.; Vekszler, G.; Trattnig, S.; Marlovits, S.; Aldrian, S. Results 2 years after matrix-associated autologous chondrocyte transplantation using the Novocart 3D scaffold: An analysis of clinical and radiological data. *Am. J. Sports Med.* **2014**, *42*, 1618–1627. [CrossRef]
36. Marcacci, M.; Berruto, M.; Brocchetta, D.; Delcogliano, A.; Ghinelli, D.; Gobbi, A.; Kon, E.; Pederzini, L.; Rosa, D.; Sacchetti, G.L.; et al. Articular cartilage engineering with Hyalograft C: 3-year clinical results. *Clin. Orthop. Rel. Res.* **2005**, *435*, 96–105. [CrossRef] [PubMed]
37. Niethammer, T.R.; Gallik, D.; Chevalier, Y.; Holzgruber, M.; Baur-Melnyk, A.; Müller, P.E.; Pietschmann, M.F. Effect of the defect localization and size on the success of third-generation autologous chondrocyte implantation in the knee joint. *Internat. Orthop.* **2021**, *45*, 1483–1491. [CrossRef] [PubMed]
38. McCarthy, H.S.; Roberts, S. A histological comparison of the repair tissue formed when using either Chondrogide(®) or periosteum during autologous chondrocyte implantation. *Osteoarthritis Cart.* **2013**, *21*, 2048–2057. [CrossRef]
39. Vijayan, S.; Bartlett, W.; Bentley, G.; Carrington, R.W.; Skinner, J.A.; Pollock, R.C.; Alorjani, M.; Briggs, T.W. Autologous chondrocyte implantation for osteochondral lesions in the knee using a bilayer collagen membrane and bone graft: A two- to eight-year follow-up study. *J. Bone Joint Surg.* **2012**, *94*, 488–492. [CrossRef]
40. Brix, M.O.; Stelzeneder, D.; Chiari, C.; Koller, U.; Nehrer, S.; Dorotka, R.; Windhager, R.; Domayer, S.E. Treatment of full-thickness chondral defects with Hyalograft C in the knee: Long-term results. *Am. J. Sports Med.* **2014**, *42*, 1426–1432. [CrossRef]
41. Hossain, M.A.; Adithan, A.; Alam, M.J.; Kopalli, S.R.; Kim, B.; Kang, C.W.; Hwang, K.C.; Kim, J.H. IGF-1 facilitates cartilage reconstruction by regulating PI3K/AKT, MAPK, and NF-kB signaling in rabbit osteoarthritis. *J. Infl. Res.* **2021**, *14*, 3555–3568. [CrossRef]
42. Kisiday, J.D. Expansion of chondrocytes for cartilage tissue engineering: A review of chondrocyte dedifferentiation and redifferentiation as a function of growth in expansion culture. *Regen. Med. Front.* **2020**, *2*, e200002. [CrossRef]
43. Chen, Y.; Yu, Y.; Wen, Y.; Chen, J.; Lin, J.; Sheng, Z.; Zhou, W.; Sun, H.; An, C.; Chen, J.; et al. A high-resolution route map reveals distinct stages of chondrocyte dedifferentiation for cartilage regeneration. *Bone Res.* **2022**, *10*, 38. [CrossRef] [PubMed]
44. Enochson, L.; Brittberg, M.; Lindahl, A. Optimization of a chondrogenic medium through the use of factorial design of experiments. *BioRes Open Access* **2012**, *1*, 306–313. [CrossRef]
45. Martinez, I.; Elvenes, J.; Olsen, R.; Bertheussen, K.; Johansen, O. Redifferentiation of in vitro expanded adult articular chondrocytes by combining the hanging-drop cultivation method with hypoxic environment. *Cell Transplant.* **2008**, *17*, 987–996. [CrossRef] [PubMed]
46. Lin, Z.; Fitzgerald, J.B.; Xu, J.; Willers, C.; Wood, D.; Grodzinsky, A.J.; Zheng, M.H. Gene expression profiles of human chondrocytes during passaged monolayer cultivation. *J. Orthop. Res.* **2008**, *26*, 1230–1237. [CrossRef] [PubMed]
47. Tallheden, T.; Karlsson, C.; Brunner, A.; Van Der Lee, J.; Hagg, R.; Tommasini, R.; Lindahl, A. Gene expression during redifferentiation of human articular chondrocytes. *Osteoarthritis Cart.* **2004**, *12*, 525–535. [CrossRef]
48. Philippe, V.; Laurent, A.; Hirt-Burri, N.; Abdel-Sayed, P.; Scaletta, C.; Schneebeli, V.; Michetti, M.; Brunet, J.-F.; Applegate, L.A.; Martin, R. Retrospective analysis of autologous chondrocyte-based cytotherapy production for clinical use: GMP process-based manufacturing optimization in a Swiss university hospital. *Cells* **2022**, *11*, 1016. [CrossRef]
49. Darwiche, S.E.; Scaletta, C.; Raffoul, W.; Pioletti, D.P.; Applegate, L.A. Epiphyseal chondroprogenitors provide a stable cell source for cartilage cell therapy. *Cell Med.* **2012**, *4*, 23–32. [CrossRef]
50. Laurent, A.; Abdel-Sayed, P.; Ducrot, A.; Hirt-Burri, N.; Scaletta, C.; Jaccoud, S.; Nuss, K.; de Buys Roessingh, A.S.; Raffoul, W.; Pioletti, D.P.; et al. Development of standardized fetal progenitor cell therapy for cartilage regenerative medicine: Industrial transposition and preliminary safety in xenogeneic transplantation. *Biomolecules* **2021**, *11*, 250. [CrossRef]
51. Studer, D.; Cavalli, E.; Formica, F.A.; Kuhn, G.A.; Salzmann, G.; Mumme, M.; Steinwachs, M.R.; Applegate, L.A.; Maniura-Weber, K.; Zenobi-Wong, M. Human chondroprogenitors in alginate-collagen hybrid scaffolds produce stable cartilage in vivo. *J. Tissue Eng. Regen. Med.* **2017**, *11*, 3014–3026. [CrossRef]
52. Cavalli, E.; Fisch, P.; Formica, F.A.; Gareus, R.; Linder, T.; Applegate, L.A.; Zenobi-Wong, M. A comparative study of cartilage engineered constructs in immunocompromised, humanized and immunocompetent mice. *J. Immunol. Regen. Med.* **2018**, *2*, 36–46. [CrossRef]
53. Levinson, C.; Lee, M.; Applegate, L.A.; Zenobi-Wong, M. An injectable heparin-conjugated hyaluronan scaffold for local delivery of transforming growth factor β1 promotes successful chondrogenesis. *Acta Biomater.* **2019**, *99*, 168–180. [CrossRef]
54. Porcello, A.; Gonzalez-Fernandez, P.; Jeannerat, A.; Peneveyre, C.; Abdel-Sayed, P.; Scaletta, C.; Raffoul, W.; Hirt-Burri, N.; Applegate, L.A.; Allémann, E.; et al. Thermo-responsive hyaluronan-based hydrogels combined with allogeneic cytotherapeutics for the treatment of osteoarthritis. *Pharmaceutics* **2023**, *15*, 1528. [CrossRef]

55. Tritschler, H.; Fischer, K.; Seissler, J.; Fiedler, J.; Halbgebauer, R.; Huber-Lang, M.; Schnieke, A.; Brenner, R.E. New insights into xenotransplantation for cartilage repair: Porcine multi-genetically modified chondrocytes as a promising cell source. *Cells* **2021**, *10*, 2152. [CrossRef]
56. Cherian, J.J.; Parvizi, J.; Bramlet, D.; Lee, K.H.; Romness, D.W.; Mont, M.A. Preliminary results of a phase II randomized study to determine the efficacy and safety of genetically engineered allogeneic human chondrocytes expressing TGF-B1 in patients with grade 3 chronic degenerative joint disease of the knee. *Osteoarthritis Cart.* **2015**, *23*, 2109–2118. [CrossRef]
57. Asnaghi, M.A.; Power, L.; Barbero, A.; Haug, M.; Köppl, R.; Wendt, D.; Martin, I. Biomarker signatures of quality for engineering nasal chondrocyte-derived cartilage. *Front. Bioeng. Biotechnol.* **2020**, *8*, 283. [CrossRef]
58. Teo, A.Q.A.; Wong, K.L.; Shen, L.; Lim, J.Y.; Wei, S.T.; Lee, H.; Hui, J.H.P. Equivalent 10-year outcomes after implantation of autologous bone marrow-derived mesenchymal stem cells versus autologous chondrocyte implantation for chondral defects of the knee. *Am. J. Sports Med.* **2019**, *47*, 2881–2887. [CrossRef]
59. Dhollander, A.A.; Verdonk, P.C.; Lambrecht, S.; Verdonk, R.; Elewaut, D.; Verbruggen, G.; Almqvist, K.F. Midterm results of the treatment of cartilage defects in the knee using alginate beads containing human mature allogenic chondrocytes. *Am. J. Sports Med.* **2012**, *40*, 75–82. [CrossRef] [PubMed]
60. Park, D.Y.; Min, B.H.; Park, S.R.; Oh, H.J.; Truong, M.D.; Kim, M.; Choi, J.Y.; Park, I.S.; Choi, B.H. Engineered cartilage utilizing fetal cartilage-derived progenitor cells for cartilage repair. *Sci. Rep.* **2020**, *10*, 5722. [CrossRef] [PubMed]
61. Ha, C.-W.; Noh, M.J.; Choi, K.B.; Lee, K.H. Initial phase I safety of retrovirally transduced human chondrocytes expressing transforming growth factor-beta-1 in degenerative arthritis patients. *Cytotherapy* **2012**, *14*, 247–256. [CrossRef] [PubMed]
62. Pelttari, K.; Pippenger, B.; Mumme, M.; Feliciano, S.; Scotti, C.; Mainil-Varlet, P.; Procino, A.; von Rechenberg, B.; Schwamborn, T.; Jakob, M.; et al. Adult human neural crest-derived cells for articular cartilage repair. *Sci. Transl. Med.* **2014**, *6*, 251ra119. [CrossRef] [PubMed]
63. Akgun, I.; Unlu, M.C.; Erdal, O.A.; Ogut, T.; Erturk, M.; Ovali, E.; Kantarci, F.; Caliskan, G.; Akgun, Y. Matrix-induced autologous mesenchymal stem cell implantation versus matrix-induced autologous chondrocyte implantation in the treatment of chondral defects of the knee: A 2-year randomized study. *Arch. Orthop. Trauma Surg.* **2015**, *135*, 251–263. [CrossRef] [PubMed]
64. Mortazavi, F.; Shafaei, H.; Soleimani Rad, J.; Rushangar, L.; Montaceri, A.; Jamshidi, M. High quality of infant chondrocytes in comparison with adult chondrocytes for cartilage tissue engineering. *World J. Plast. Surg.* **2017**, *6*, 183–189.
65. Laurent, A.; Rey, M.; Scaletta, C.; Abdel-Sayed, P.; Michetti, M.; Flahaut, M.; Raffoul, W.; de Buys Roessingh, A.; Hirt-Burri, N.; Applegate, L.A. Retrospectives on three decades of safe clinical experience with allogeneic dermal progenitor fibroblasts: High versatility in topical cytotherapeutic care. *Pharmaceutics* **2023**, *15*, 184. [CrossRef] [PubMed]
66. Philippe, V.; Laurent, A.; Abdel-Sayed, P.; Hirt-Burri, N.; Applegate, L.A.; Martin, R. Human platelet lysate as an alternative to autologous serum for human chondrocyte clinical use. *Cartilage* **2021**, *13*, 509S–518S. [CrossRef] [PubMed]
67. Chuma, H.; Mizuta, H.; Kudo, S.; Takagi, K.; Hiraki, Y. One day exposure to FGF-2 was sufficient for the regenerative repair of full-thickness defects of articular cartilage in rabbits. *Osteoarthritis Cart.* **2004**, *12*, 834–842. [CrossRef]
68. Tonomura, H.; Nagae, M.; Takatori, R.; Ishibashi, H.; Itsuji, T.; Takahashi, K. The potential role of hepatocyte growth factor in degenerative disorders of the synovial joint and spine. *Int. J. Mol. Sci.* **2020**, *21*, 8717. [CrossRef]
69. Muthu, S.; Korpershoek, J.V.; Novais, E.J.; Tawy, G.F.; Hollander, A.P.; Martin, I. Failure of cartilage regeneration: Emerging hypotheses and related therapeutic strategies. *Nat. Rev. Rheumatol.* **2023**, *19*, 403–416. [CrossRef]
70. Stampoultzis, T.; Guo, Y.; Nasrollahzadeh, N.; Karami, P.; Pioletti, D.P. Mimicking loading-induced cartilage self-heating in vitro promotes matrix formation in chondrocyte-laden constructs with different mechanical properties. *ACS Biomat. Sci. Eng.* **2023**, *9*, 651–661. [CrossRef]
71. Tran, N.T.; Truong, M.D.; Yun, H.W.; Min, B.H. Potential of secretome of human fetal cartilage progenitor cells as disease modifying agent for osteoarthritis. *Life Sci.* **2023**, *324*, 121741. [CrossRef]
72. Haeusner, S.; Herbst, L.; Bittorf, P.; Schwarz, T.; Henze, C.; Mauermann, M.; Ochs, J.; Schmitt, R.; Blache, U.; Wixmerten, A.; et al. From single batch to mass production-Automated platform design concept for a phase II clinical trial tissue engineered cartilage product. *Front. Med.* **2021**, *8*, 712917. [CrossRef] [PubMed]
73. Wixmerten, A.; Miot, S.; Bittorf, P.; Wolf, F.; Feliciano, S.; Hackenberg, S.; Häusner, S.; Krenger, W.; Haug, M.; Martin, I.; et al. Good Manufacturing Practice-compliant change of raw material in the manufacturing process of a clinically used advanced therapy medicinal product-A comparability study. *Cytotherapy* **2023**, *25*, 548–558. [CrossRef] [PubMed]
74. Hulme, C.H.; Garcia, J.; Mennan, C.; Perry, J.; Roberts, S.; Norris, K.; Baird, D.; Rix, L.; Banerjee, R.; Meyer, C.; et al. The up-scale manufacture of chondrocytes for allogeneic cartilage therapies. *Tissue Eng. Part C* **2023**. *online ahead of print*. [CrossRef] [PubMed]
75. Kutaish, H.; Tscholl, P.M.; Cosset, E.; Bengtsson, L.; Braunersreuther, V.; Mor, F.M.; Laedermann, J.; Furfaro, I.; Stafylakis, D.; Hannouche, D.; et al. Articular cartilage repair after implantation of hyaline cartilage beads engineered from adult dedifferentiated chondrocytes: Cartibeads preclinical efficacy study in a large animal model. *Am. J. Sports Med.* **2023**, *51*, 237–249. [CrossRef]
76. Marlovits, S.; Aldrian, S.; Wondrasch, B.; Zak, L.; Albrecht, C.; Welsch, G.; Trattnig, S. Clinical and radiological outcomes 5 years after matrix-induced autologous chondrocyte implantation in patients with symptomatic, traumatic chondral defects. *Am. J. Sports Med.* **2012**, *40*, 2273–2280. [CrossRef]
77. Nawaz, S.Z.; Bentley, G.; Briggs, T.W.; Carrington, R.W.; Skinner, J.A.; Gallagher, K.R.; Dhinsa, B.S. Autologous chondrocyte implantation in the knee: Mid-term to long-term results. *J. Bone Joint Surg.* **2014**, *96*, 824–830. [CrossRef]

78. Harris, J.D.; Siston, R.A.; Pan, X.; Flanigan, D.C. Autologous chondrocyte implantation: A systematic review. *J. Bone Joint Surg.* **2010**, *92*, 2220–2233. [CrossRef]
79. Aldrian, S.; Zak, L.; Wondrasch, B.; Albrecht, C.; Stelzeneder, B.; Binder, H.; Kovar, F.; Trattnig, S.; Marlovits, S. Clinical and radiological long-term outcomes after matrix-induced autologous chondrocyte transplantation: A prospective follow-up at a minimum of 10 years. *Am. J. Sports Med.* **2014**, *42*, 2680–2688. [CrossRef]
80. Basad, E.; Wissing, F.R.; Fehrenbach, P.; Rickert, M.; Steinmeyer, J.; Ishaque, B. Matrix-induced autologous chondrocyte implantation (MACI) in the knee: Clinical outcomes and challenges. *Knee Surg. Sports Traumatol. Arthrosc.* **2015**, *23*, 3729–3735. [CrossRef]
81. Tosoratti, E.; Fisch, P.; Taylor, S.; Laurent-Applegate, L.A.; Zenobi-Wong, M. 3D-printed reinforcement scaffolds with targeted biodegradation properties for the tissue engineering of articular cartilage. *Adv. Healthcare Mat.* **2021**, *10*, e2101094. [CrossRef]
82. Mumme, M.; Steinitz, A.; Nuss, K.M.; Klein, K.; Feliciano, S.; Kronen, P.; Jakob, M.; von Rechenberg, B.; Martin, I.; Barbero, A.; et al. Regenerative potential of tissue-engineered nasal chondrocytes in goat articular cartilage defects. *Tissue Eng. Part A* **2016**, *22*, 1286–1295. [CrossRef] [PubMed]
83. Mantripragada, V.P.; Muschler, G.F. Improved biological performance of human cartilage-derived progenitors in platelet lysate xenofree media in comparison to fetal bovine serum media. *Cur. Res. Transl. Med.* **2022**, *70*, 103353. [CrossRef] [PubMed]
84. Sykes, J.G.; Kuiper, J.H.; Richardson, J.B.; Roberts, S.; Wright, K.T.; Kuiper, N.J. Impact of human platelet lysate on the expansion and chondrogenic capacity of cultured human chondrocytes for cartilage cell therapy. *Eur. Cell Mater.* **2018**, *35*, 255–267. [CrossRef] [PubMed]
85. Kachroo, U.; Zachariah, S.M.; Thambaiah, A.; Tabasum, A.; Livingston, A.; Rebekah, G.; Srivastava, A.; Vinod, E. Comparison of human platelet lysate versus fetal bovine serum for expansion of human articular cartilage-derived chondroprogenitors. *Cartilage* **2021**, *13*, 107S–116S. [CrossRef] [PubMed]
86. Liau, L.L.; bin Hassan, M.N.F.; Tang, Y.L.; Ng, M.H.; Law, J.X. Feasibility of human platelet lysate as an alternative to fetal bovine serum for in vitro expansion of chondrocytes. *Int. J. Mol. Sci.* **2021**, *22*, 1269. [CrossRef]
87. Rikkers, M.; Levato, R.; Malda, J.; Vonk, L.A. Importance of timing of platelet lysate-supplementation in expanding or redifferentiating human chondrocytes for chondrogenesis. *Front. Bioeng. Biotechnol.* **2020**, *8*, 804. [CrossRef]
88. Gaissmaier, C.; Fritz, J.; Krackhardt, T.; Flesch, I.; Aicher, W.K.; Ashammakhi, N. Effect of human platelet supernatant on proliferation and matrix synthesis of human articular chondrocytes in monolayer and three-dimensional alginate cultures. *Biomaterials* **2005**, *26*, 1953–1960. [CrossRef]
89. Hildner, F.; Eder, M.J.; Hofer, K.; Aberl, J.; Redl, H.; van Griensven, M.; Gabriel, C.; Peterbauer-Scherb, A. Human platelet lysate successfully promotes proliferation and subsequent chondrogenic differentiation of adipose-derived stem cells: A comparison with articular chondrocytes. *J. Tissue Eng. Regen. Med.* **2015**, *9*, 808–818. [CrossRef]
90. Textor, M.; Hoburg, A.; Lehnigk, R.; Perka, C.; Duda, G.N.; Reinke, S.; Blankenstein, A.; Hochmann, S.; Stockinger, A.; Resch, H.; et al. Chondrocyte isolation from loose bodies—An option for reducing donor site morbidity for autologous chondrocyte implantation. *Int. J. Mol. Sci.* **2023**, *24*, 1484. [CrossRef]
91. Kim, J.; Park, J.; Song, S.Y.; Kim, E. Advanced therapy medicinal products for autologous chondrocytes and comparison of regulatory systems in target countries. *Regen. Ther.* **2022**, *20*, 126–137. [CrossRef]
92. Nordberg, R.C.; Otarola, G.A.; Wang, D.; Hu, J.C.; Athanasiou, K.A. Navigating regulatory pathways for translation of biologic cartilage repair products. *Sci. Transl. Med.* **2022**, *14*, eabp8163. [CrossRef] [PubMed]
93. Evans, C.H.; Ghivizzani, S.C.; Robbins, P.D. Orthopaedic gene therapy: Twenty-five years on. *JBJS Rev.* **2021**, *9*, e20. [CrossRef] [PubMed]
94. Salem, H.S.; Parvizi, J.; Ehiorobo, J.O.; Mont, M.A. The safety and efficacy of a novel cell-based gene therapy for knee osteoarthritis. *Surg. Technol. Int.* **2019**, *35*, 370–376.
95. Sadri, B.; Tamimi, A.; Nouraein, S.; Bagheri Fard, A.; Mohammadi, J.; Mohammadpour, M.; Hassanzadeh, M.; Bajouri, A.; Madani, H.; Barekat, M.; et al. Clinical and laboratory findings following transplantation of allogeneic adipose-derived mesenchymal stromal cells in knee osteoarthritis, a brief report. *Connect. Tissue Res.* **2022**, *63*, 663–674. [CrossRef]
96. Sadri, B.; Hassanzadeh, M.; Bagherifard, A.; Mohammadi, J.; Alikhani, M.; Moeinabadi-Bidgoli, K.; Madani, H.; Diaz-Solano, D.; Karimi, S.; Mehrazmay, M.; et al. Cartilage regeneration and inflammation modulation in knee osteoarthritis following injection of allogeneic adipose-derived mesenchymal stromal cells: A phase II, triple-blinded, placebo controlled, randomized trial. *Stem Cell Res. Ther.* **2023**, *14*, 162. [CrossRef] [PubMed]
97. Ikawa, T.; Yano, K.; Watanabe, N.; Masamune, K.; Yamato, M. Non-clinical assessment design of autologous chondrocyte implantation products. *Regen. Ther.* **2015**, *1*, 98–108. [CrossRef] [PubMed]
98. Kuah, D.; Sivell, S.; Longworth, T.; James, K.; Guermazi, A.; Cicuttini, F.; Wang, Y.; Craig, S.; Comin, G.; Robinson, D.; et al. Safety, tolerability and efficacy of intra-articular Progenza in knee osteoarthritis: A randomized double-blind placebo-controlled single ascending dose study. *J. Transl. Med.* **2018**, *16*, 49. [CrossRef] [PubMed]
99. Hamahashi, K.; Toyoda, E.; Ishihara, M.; Mitani, G.; Takagaki, T.; Kaneshiro, N.; Maehara, M.; Takahashi, T.; Okada, E.; Watanabe, A.; et al. Polydactyly-derived allogeneic chondrocyte cell-sheet transplantation with high tibial osteotomy as regenerative therapy for knee osteoarthritis. *NPJ Regen. Med.* **2022**, *7*, 71. [CrossRef]

100. Chijimatsu, R.; Kobayashi, M.; Ebina, K.; Iwahashi, T.; Okuno, Y.; Hirao, M.; Fukuhara, A.; Nakamura, N.; Yoshikawa, H. Impact of dexamethasone concentration on cartilage tissue formation from human synovial derived stem cells in vitro. *Cytotechnology* **2018**, *70*, 819–829. [CrossRef]
101. Oseni, A.O.; Butler, P.E.; Seifalian, A.M. Optimization of chondrocyte isolation and characterization for large-scale cartilage tissue engineering. *J. Surg. Res.* **2013**, *181*, 41–48. [CrossRef]
102. Albrecht, C.; Tichy, B.; Nürnberger, S.; Hosiner, S.; Zak, L.; Aldrian, S.; Marlovits, S. Gene expression and cell differentiation in matrix-associated chondrocyte transplantation grafts: A comparative study. *Osteoarthritis Cart.* **2011**, *19*, 1219–1227. [CrossRef] [PubMed]
103. Brun, P.; Dickinson, S.C.; Zavan, B.; Cortivo, R.; Hollander, A.P.; Abatangelo, G. Characteristics of repair tissue in second-look and third-look biopsies from patients treated with engineered cartilage: Relationship to symptomatology and time after implantation. *Arthritis Res. Ther.* **2008**, *10*, R132. [CrossRef] [PubMed]
104. Kon, E.; Di Martino, A.; Filardo, G.; Tetta, C.; Busacca, M.; Iacono, F.; Delcogliano, M.; Albisinni, U.; Marcacci, M. Second-generation autologous chondrocyte transplantation: MRI findings and clinical correlations at a minimum 5-year follow-up. *Europ. J. Radiol.* **2011**, *79*, 382–388. [CrossRef]
105. Harris, J.D.; Siston, R.A.; Brophy, R.H.; Lattermann, C.; Carey, J.L.; Flanigan, D.C. Failures, re-operations, and complications after autologous chondrocyte implantation—A systematic review. *Osteoarthritis Cart.* **2011**, *19*, 779–791. [CrossRef] [PubMed]
106. World Medical Association. Declaration of Helsinki: Ethical principles for medical research involving human subjects. *JAMA* **2013**, *310*, 2191–2194. [CrossRef] [PubMed]
107. Bukovac, P.K.; Hauser, M.; Lottaz, D.; Marti, A.; Schmitt, I.; Schochat, T. The regulation of cell therapy and gene therapy products in Switzerland. *Adv. Exp. Med. Biol.* **2023**, *1430*, 41–58. [CrossRef]

pharmaceutics

*Article*

# Cutaneous Cell Therapy Manufacturing Timeframe Rationalization: Allogeneic Off-the-Freezer Fibroblasts for Dermo-Epidermal Combined Preparations (DE-FE002-SK2) in Burn Care

**Xi Chen [1,†], Alexis Laurent [1,2,3,†], Zhifeng Liao [1], Sandra Jaccoud [1,4], Philippe Abdel-Sayed [1,5,6], Marjorie Flahaut [1,6], Corinne Scaletta [1], Wassim Raffoul [1,6], Lee Ann Applegate [1,6,7,8,*,‡] and Nathalie Hirt-Burri [1,*,‡]**

1 Plastic, Reconstructive and Hand Surgery Service, Lausanne University Hospital, University of Lausanne, CH-1011 Lausanne, Switzerland; xi.chen.1@unil.ch (X.C.); alexis.laurent@unil.ch (A.L.); liao.zhifeng@unil.ch (Z.L.); sandra.jaccoud@chuv.ch (S.J.); philippe.abdel-sayed@chuv.ch (P.A.-S.); marjorie.flahaut@chuv.ch (M.F.); corinne.scaletta@chuv.ch (C.S.); wassim.raffoul@chuv.ch (W.R.)
2 Manufacturing Department, TEC-PHARMA SA, CH-1038 Bercher, Switzerland
3 Manufacturing Department, LAM Biotechnologies SA, CH-1066 Epalinges, Switzerland
4 Laboratory of Biomechanical Orthopedics, Federal Polytechnic School of Lausanne, CH-1015 Lausanne, Switzerland
5 STI School of Engineering, Federal Polytechnic School of Lausanne, CH-1015 Lausanne, Switzerland
6 Lausanne Burn Center, Lausanne University Hospital, University of Lausanne, CH-1011 Lausanne, Switzerland
7 Center for Applied Biotechnology and Molecular Medicine, University of Zurich, CH-8057 Zurich, Switzerland
8 Oxford OSCAR Suzhou Center, Oxford University, Suzhou 215123, China
* Correspondence: lee.laurent-applegate@chuv.ch (L.A.A.); nathalie.burri@chuv.ch (N.H.-B.); Tel.: +41-21-314-35-10 (L.A.A. & N.H.-B.)
† These authors contributed equally to this work.
‡ These authors also contributed equally to this work.

**Abstract:** Autologous cell therapy manufacturing timeframes constitute bottlenecks in clinical management pathways of severe burn patients. While effective temporary wound coverings exist for high-TBSA burns, any means to shorten the time-to-treatment with cytotherapeutic skin grafts could provide substantial therapeutic benefits. This study aimed to establish proofs-of-concept for a novel combinational cytotherapeutic construct (autologous/allogeneic DE-FE002-SK2 full dermo-epidermal graft) designed for significant cutaneous cell therapy manufacturing timeframe rationalization. Process development was based on several decades (four for autologous protocols, three for allogeneic protocols) of in-house clinical experience in cutaneous cytotherapies. Clinical grade dermal progenitor fibroblasts (standardized FE002-SK2 cell source) were used as off-the-freezer substrates in novel autologous/allogeneic dermo-epidermal bilayer sheets. Under vitamin C stimulation, FE002-SK2 primary progenitor fibroblasts rapidly produced robust allogeneic dermal templates, allowing patient keratinocyte attachment in co-culture. Notably, FE002-SK2 primary progenitor fibroblasts significantly outperformed patient fibroblasts for collagen deposition. An ex vivo de-epidermalized dermis model was used to demonstrate the efficient DE-FE002-SK2 construct bio-adhesion properties. Importantly, the presented DE-FE002-SK2 manufacturing process decreased clinical lot production timeframes from 6–8 weeks (standard autologous combined cytotherapies) to 2–3 weeks. Overall, these findings bear the potential to significantly optimize burn patient clinical pathways (for rapid wound closure and enhanced tissue healing quality) by combining extensively clinically proven cutaneous cell-based technologies.

**Keywords:** autologous keratinocytes; burn center; cutaneous cell therapy; dermal template; dermo-epidermal grafts; early coverage solutions; FE002 dermal progenitor fibroblasts; manufacturing optimization; severe burns; standardized skin grafts

## 1. Introduction

Despite considerable constitutive regenerative potential, human skin is often incapable of managing serious burn injuries without exogenous interventions [1,2]. Thermal burns cause necrosis of the epidermis and of underlying tissues and structures. The extent of the related damage depends on the temperature to which the cutaneous cells and tissues are exposed and on the duration of said exposure [1]. The resulting high morbidity is intrinsically modulated by the wound depth and surface (i.e., burn degree) or by the severity of inhalation co-injuries [1,2]. Specifically, major burn victims are qualified upon initial presentation of $\geq$20% total body surface area (TBSA) lesions for adults and $\geq$10% TBSA lesions for pediatric patients [1–3]. Overall, severe burn patient care, remission, and rehabilitation are often long and painful [2,3].

Highly specialized therapeutic care centers are necessary for the effective management of severe burn victims [3]. With a yearly incidence of around 100 adult and pediatric burn cases, Switzerland is served by three specialized and multidisciplinary university hospital platforms (i.e., combined adult and pediatric pathway in Western Switzerland; separate centers in Eastern Switzerland) [3–5]. When considering the acute phase of burn victim care, patient resuscitation is followed by lesion characterization and escharotomies, as required (Figure S1). During the subsequent cardiorespiratory stabilization phase, the affected area is debrided, and a topical antiseptic (e.g., Ialugen Plus, Aquacel Ag) is applied [3]. Rapid wound coverage may be attained using appropriate bandages such as Mepitel, Polymem, Kaltostat, or DuoDerm. In severe cases, cadaver skin (i.e., human or porcine) or advanced coverage solutions (e.g., TransCyte, Lyphoderm, Apligraf, ReCell, OrCel, Epicel, Allox) can be deployed to prevent catastrophic fluid loss and to stimulate structural/functional restauration [6–12]. Thereafter, cutaneous stabilization is addressed by permanent wound closure using various surgical and/or grafting procedures [2–5,10].

From a cytotherapeutic viewpoint, burn wound stabilization and closure have been successfully performed using stratified autologous keratinocyte cultures (i.e., cultured epithelial autografts, CEA, Figure S2) [13–16]. In addition to half a century of available clinical hindsight, this approach is characterized by limited iatrogenesis related to autologous skin harvests, contrasting with split-thickness grafting [17–24]. While constituting a therapeutic breakthrough, classical CEA-based protocols are inherently technically limited by the in vitro graft manufacturing timeframes of 2–3 weeks [3,4,21]. Despite the commercial availability of various autologous keratinocyte preparation types (i.e., cell sheets or spray formats, e.g., EpicelT, ReCell), widespread clinical adoption has not yet been achieved. Notably, dependency towards the use of embryonic 3T3 murine feeder layers (i.e., for autologous keratinocyte culture) and the extensive manufacturing temporal constraints have not yet been satisfactorily addressed [25,26].

Furthermore, it has been reported for severe burn patients that CEA-treated cutaneous structures are often characterized by sub-optimal quality and by mechanical fragility due to the absence of a dermis to support the epidermal layer or due to poor graft integration [18]. To enhance the efficacy of the intervention, the tissue engineering technique has evolved to include a co-cultured basal dermal component (i.e., functionally stimulated patient fibroblasts), forming cultured dermo-epidermal autografts (CDEAs, Figure S3) [18,20,27]. However, the major technical drawback incurred by this combinational approach is the additionally extended manufacturing timeframe of 6–8 weeks for clinical grade CDEA production [28–31]. Notwithstanding, available clinical reports on CDEA use in burn care have confirmed the superior efficacy and enhanced tissular repair quality compared to CEA treatment [27–32]. Mechanistically, human dermal fibroblasts have notably been functionally characterized to aid in modeling collagen fibers and in secreting factors for epidermalization. Therefore, the presence of functional fibroblasts in modern cutaneous cytotherapies was considered necessary to promote epidermal outgrowth [33,34].

Clinically applied in the Lausanne Burn Center for over twenty years, CDEA constructs were shown to enhance the quality of skin repairs in burn victims compared to CEAs, themselves clinically used locally since 1985 [27]. However, the lack of an optimal early wound coverage solution for transient wound management prior to CDEA application was assessed as a major clinical bottleneck [5,10]. Therefore, in order to mitigate risks for the patient and to optimally prepare the wound bed before CDEA grafting, Integra membranes were locally used as temporary coverings [21,27]. As an alternative and bioactive early wound coverage solution, allogeneic progenitor biological bandages (PBBs) were developed and have been clinically applied in Lausanne since 2004 [35–39]. Designed and manufactured under the Swiss progenitor cell transplantation program, PBBs consist of banked allogeneic dermal progenitor fibroblasts (i.e., clinical grade FE002-SK2 cell source) formulated for topical delivery on resorbable equine collagen sheets (Figure S4, Table S1) [35–39]. Over two decades, viable allogeneic dermal progenitor fibroblasts have been cytotherapeutically applied on over 160 patients in Lausanne, where no safety-related concerns have been raised and an enhanced repair tissue quality was clearly evidenced [37,39]. Importantly, PBBs were found to optimally act as a "first cover" solution in view of early wound bed preparation (i.e., biological stimulation over the first 10–12 days) for eventual autologous skin grafting [37]. In several reported clinical cases, the use of PBBs alone drastically reduced or even negated the need for subsequent skin grafting, CEA use, or CDEA use [36–39].

Based on the combined translational and clinical experience gained in the Lausanne Burn Center with CEAs, CDEAs, and PBBs, a new generation of autologous/allogeneic constructs was devised for significant manufacturing and clinical workflow rationalization. Therefore, the objective of this study consisted in the establishment of in vitro and ex vivo functional proofs-of-concept for the DE-FE002-SK2 dermo-epidermal construct based on allogeneic dermal progenitor fibroblasts and autologous keratinocytes. Clinical grade FE002-SK2 cells were firstly used as standardized off-the-freezer allogeneic substrates and were stimulated with vitamin C for rapid preparation of a collagen-rich dermal template [40]. Secondly, patient primary keratinocytes were co-cultured on the allogeneic dermal template to form a stratified epidermal layer. Importantly, the presented multiphasic process for DE-FE002-SK2 dermo-epidermal construct preparation decreased the cutaneous graft manufacturing timeframes from 6–8 weeks (i.e., standard CDEA protocol) to 2–3 weeks. Finally, an ex vivo de-epidermalized dermis (DED) model was used to functionally characterize the DE-FE002-SK2 construct and validate its applicability in a clinical setting. Overall, this work sets the technical basis for potentially significantly optimized burn patient clinical care using clinically proven and standardized biologicals with rationalized manufacturing resources.

## 2. Materials and Methods

### *2.1. Ethical Compliance of the Study*

Obtention and use of patient primary cellular materials (i.e., primary fibroblast and keratinocyte cell types) followed the regulations of the Biobank of the Department of Musculoskeletal Medicine at the CHUV (Lausanne University Hospital, Lausanne, Switzerland). Biological materials and anonymous patient information materials were included in the biobank following patient consent documentation and protocol validation by the Vaud Cantonal Ethics Committee (University Hospital of Lausanne, Ethics Committee Protocol N°264/12). The clinical grade primary progenitor cell source used in the present study (i.e., FE002-SK2 primary progenitor fibroblasts) was established from the FE002 organ donation, as approved by the Vaud Cantonal Ethics Committee (University Hospital of Lausanne, Ethics Committee Protocol N°62/07). The FE002 organ donation was registered under a federal cell transplantation program (i.e., Swiss progenitor cell transplantation program). Appropriate material traceability and anonymity maintenance protocols were applied during the study.

### *2.2. Materials and Consumables Used for the Study*

The reagents and consumables which were used in this study are listed hereafter: purified water, PBS buffer, and NaCl 0.9% solutions (Bichsel, Unterseen, Switzerland); high-glucose DMEM cell culture medium, L-glutamine, D-PBS, TrypLE dissociation reagent, MTT, and antibodies (Thermo Fisher Scientific, Waltham, MA, USA); penicillin-streptomycin and trypsin (Life Technologies, Paisley, UK); CnT-PR medium (CellnTec, Bern, Switzerland); C-Chip Neubauer hemocytometers (NanoEntek, Seoul, Republic of Korea); ethanol and HCl (Chemie Brunschwig, Basel, Switzerland); methanol (Fluka, Buchs, Switzerland); EDTA and gentamycin (Lausanne University Hospital, Lausanne, Switzerland); mitomycin C (Medac Pharma, Chicago, IL, USA); cholera toxin (Lubio Science, Zurich, Switzerland); hydrocortisone (Pfizer, New York, NY, USA); insulin (Novo Nordisk Pharma, Bagsværd, Danemark); Millipore Stericup with 0.22 μm pores, milliQ water, Ham's F12 medium, EGF, vitamin C, picric acid, sodium hydroxide, sodium chloride, Trypan Blue solution, and FBS (Merck, Darmstadt, Germany); formalin-buffered solution, dispase, paraffin, H&E stain, xylene, and $H_2O_2$ (Sigma Aldrich, Buchs, Switzerland); Sirius Red solution and antibodies (Abcam, Cambridge, UK); antibodies (Vector Laboratories, Newark, CA, USA); a ChromoMap DAB kit (Roche Diagnostics, Rotkreuz, Switzerland); rat tail collagen and agar (Corning Life Sciences, Tewksbury, MA, USA); cell culture vessels and plastic assay surfaces (Greiner BioOne, Frickenhausen, Germany; Corning, New York, NY, USA; and TPP Techno Plastic Products, Trasadingen, Switzerland); and Vaseline gauze (Smith and Nephew, Watford, UK).

### 2.3. Equipment Used for the Study

Component weighing was performed on a laboratory scale (Ohaus, Parsippany, NJ, USA). Sample centrifugation was performed on a Sorvall Legend Micro 21R microcentrifuge (Thermo Fisher Scientific, Waltham, MA, USA). Absorbance measurements were performed on a Varioskan LUX multimode plate reader (Thermo Fisher Scientific, Waltham, MA, USA). Absorbance data were analyzed using the Skanit-RE software v5.0 (Thermo Fisher Scientific, Waltham, MA, USA). Immunohistology sample preparation was performed using a Ventana Discovery ULTRA system (Roche Diagnostics, Rotkreuz, Switzerland). Immunohistochemistry imaging was performed on an inverted IX81 fluorescence microscope (Olympus, Tokyo, Japan). Macroscopic imaging was performed on an iPhone 12 (Apple, Cupertino, CA, USA).

### 2.4. Primary Cell Sourcing and Cellular Raw Material Manufacture

Patient primary fibroblasts and keratinocytes were isolated and cultured from skin tissue designated as medical waste following routine abdominoplasties at the Lausanne University Hospital. At reception, each skin biopsy was washed several times in PBS with 1% penicillin–streptomycin to remove the residual blood cells. Subcutaneous fat was completely ablated using a scalpel. Then, the skin biopsies were incubated in DMEM with 10 mg/mL dispase overnight at 4 °C and then in 0.05% trypsin–EDTA for 30 min at 37 °C, after which the dermis was mechanically separated from the epidermis using forceps.

For primary keratinocyte isolation by enzymatic digestion, the epidermis was cut into small fragments and was transferred to a tube containing EDTA 0.02% and trypsin 0.25% in 1:1 proportion. The digestion tubes were incubated for 30 min at 37 °C on a rotational shaker. This step was repeated at least twice to obtain a maximal cell yield. Then, keratinocytes were enumerated and were seeded in vitro at a density of $2–3 \times 10^4$ cells/cm$^2$. The cells were either seeded in CnT-PR medium and incubated at 37 °C under 5% $CO_2$ or they were cultured on a feeder layer of proprietary 3T3-J2 mouse fibroblasts. The 3T3-J2 feeder fibroblasts were inactivated for 2 h using 4 μg/mL mitomycin C. In the feeder layer group, the keratinocyte proliferation medium was composed of DMEM and Ham's F12 with a 3:1 proportion, with 20 μg/mL gentamycin, 0.14 nM cholera toxin, 400 ng/mL hydrocortisone, 8.3 ng/mL EGF, 832.2 μM L-glutamine, 0.12 U/mL insulin, and 10% FBS. All the cultures were maintained in humidified incubators at 37 °C with 5% $CO_2$ and the cell proliferation medium was exchanged three times per week. Primary keratinocytes were serially expanded in vitro and were used for experiments at passage levels 3–6. The cells were cryopreserved in a solution of 50% DMEM, 40% FBS, and 10% DMSO at a cellular density of $10^6$ viable cells/vial.

For primary fibroblast isolation by explanting, the dermis was cut into small fragments and was transferred to a tissue culture dish. The tissue fragments were minced and placed within a checkboard pattern created on the culture surface by mechanical scoring. The fibroblast proliferation medium was composed of high-glucose DMEM supplemented with 2 mM L-glutamine and 10% FBS. The cultures were maintained in humidified incubators at 37 °C with 5% $CO_2$ and the cell proliferation medium was exchanged twice per week. Once the cells reached 50–70% confluency, they were transferred and expanded in culture flasks, with medium exchange procedures performed twice per week. Primary fibroblasts were serially expanded in vitro and were used for experiments at passage levels 3–6. The cells were cryopreserved as described hereabove.

For primary dermal progenitor fibroblast use, cryopreserved cellular materials were procured under the Swiss progenitor cell transplantation program. Clinical grade FE002-SK2 primary progenitor fibroblast vials were used as cellular starting materials and were serially expanded in vitro. The cells were seeded at viable densities of $1.5 \times 10^3$, $3 \times 10^3$, $5 \times 10^3$, and $20 \times 10^3$ cells/cm$^2$ and were maintained in culture until the monolayers attained confluency. The progenitor fibroblast proliferation medium was composed of high-glucose DMEM supplemented with 2 mM L-glutamine and 10% FBS. The cultures were maintained in humidified incubators at 37 °C with 5% $CO_2$ and the cell proliferation medium was exchanged twice per week. Primary progenitor fibroblasts were serially expanded in vitro and were used for experiments at passage levels 5–12. The cells were cryopreserved as described hereabove.

### 2.5. Dermal Template Preparation: In Vitro Collagen Synthesis Induction Conditions

In order to prepare the basal component of standard CDEAs or of DE-FE002-SK2 constructs, primary fibroblasts were used to synthesize extracellular matrix components (e.g., collagens). For the autologous group, primary patient fibroblasts were used according to the standard CDEA manufacturing protocols [3]. For the allogeneic group, clinical grade FE002-SK2 primary progenitor fibroblasts were used following the same protocol. Briefly, confluent fibroblast cultures were harvested and the cells were seeded in 12-well culture plates at a viable density of $3 \times 10^3$ cells/cm$^2$. The cultures were maintained as described hereabove. When the cells reached 100% confluency, the fibroblast proliferation medium was exchanged for fibroblast induction medium supplemented with $10^{-4}$ M vitamin C to induce collagen production. The induction medium was replaced every 2 days for 1 week. Then, the treated cell monolayers were washed with 1× PBS, fixed with −20 °C methanol for 10 min, rinsed 3 times with 1× PBS, and stored at −80 °C until further use.

### 2.6. Allogeneic Dermal Template Preparation: In Vitro Manufacturing Optimization

As global manufacturing timeframe rationalization constituted the main objective of this study, specific technical optimization work aimed to reduce the time necessary for allogeneic dermal template preparation for the DE-FE002-SK2 constructs to a minimum. Specific process design elements were taken into consideration, such as cellular material availability, GMP manufacturing suite occupation, and targeted production timelines [3]. Within the allogeneic protocol, cryopreserved vials of FE002-SK2 primary progenitor fibroblasts were thawed and used at various cell seeding densities (i.e., 1.5–20 $\times 10^3$ cells/cm$^2$) to determine optimal and condensed culture technical specifications (i.e., shortest culture time with sparing use of cell stocks). The cultures were otherwise maintained as described hereabove. The time to confluency was monitored for each seeding cellular density group. Operator assessments were independently performed by 3 experienced cellular biologists (i.e., trained in the development and release of cutaneous grafts produced for severe burn patients) in standardized blind experimental set-ups.

### 2.7. Dermal Template Characterization Assay: Sirius Red Staining and Collagen Quantification

In order to quantitatively and comparatively assess the production of collagens by the prepared dermal templates, Sirius Red staining and subsequent quantification were performed at various timepoints of the primary fibroblast induction phase (i.e., after 0, 2, 4, and 7 days). To prepare a standard curve, serial dilutions of rat tail collagen (i.e., at 3200, 1600, 800, 400, 200, 100, 50, 25, 12.5, 6.25, and 0 µg/mL) were performed in 1× PBS. Equal 150 µL volumes of collagen standard were dispensed in triplicate in a 96-well microplate. The plates were incubated at 37 °C overnight to evaporate the liquid phase. Each well was then gently rinsed 4 times with milliQ water. The collagen standards were stained with 150 µL of 0.1% Sirius Red in 1.3% picric acid aqueous solution for 1 h at ambient temperature and under agitation. Macroscopic and microscopic imaging were performed. For Sirius Red stain quantification, 150 µL of 0.1 M NaOH was added to the wells and the plates were incubated for 30 min at ambient temperature under agitation. The samples were then transferred to a new 96-well microplate and absorbance measurements were performed at a wavelength of 560 nm. For the analysis of the prepared dermal template samples, the corresponding 12-well plates were thawed at ambient temperature. The same Sirius Red staining and quantification steps were performed as described hereabove for the reference standards. The data were analyzed using the Skanit-RE software with a linear regression curve.

### 2.8. Combined DE-FE002-SK2 Construct Manufacturing Process

In order to prepare DE-FE002-SK2 dermo-epidermal constructs, FE002-SK2 primary progenitor fibroblasts were seeded in 6-well plates at a viable density of $3 \times 10^3$ cells/cm$^2$ and the cultures were maintained with medium exchanges performed twice weekly. Once confluency was reached after one week of culture, the cells were treated with fibroblast induction medium, which was exchanged every 2 days for one week. Primary patient keratinocytes were grown in parallel in CnT-PR medium or on 3T3-J2 feeder layers with keratinocyte proliferation medium. Upon reaching 60–80% confluency, the keratinocytes were enzymatically harvested to form a cell suspension and were transferred by cell seeding on top of the induced fibroblasts (i.e., 5–10 $\times 10^5$ keratinocytes/well). Then, the fibroblast–keratinocyte co-cultures were maintained for one week in keratinocyte proliferation medium.

At the end of the bilayer construct manufacturing phase, a part of the obtained samples was transferred onto a Vaseline gauze and was then deposited on top of a de-epidermalized dermis model (DED, see Section 2.10 for a process description of model preparation/validation) to mimic burned skin treatment. The other part of the obtained samples was washed in 1× PBS and was fixed with formalin-buffered solution for 15 min. Then, the sheets were gently detached from the wells with a brush, and 1% agar was poured in the wells. The samples were conserved at 4 °C for 3 days before being embedded in paraffin for histology assays.

In order to prepare epidermal constructs as controls, the standard CEA manufacturing protocol was used [3]. Briefly, primary patient keratinocytes were cultured on 3T3-J2 feeder layers until reaching hyperconfluency. Then, the stratified keratinocyte sheets were transferred onto a Vaseline gauze and were used for the DED or the histology assays.

### 2.9. Combined DE-FE002-SK2 Construct Structural Characterization: Histology and Immunohistochemistry Assays

In order to process the obtained constructs for histological analysis, a standard protocol was used. Briefly, the tissues were embedded in paraffin wax blocks and were sectioned to 7 µm in thickness with a microtome before being placed on glass slides. The slides were stained with hematoxylin and eosin (H&E) and Haris hematoxylin.

P63 immunohistochemistry was performed on the samples to assess the presence of keratinocytes in the different constructs. Therefore, the embedded sample sections were deparaffinized in xylene (i.e., twice for 10 min) and were sequentially passed through 100%

ethanol (i.e., twice for 10 min), 90% ethanol (i.e., once for 10 min), and 74% ethanol (i.e., once for 10 min). Then, a 30 min incubation step in $H_2O_2$ (i.e., 10% in 1× PBS) was performed to block endogenous peroxidase activity. Subsequently, the sections were washed and then incubated with 2.5% horse serum for 1 h. The slides were then incubated overnight at 4 °C with a rabbit anti-p63 antibody (i.e., 1:2000 dilution, N°ab124762, Abcam) for human keratinocyte visualization. The following day, after the washing steps, the appropriate secondary antibody (i.e., horse anti-rabbit) was added to the slides and the samples were incubated for 1 h. The revelation step using ImmPact DAB was performed under the microscope for less than 2 min. Following immunohistochemical staining, the slides were counterstained with fastRed and mounted on resin with glass coverslips. The negative controls were obtained by omitting the addition of the primary antibodies.

Ki67 immunohistochemistry was performed on the samples to assess the presence of proliferating cells in the different constructs. Detection of cell proliferation was performed using a rabbit α-Ki67 antibody (i.e., 1:100 dilution, SP6, N°MA5-14520, Thermo Fisher Scientific) and the fully automated Ventana Discovery ULTRA system (Roche Diagnostics, Rotkreuz, Switzerland). Briefly, dewaxed and rehydrated paraffin sections were pre-treated with heat using standard conditions (40 min) in the CC1 solution. The samples were incubated with the primary antibodies at 37 °C for 1 h. After incubation with a secondary rabbit HRP antibody (i.e., N°MP 7401, Vector Laboratories), chromogenic revelation was performed with a ChromoMap DAB kit. The sections were counterstained with Harris hematoxylin and permanently mounted. Ki67 immunohistochemistry was performed at the Histology Core Facility of the Swiss Federal Institute of Technology in Lausanne (EPFL, Lausanne, Switzerland).

### *2.10. Combined DE-FE002-SK2 Construct Functional Characterization: Ex Vivo De-Epidermalized Dermis Model*

The protocol for establishing the ex vivo DED model was adapted from MacNeil et al. [41]. Briefly, the DED model was prepared by cutting abdominoplasty skin sections into 1–2 $cm^2$ pieces, which were then incubated at 37 °C for at least 24 h and up to 72 h in 1 M NaCl, where the duration of the incubation step was dependent on the treated sample. The incubation step in NaCl (i.e., 24 h in general) was sufficient to enable epidermis detachment, but without causing damage or destruction to the dermal component. The epidermis was delicately removed from the dermis using forceps to obtain a decellularized, de-epidermalized dermis (DED) section. The DED samples were washed several times with 1× PBS and were stored at 4 °C until use. For validation of the DED model (i.e., to verify the absence of keratinocytes on the dermal component following NaCl incubation), the experimental materials were qualified using histology, immunohistochemistry, and MTT controls (i.e., following treatment and after a recovery period in culture medium), for general exclusion of the presence of metabolically active cells and specific exclusion of the presence of keratinocytes on the dermal structures.

For the assays, DED samples were transferred into 12-well plates with 1 mL of keratinocyte proliferation medium and were incubated at 37 °C under 5% $CO_2$ for 24 h. Then, the cultured DE-FE002-SK2 constructs (i.e., on Vaseline gauze) were transferred to the top of the DED sections and the plates were incubated for one week. The culture medium was exchanged twice weekly. After one week, a part of the samples was fixed in formalin for 24 h at ambient temperature, rinsed with 1× PBS, and placed in 70% ethanol at 4 °C until paraffin inclusion. Another part of the samples was stained with MTT to assess cellular viability and homogeneity. Therefore, DED samples were stained with 0.5 mg/mL MTT in PBS for 2 h at 37 °C and then washed twice with PBS.

Control samples were prepared using different combinations of cultured cells (i.e., FE002-SK2 fibroblasts and patient keratinocytes), which were deposited on the DED model. Therefore, 8-mm diameter glass inserts were placed on the surface of the DED sections and 100 μL of cell suspensions in proliferation medium was dispensed in the insert. The plates were incubated for 3 days to enable cellular attachment. Then, the glass inserts were removed and the DED samples were deposited on a plastic grid to constitute an air–liquid interface.

*2.11. Statistical Analyses and Data Presentation*

The presented experiments were performed in triplicate and using three experimental repetitions unless specified otherwise. For statistical comparison of average values from two sets of data, a paired Student's *t*-test was applied after appropriate evaluation of the normal distribution of the data. For a statistical comparison of values from multiple quantitative datasets from experiments where multiple variables applied, a one-way ANOVA test or a two-way repeated measures ANOVA test was performed and was followed by a post hoc Tukey's multiple comparison test. A $p$-value < 0.05 was retained as a base for statistical significance determination. The calculations were performed using Microsoft Excel (Microsoft Corporation, Redmond, WA, USA) and GraphPad Prism version 8.0.2 (GraphPad Software, San Diego, CA, USA). Data were presented using Microsoft PowerPoint and GraphPad Prism version 8.0.2.

## 3. Results

*3.1. FE002-SK2 Primary Progenitor Fibroblasts Are Functionally Superior to Patient Fibroblasts for In Vitro Collagen Synthesis*

For tangible consideration of an autologous to allogeneic substitution of the fibroblast cell source in CDEAs, in vitro benchmarking of critical functional attributes was necessary. Therefore, the potential of both primary fibroblast types for in vitro collagen synthesis under vitamin C induction was comparatively assessed in two types of culture media (i.e., fibroblast and keratinocyte proliferation medium, respectively). The results indicated that patient fibroblasts and FE002-SK2 primary progenitor fibroblasts were functionally stimulated (i.e., significantly increased collagen synthesis after 7 days) by the addition of vitamin C in all conditions (Figure 1, Table S2).

Overall, a trend of higher collagen synthesis was exhibited in the groups of primary cells which were induced in keratinocyte proliferation medium compared to the fibroblast proliferation medium (Figure 1B). Additionally, the differences in endpoint collagen levels between the cell types were less pronounced in the keratinocyte proliferation medium (Figure 1B). Furthermore, it was noted that the baseline collagen synthesis levels of the FE002-SK2 primary progenitor fibroblasts were systematically higher than those of the primary patient fibroblasts (i.e., all experimental groups and conditions, Figure 1). The results indicated that the FE002-SK2 primary progenitor fibroblasts synthesized more than twice the amount of collagen in 7 days of culture/induction in fibroblast medium compared to patient fibroblasts (Figure 1(A5)). The optimal technical specifications for dermal template manufacture (i.e., maximization of collagen synthesis) comprised vitamin C induction of FE002-SK2 primary progenitor fibroblasts for 7 days in keratinocyte proliferation medium (Figure 1). Therefore, these specifications were used for the manufacture of the functional allogeneic dermal template component in DE-FE002-SK2 constructs.

*3.2. DE-FE002-SK2 Constructs Can Be Manufactured for Clinical Use in Three Weeks*

In addition to collagen-producing functions, another main advantage of using an off-the-freezer allogeneic cell source resides in the temporal decoupling of lengthy cell manufacturing phases from the clinical workflow. Clinical grade cryopreserved FE002-SK2 cell stocks (e.g., for PBB batches) were used for a brief monolayer expansion phase before vitamin C stimulation for rapid allogeneic dermal template preparation [37]. With a targeted cellular expansion time of 7 days, various culture technical specifications were tested. The various culture groups were monitored by three experienced operators and were maintained until confluency levels of 95–100% were reached. The results indicated that a cell seeding density of 6000 cells/cm$^2$ produced confluent monolayers after 7 days of culture (Table 1).

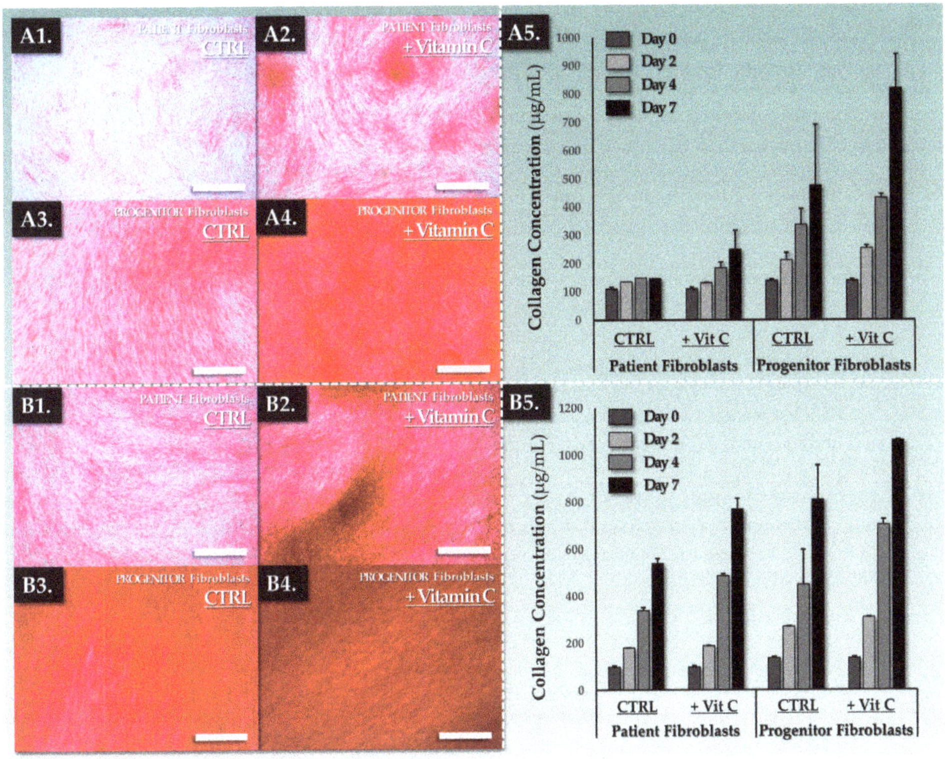


**Figure 1.** In vitro comparative functional characterization of primary patient fibroblasts and FE002-SK2 primary progenitor fibroblasts. (**A1–A4**) Endpoint imaging of Sirius Red staining for both primary fibroblast types following 7 days of vitamin C induction in fibroblast proliferation medium. Scale bars = 400 µm for patient fibroblasts and 200 µm for progenitor fibroblasts. (**A5**) Time-course of collagen synthesis during vitamin C induction in fibroblast proliferation medium. (**B1–B4**) Endpoint imaging of Sirius Red staining for both primary fibroblast types following 7 days of vitamin C induction in keratinocyte proliferation medium. Scale bars = 400 µm for patient fibroblasts and 200 µm for progenitor fibroblasts. (**B5**) Time-course of collagen synthesis during vitamin C induction in keratinocyte proliferation medium. Results of the statistical analyses relative to collagen quantification experiments under vitamin C stimulation are presented in Table S2. CTRL, control group; Vit C, vitamin C.

**Table 1.** Quantitative results of the optimization study for the allogeneic FE002-SK2 primary progenitor fibroblast expansion phase. For the needs of the experiments, cryopreserved FE002-SK2 primary progenitor fibroblasts at passage level 10 were used as cell seeding materials.

| Parameters | Values/Results | | | |
|---|---|---|---|---|
| Cell seeding density (viable cells/cm$^2$) | 1500 | 3000 | 6000 | 20,000 |
| Time to confluency (days) | $12 \pm 2$ | $10 \pm 2$ | $7 \pm 1$ | $4 \pm 0.5$ |
| Medium exchange procedures (n) | 5 | 4 | 3 | 2 |
| Seeding lot size [1] ($10^6$ cells) | 2.8 | 5.6 | 11.3 | 37.5 |

[1] Calculated for 25 units of T75 cell culture flasks.

Notably, preliminary experiments had shown that a confluency level of 95–100% was optimal before the initiation of vitamin C induction in order to obtain maximized collagen synthesis. Therein, FE002-SK2 primary progenitor fibroblasts were found to spontaneously form multilayer sheets, which were assessed to optimally conform to the considered subsequent use as a dermal template. The obtention of 95–100% confluent cultures in 7 days was consistently achieved throughout passages 5–10 in the retained experimental setup and up to passage 12 in GMP manufacturing campaigns (i.e., end of production cell banks, EOPCB, Figure S4).

As previously reported, appropriate multi-tiered FE002 primary progenitor cell banking strategies enable the potential obtention of sufficient clinical grade materials to sustainably produce hundreds of millions of cell-based therapies, largely outweighing the number of patients that could practically be treated with such biologicals [39]. Within clinical investigation protocols for PBB lot preparation, FE002-SK2 progenitor fibroblasts are extemporaneously thawed to constitute the topical PBB constructs [37]. The cell-bearing constructs are made available after 18–24 h for clinical application over the first two weeks of patient treatment [37]. Therefore, additional FE002-SK2 primary progenitor fibroblasts may be simultaneously initiated from storage, in view of parallel DE-FE002-SK2 construct lot preparation for subsequent application.

The optimized FE002-SK2 primary progenitor fibroblast expansion data and the identified bottlenecks for CEA and CDEA production allowed for the establishment of a process for DE-FE002-SK2 construct preparation under GMP (Table 1, Figure 2).

Specifically, initiation of FE002-SK2 cells for allogeneic dermal template preparation may be performed at the same time as autologous epidermal biopsy harvesting (Figure 2). As no dermal biopsy harvesting is necessary within the novel combinational protocol (i.e., use of allogeneic fibroblasts), the patient donor site morbidity factor is reduced (Figure 2). Then, from a 4–10 cm$^2$ epidermal biopsy, autologous keratinocytes may be isolated and expanded in vitro over a period of two weeks. This timeframe is sufficient for the parallel preparation of the allogeneic dermal template component (i.e., allogeneic fibroblast proliferation and functional induction, Figure 2(A1,A2)). Once both components have appropriately reached maturity, the expanded autologous keratinocytes are transferred via cell seeding to the top of the allogeneic dermal template and the co-cultures are maintained for one week before clinical delivery (Figure 2(C1)). In detail, DE-FE002-SK2 construct delivery can be arranged after 4–7 days of the final co-culture to allow for flexible organization of the reconstructive surgery. Overall and importantly, the optimized DE-FE002-SK2 manufacturing process enables clinical delivery within 16–21 days of autologous epidermal biopsy harvest, which constitutes a significant improvement over the 6–8-week delay of the standard CDEA manufacturing protocol (Figure 2).

### 3.3. DE-FE002-SK2 Constructs Display Structural Attributes Which Are Equivalent or Superior to Fully Autologous CDEAs

Parallel preparation of CDEAs using the standard protocol and of DE-FE002-SK2 constructs using the established protocol enabled us to technically benchmark both complex graft types using parametric gradings (Figure 2, Table 2).

Illustrated records of these assessments are presented in Figure 3. In the allogeneic dermal template group, vitamin C-induced FE002-SK2 primary progenitor fibroblasts formed homogeneous multi-layers (Figure 3(A1)). The resulting sheets could then be detached and were processed for analysis, which confirmed the homogeneity of important structural attributes (Figure 3(A2,A3)).

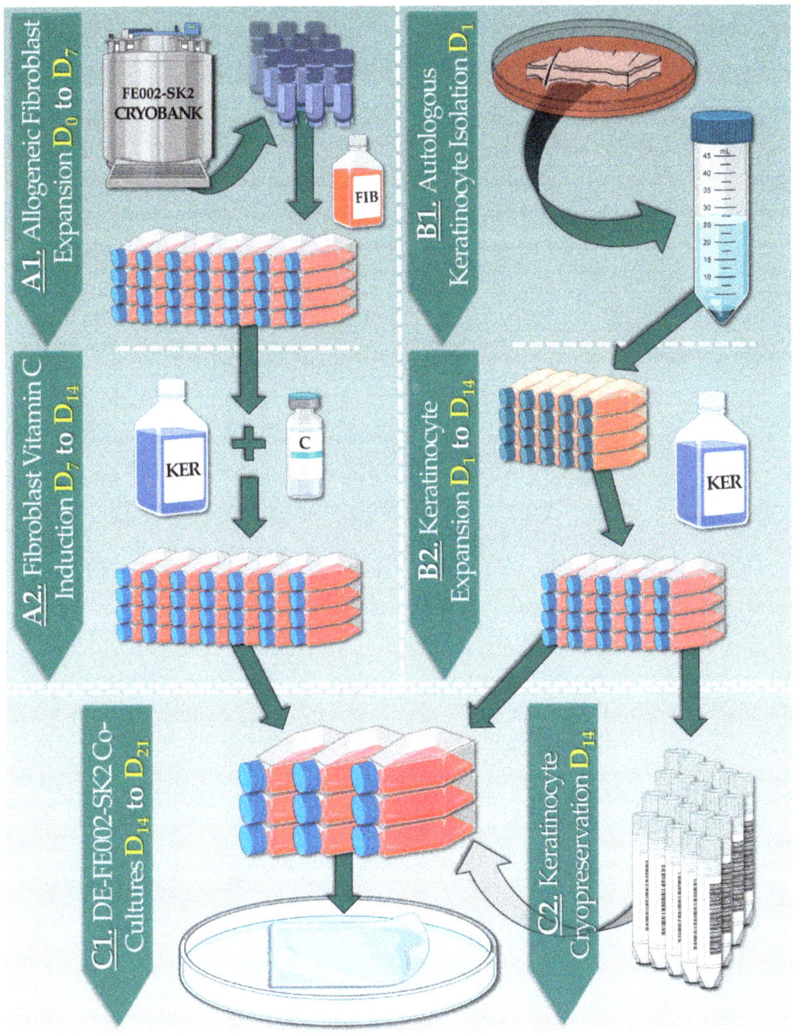


**Figure 2.** Schematic process detailing the parallel and sequential phases of DE-FE002-SK2 construct preparation. (**A1**) Using optimized technical specifications, allogeneic FE002-SK2 fibroblasts are expanded to confluency. (**A2**) For stimulation of collagen production, fibroblast cultures are treated with vitamin C. (**B1**) Upon epidermal biopsy reception, autologous keratinocyte isolation is rapidly performed. (**B2**) Autologous keratinocytes are cultured until the allogeneic dermal template is formed. (**C1**) The allogeneic dermal template and the autologous epidermal components are combined and further co-cultured in view of finished DE-FE002-SK2 construct formation. (**C2**) The excess autologous keratinocytes are cryopreserved and may be subsequently used to rapidly prepare new batches of DE-FE002-SK2 constructs. C, vitamin C; D, day; FIB, fibroblast proliferation medium; KER, keratinocyte proliferation medium.

**Table 2.** Comparative assessment of the attributes of autologous CDEAs and of autologous/allogeneic DE-FE002-SK2 constructs. Assessments were recorded as mean multi-operator gradings at the end of the dermal template formation phase and at the end of the combined construct formation phase. CDEA, cultured dermo-epidermal autograft.

| Process Phase | Parameters | Targets | Methods | Gradings [1] | |
|---|---|---|---|---|---|
| | | | | CDEA Group | DE-FE002-SK2 Group |
| 1. Dermal Template | Manufacturing timeframe | Two weeks of culture | Operator assessment | − | +++ |
| | Fibroblast monolayer formation after expansion | Formation of a homogeneous cellular layer | Operator assessment; microscopy | ++ | +++ |
| | Dermal template sheet formation after vitamin C induction | Formation of a dermal template by collagen synthesis | Operator assessment; collagen staining | ++ | +++ |
| | Homogeneity of the dermal template sheet | Consistency of dermal template attributes over the whole surface | Operator assessment; histology | ++ | +++ |
| | Robustness of the dermal template sheet | Possibility to detach and manipulate the dermal template | Operator assessment; handling | + | +++ |
| 2. Combined Construct | Manufacturing timeframe | One week of culture | Operator assessment | + | +++ |
| | Compatibility between the dermal template and autologous keratinocytes | Passive combination of components in co-culture | Operator assessment; histology | ++ | +++ |
| | Stratification of the epidermal component | Formation of a stratified epidermal component | Operator assessment; histology | + | +++ |
| | Homogeneity of the construct | Consistency of construct attributes over the whole surface | Operator assessment; histology | + | ++ |
| | Robustness of the construct | Possibility to detach and manipulate the construct | Operator assessment; handling | + | ++ |

[1] Gradings were attributed as follows: (+++) = conforming, excellent performance; (++) = conforming, good performance; (+) = conforming; (−) = non-conforming.

Then, transfer of patient primary keratinocytes to the top of the formed dermal templates resulted in appropriate passive combination during the co-culture phase (Figure 3(B1–B3), Table 2). Importantly, it was confirmed that the epidermal component of the DE-FE002-SK2 constructs was composed of stratified keratinocytes (i.e., after 1 week of co-culture) and that the fully formed constructs could be detached and appropriately manipulated (Figure 3(B3)). Overall, the gathered experimental data enabled a thorough assessment of the DE-FE002-SK2 constructs, which display endpoint structural attributes which are equivalent or superior to autologous CDEA constructs (Table 2, Figure 3).

### *3.4. DE-FE002-SK2 Constructs Display Enhanced Bio-Adhesive Functions on DED Compared to CEAs*

The important functional attributes of complex cell-based cutaneous grafts comprise the maintenance of structural integrity during handling and administration, as well as appropriate bio-adhesion and graft take. As DE-FE002-SK2 constructs could be rapidly obtained, several construct attributes of translational and functional importance were investigated further. Multiple CEA and DE-FE002-SK2 construct lots were prepared as described hereabove. The constructs were then transferred to a Vaseline gauze (i.e., transport scaffold) and were deposited on top of 1.0–2.5 cm$^2$ DED models (Figure 4A,B). An illustrated stepwise overview of the preparation process for the DED model is presented in Figure S5.

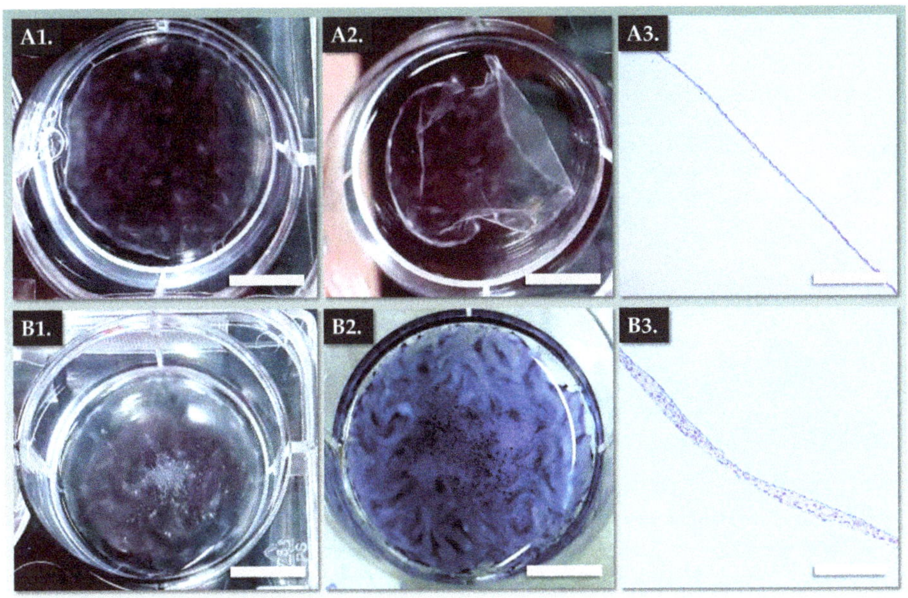


**Figure 3.** Macroscopic and microscopic records of allogeneic dermal templates and of the DE-FE002-SK2 constructs in formation. (**A1**) FE002-SK2-based dermal template following vitamin C induction. Scale bar = 5 mm. (**A2**) Detached FE002-SK2-based dermal template in PBS. Scale bar = 5 mm. (**A3**) Harris hematoxylin staining of the FE002-SK2-based dermal template. Scale bar = 300 μm. (**B1**) Fully formed FE002-SK2-based dermal template after 1 day of co-culture with patient primary keratinocytes. Scale bar = 5 mm. (**B2**) Combined DE-FE002-SK2 construct in co-culture following endpoint MTT staining. Scale bar = 5 mm. (**B3**) Harris hematoxylin staining of the fully formed combined DE-FE002-SK2 construct, showing stratified epidermal component formation. Scale bar = 300 μm. PBS, phosphate-buffered saline.

Then, the transport gauze could be easily removed and constructs could be observed on top of the DED model (Figure 4A,B). Following topical graft application, the models were maintained in air–liquid organoculture for one week. Upon endpoint MTT staining, it was shown that the DE-FE002-SK2 constructs presented significantly enhanced bio-adhesion attributes compared to the standard CEAs (Figure 4C). Specifically, construct adhesion in the CEA group was found to be partial and inhomogeneous, with important CEA detachment at the end of the organoculture phase (Figure 4(C1)). Conversely, complete and homogeneous adhesion of the DE-FE002-SK2 preparations was observed (Figure 4(C2)). Such differential results may potentially be partly explained at a molecular level by the action (i.e., mediated by the presence of dermal fibroblasts) of basement membrane components (e.g., integrins, laminins, growth factors), which are known to possess important interface modulation functionalities [42]. Finally, comparative parametric assessments of CEA and DE-FE002-SK2 constructs were performed in terms of translational and functional attributes (Table 3).

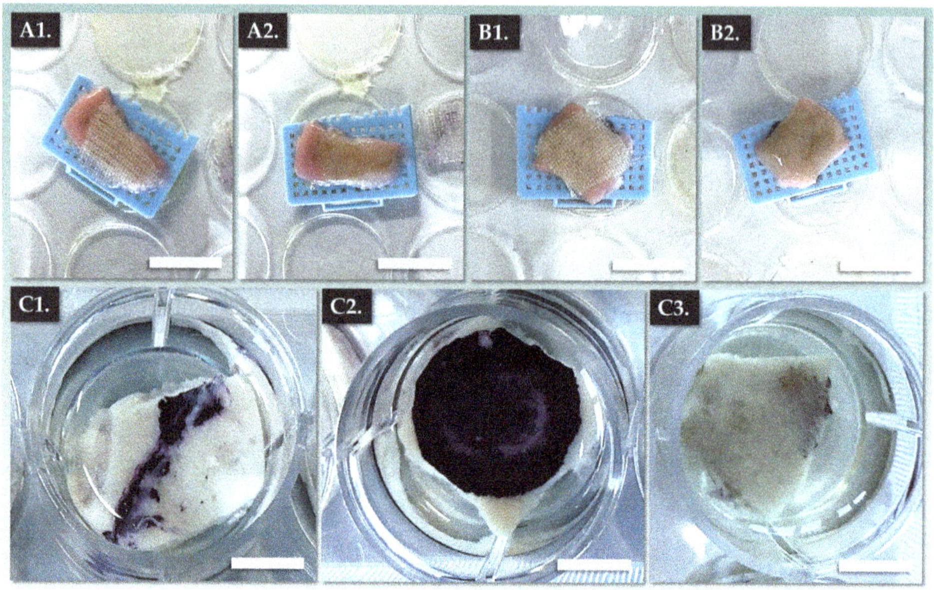


**Figure 4.** Assessment results of CEA and DE-FE002-SK2 construct adhesion capacities on a standardized ex vivo DED model. (**A1**,**A2**) Aspect of the DED model following topical CEA construct application and following gentle removal of the transport gauze. Scale bars = 10 mm. (**B1**,**B2**) Aspect of the DED model following topical DE-FE002-SK2 construct application and following gentle removal of the transport gauze. Scale bars = 10 mm. (**C1**) MTT staining of the model from the CEA group after 1 week of air–liquid organoculture, showing inhomogeneous graft take. Scale bar = 7 mm. (**C2**) MTT staining of the model from the DE-FE002-SK2 group after 1 week of air–liquid organoculture, showing homogeneous graft take. Scale bar = 7 mm. (**C3**) MTT staining of the model from the DED control group after 1 week of air–liquid organoculture. Scale bar = 7 mm. CEA, cultured epithelial autografts; DED, de-epidermalized dermis.

For further mechanistic investigation into the bio-adhesive properties of the DE-FE002-SK2 constructs, the impact of autologous keratinocyte addition on the structural and functional attributes of the allogeneic dermal template was assessed using the DED model. Therefore, allogeneic dermal templates were prepared and divided into two groups. The first group consisted of the allogeneic dermal template alone (i.e., without keratinocytes) and the second group consisted of the fully formed DE-FE002-SK2 constructs. All samples were placed on fresh DED models and maintained in organoculture for one week. Endpoint MTT staining revealed that both experimental groups showed homogeneous adhesion on the DED model (Figure 5A).

Furthermore, and importantly, H&E staining of histological sections showed that both preparations presented multiple cell layers which were integrated within the DED (Figure 5(B1,B2)). Notably, it was not possible to obtain the corresponding data for CEA preparations, as these would not adhere to the DED model. Importantly, staining with the p63 marker (which specifically identifies keratinocytes) was observed in the upper to middle layers of the DE-FE002-SK2 preparations, confirming the bilayer structure of the complex grafts (Figure 5(D2)). Finally, the results showed that Ki67-positive cells (i.e., proliferating cells) were present in both graft components, confirming the maintenance of cellular functions following application on the DED (Figure 5(F1,F2)).

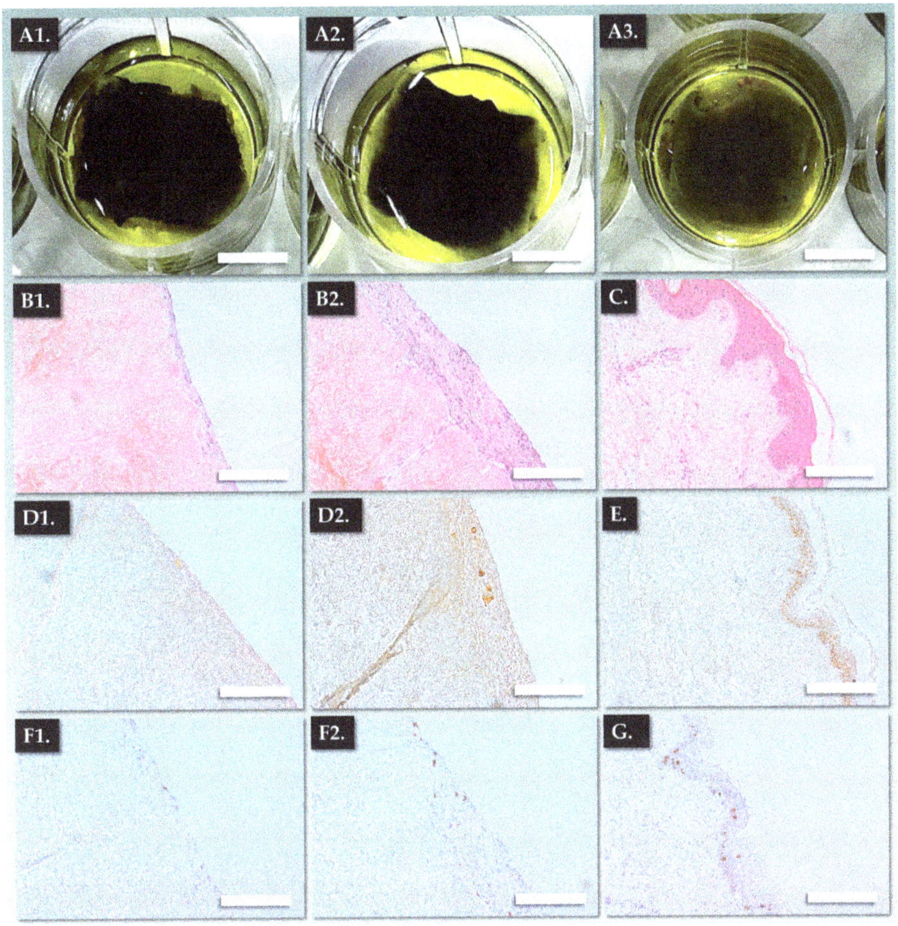


**Figure 5.** Functional investigation results for allogeneic dermal templates and fully formed DE-FE002-SK2 constructs on the ex vivo DED model. (**A1–A3**) MTT staining of the allogeneic dermal template on the DED, the DE-FE002-SK2 construct on the DED, and the DED control group following 1 week of air–liquid organoculture. Scale bars = 5 mm. (**B1**,**B2**) H&E staining of the allogeneic dermal template on the DED and the DE-FE002-SK2 construct on the DED. Scale bars = 150 μm. (**C**) H&E staining of the normal skin control group. Scale bar = 150 μm. (**D1**,**D2**) P63 staining of the allogeneic dermal template on the DED and the DE-FE002-SK2 construct on the DED. Scale bars = 150 μm. (**E**) P63 staining of the normal skin control group. Scale bar = 150 μm. (**F1**,**F2**) Ki67 staining of the allogeneic dermal template on the DED and the DE-FE002-SK2 construct on the DED. Scale bars = 150 μm. (**G**) Ki67 staining of the normal skin control group. DED, de-epidermalized dermis; H&E, hematoxylin and eosin.

**Table 3.** Comparative assessment of translational and functional attributes of CEAs and DE-FE002-SK2 constructs within the ex vivo DED model. Assessments were recorded as mean multi-operator gradings at the time of construct topical application on the DED model and at the end of the organoculture phase. CEA, cultured epithelial autograft; DED, de-epidermalized dermis.

| Attribute Type | Parameters | Targets | Methods | Gradings [1] | |
|---|---|---|---|---|---|
| | | | | CEA Group | DE-FE002-SK2 Group |
| 1. Translational Attributes | Transfer of the construct to a Vaseline gauze | Possibility to manipulate and transport the construct using the gauze | Operator assessment | ++ | +++ |
| | Application of the construct on the DED model | Simple topical application on the DED surface | Operator assessment | +++ | +++ |
| | Applied construct structural integrity maintenance | Maintenance of construct structural integrity on the DED model | Operator assessment | ++ | ++ |
| 2. Functional Attributes | Initial adhesion of the construct to the DED model | Construct adheres rapidly to the DED model | Operator assessment | ++ | ++ |
| | Endpoint homogeneous adhesion of the construct to the DED model | Construct adheres homogeneously to the DED model | Operator assessment; MTT | − | ++ |
| | Endpoint homogeneous metabolic activity throughout of the construct on the DED model | Cellular metabolic activity is significant and homogeneous throughout the construct on the DED model | Operator assessment; MTT | ± | +++ |

[1] Gradings were attributed as follows: (+++) = conforming, excellent performance; (++) = conforming, good performance; (±) = unclear, additional data required; (−) = non-conforming.

Overall, it was confirmed that the bio-adhesive functions of DE-FE002-SK2 constructs were conferred by the allogeneic dermal template, which enabled a significantly enhanced graft take (Figures 4 and 5). Importantly, the results of ex vivo adhesion assays showed that allogeneic dermal templates based on functionally induced FE002-SK2 primary progenitor fibroblasts could potentially serve as standalone, rapidly obtainable under GMP, and universal dermal coverings for subsequent overlaying with a variety of epidermal substrates (Figure 5).

## 4. Discussion

### *4.1. Historical Evolution and Technical Bottlenecks in Burn Patient Cytotherapeutic Care*

Notable advances in burn care and plastic surgery and specific improvements to techniques to assure tegument cover and quality have recently been emphasized [1–6]. Therein, a critical clinical objective is to cover the patient as rapidly as possible for optimized infection control. Secondly, esthetic and functional outcomes have become key components of modern rehabilitation pathways, as increasing numbers of severely burned patients return to regular activities [27].

From a skin transplant point-of-view, early allotransplantation began over 60 years ago, with hallmark advances made by Medawar in treating WWII burn victims [43]. He was able to present data on immune tolerance and transplantation, which provided the notion of immune privilege. He was awarded the Nobel Prize in 1960 for modern transplantation immunology and for providing the fundamental basis for showing that skin from one patient cannot be readily grafted to another patient [44]. Despite this described rejection process, allogeneic skin is still widely used as a functional biological dressing for temporary wound cover, assuring the necessary fluid balance and preparing the wound bed for subsequent autologous grafting and burn wound closure [17–19]. Conversely, allogeneic skin grafts are not advantageous for long-term cover due to secondary graft rejection, infection, and scar tissue formation [12,17,18].

Due to the lack of availability of human cadaver skin, development efforts have been directed toward temporary skin covers using artificial or xenogeneic products. Widely clinically applied porcine skin grafts (e.g., sterile and viable split-skin grafts from neonatal pigs) have been continuously developed as a source of high-quality and functional coverings for clinical use in human medicine [45,46]. More recently, natural sourcing of clinical grade biological coverage materials has been demonstrated from Nile Tilapia fish (i.e., *Orechromis niloticus*) skin. Similarly, North Atlantic cod (i.e., *Gadus morhua*) skin was first approved by the US FDA in 2013 (i.e., Kerecis Omega 3 dressings) despite the higher costs if used to treat high-TBSA burn patients [47–49]. From a cytotherapeutic viewpoint, several literature reviews have described the evolution of autologous keratinocyte culture use for severe burn wound management [1–4,21–24]. Despite the availability of formulation options (e.g., cell sheets and cell sprays), several weeks of culture remain necessary for therapeutic cell manufacture [24,27–30]. Notably, several clinical groups have studied the use of allogeneic keratinocytes (i.e., cultured and frozen) for initial treatments, yet these preparations tended to behave like cadaver skin and had to be replaced rapidly with autologous preparations [18].

Alternative projects have focused on genetically modified keratinocytes isolated from allogeneic sources [50]. Despite substantial progress in understanding immune competence and graft rejection, it is not yet possible to achieve immune compatibility [51]. Further understanding of immunological responses to modified allogeneic keratinocytes will help to develop potential clinical applications. Therefore, a variety of experimental methods are currently studied to obtain allogeneic keratinocytes which can be used universally and that may overcome host cellular immune responses [52]. However, depending on the experimental methods (e.g., use of viral vectors), other safety issues arise, such as the duration of transgene expression, vector immunogenicity, and vector tropism.

### 4.2. Transitioning to Complex Cutaneous Grafts for Enhanced Burn Victim Clinical Outcomes

Translational research groups have focused on artificial dermal matrices developed with collagens, polymers, and foams, which are adapted for association with therapeutic cell sources [2,4,6–8,10]. Therein, degradation of exogeneous substrates and parallel remodeling of autologous tissues are key factors. The overall performance in esthetics, functionality, and immune compatibility determines the level of success of allogeneic skin graft approaches [27,29–31]. Notably, there have been many efforts directed toward the development of dermal substitutes [2,11]. While several products are clinically investigated and marketed, there is no commercially available substrate which can sufficiently restore the functions of the skin. Specifically, an optimal substitute should ensure early restoration of anatomical and physiological skin functions, a feat which can currently only be provided by using a full-thickness skin graft or flap reconstruction protocols [11,12].

Therefore, strong emphasis has been placed on cultured cells to reconstitute an optimized tegument, with or without a dermal substrate or template [3–5,9,12,22]. From a functional and esthetic standpoint, it is generally accepted that including a dermal component (i.e., such as dermal fibroblasts) would significantly aid in graft take. This combinational approach has been studied using various allogeneic tissues and autologous cells, yet technical bottlenecks remain (i.e., differences in manufacturing timeframe requirements) [21–24,26,27,33]. Therefore, much room remains for further cutaneous cell therapy optimization, primarily to ensure full wound closure in a short time-period following injury to decrease the risk of infection.

As regards the use of allogeneic skin grafting materials in the Lausanne Burn Center, initial case studies date back to 1992 [17]. These cases were managed using the Cuono technique, with allogeneic cadaver skin bearing cultured autologous keratinocytes. The need for immunosuppressive therapy was evident due to the grafting of cadaver skin.

Similarly, Damour et al. employed cultured allogeneic keratinocytes (i.e., the adapted Cuono technique) in 18 burn patients from 1998 to 2000 in France [18,19]. Namely, from one single cadaver, they were able to culture 30 $m^2$ of epidermis [18]. Based on these advances, the standard CDEA protocols were developed and implemented in the CHUV in 1998, enabling the elimination of cadaver skin and the inclusion of functionally induced fibroblasts as dermal template components [20,27]. As the original protocols of Reinwald and Green for CEA preparation had already been implemented in the CHUV in 1985, early and rapid clinical adoption of novel topical cell therapies has constituted a landmark in Lausanne [13–17].

From a technical standpoint, a major drawback linked to the inclusion of autologous dermal fibroblasts in the CDEA manufacturing process is the lengthy manufacturing timeframe (i.e., practically doubled compared to CEAs). Of note, CEA manufacture was reported to require an average of 22.9 $\pm$ 4.2 days, while CDEA manufacture required an average of 50.0 $\pm$ 8.5 days in a patient cohort study from 2016 to 2018 (Table S1) [27]. Therefore, patients were transiently covered with Integra matrices before the CDEA cultures were ready for use. Additionally, clinically available cell therapy quantities are technically limited by the respective manufacturing lot sizes. Therein, a maximum of 0.4 $m^2$ of skin grafts may be manufactured at one given time (i.e., approximately 50 units of T75 culture flasks for CEAs and 40 units of T75 culture flasks for CDEAs, Table S1) [27]. Therefore, alternative and readily available (e.g., off-the-freezer) therapeutic cell sources would be of particular importance in the early management of severe burn trauma and could potentially help save lives.

### *4.3. Dermal Components Are Necessary for High-Quality Closure of Extensive and Deep Burns*

Skin grafting is mandatory in extensive, deep second and third degree burns because the endogenous cellular components necessary for cutaneous regeneration are damaged. Extensive burns generate a disturbance of tissue oxygenation as well as fluid and protein losses, which increase the risk of dehydration and infections. This is why it is important to rapidly cover the wounds to support their repair and limit the related consequences. We have previously reported the surgical management of two seriously burned patients (i.e., 92% and 90% TBSA, respectively) with a 17-year interval [27]. Differences in treatment regimens led to a significant difference in hospitalization stay. Therein, the first patient benefited from both CEA and CDEA preparations at various stages of surgical reconstruction [27]. The second patient was able to benefit from early allogeneic cellular therapies with the use of PBBs to replace cadaver skin and to prepare the wound beds [27].

The second patient was subsequently treated with CEA preparations only (i.e., no CDEAs), as his hospital stay in the ICU was reduced to 76 days compared to 162 days for the first patient [27]. Standardized monitoring of skin reconstruction quality revealed that the use of CDEAs resulted in a markedly superior cosmetic appearance and a significantly higher elastic recovery as compared to CEA use only (Figure S6). These findings indicated that by reconstructing dermal and epidermal structures, both esthetic and significant functional improvements could additionally be obtained over time. These in-house clinical observations were in line with those of Lamme et al., who noted that the improvement in wound healing was correlated with higher numbers of fibroblasts within the applied dermal substitute [34]. Therefore, the use of appropriate dermal components in complex wound care may demonstrably enhance quality-related clinical outcomes.

### *4.4. Allogeneic FE002-SK2 Primary Progenitor Fibroblasts Have Been Extensively Clinically Tested*

Primary progenitor cells are differentiated cells, notably differing from stem cells in terms of differentiation potential [35]. They are highly resistant to oxidative stress and have minimal nutritional requirements, while having high proliferation potentials and low immunogenic properties [39]. Formulated in temporary topical PBB constructs, such cells are thought to mainly act by means of tissue repair/regeneration mediation [35,37,39].

The absence of therapeutic cell engraftment was evidenced in early clinical studies, where biopsies were harvested from a female patient having received multiple male progenitor cell topical applications [35]. Such elements were considered positively from a safety viewpoint, in conjunction with the fact that no clinical evidence of immunological rejection of primary FE002 cells was reported to date [37,53]. Specifically, the immune privilege of FE002 primary progenitor cells and of similar cell sources was studied in vitro (e.g., optimal HLA marker panels) and using various immunological settings in vivo (e.g., use of FE002 primary chondroprogenitors in caprine and mice models) [35,39,54,55]. However, while the considered DE-FE002-SK2 constructs (i.e., tissue engineering products) are designed to engraft in the host, further long-term in vivo studies would be warranted to optimally document safety attributes, building on the existing body of knowledge around FE002 allogeneic biologicals [53].

The main therapeutic objective of using PBBs is to stimulate the natural cutaneous healing process of treated burn wounds during the first ten to twelve days, and thus potentially avoid the need for an autograft or at least reduce the size of the grafted area. Subsequently, in cases where skin autografts are required, PBBs may be further applied for promoting re-epithelialization of donor site wounds. It was shown that the early use of PBBs resulted in the promotion of a qualitatively enhanced cutaneous healing process, with drastically improved esthetic and functional outcomes, and reduced the need for subsequent corrective interventions [4,5,37]. From a therapeutic viewpoint, PBBs were developed and have been clinically applied in Lausanne since 2000–2005 [37]. Therein, no safety-related concerns have been raised and an enhanced repair tissue quality was evidenced [37]. From a regulatory standpoint, the use of FE002-SK2-based therapeutic materials in clinical investigation settings has thus far been approved by the US FDA, the Taiwanese FDA, the Japanese PMDA, and Swissmedic [39].

Based on the available scientific, technical, and clinical hindsight on the clinical grade FE002-SK2 primary progenitor cell source, its inclusion as a dermal component of a novel combinational cutaneous graft (e.g., DE-FE002-SK2 construct) may tangibly be considered [35–39]. Notably, in vitro functional induction of dermal fibroblast sources has been reported since the early 1970s, when it was shown that vitamin C could enhance collagen synthesis [40]. Individual experiments comparing adult fibroblasts to FE002-SK2 primary progenitor cells showed that the FE002 progenitor cells possess significant innate collagen synthesis capacities (Figure 1). Such attributes were further studied, harnessed, and potentiated in the present study for the obtention of standardized and optimized functionality within allogeneic dermal template manufacturing (Figure 2).

### *4.5. DE-FE002-SK2 Constructs: Technically Enhanced Modern Alternatives to Standard CDEA Protocols*

Vitamin C is known to functionally enhance extracellular matrix formation in vitro, whereas the FE002-SK2 cells constitutively possessed higher collagen production and deposition activities compared to patient fibroblasts (Figure 1). Stimulation with vitamin C potentiated extracellular matrix formation by the allogeneic cells, and enhanced bio-adhesion attributes of the DE-FE002-SK2 constructs were recorded (Figures 1, 4 and 5). Notably, the ex vivo DED model suggested an enhanced DE-FE002-SK2 graft take over CEAs, which have been used locally and internationally (supplied by the Lausanne Burn Center, e.g., Zurich-based clinical centers, UK, or Finland) as a standard of care. From a technical standpoint, while the retained MTT readout provided only basic information about the mitochondrial activity of the cells, the simplicity of the assay and the visual assessment of cellular presence and cellular homogeneity were assessed to be appropriate within the scope of the present proof-of-concept work (i.e., functionality optimization at the construct level).

Multiparametric advantages were set forth herein around the use of FE002-SK2 cells over autologous fibroblasts (i.e., sustainable off-the-freezer cell source, rapid production, constitutive collagen synthesis, and enhanced bio-adhesiveness). Comparative parametric assessments of CEAs or CDEAs and DE-FE002-SK2 constructs were performed in terms of translational and functional attributes (Tables 2 and 3). Importantly, the structural integrity maintenance of the DE-FE002-SK2 constructs during standard handling (i.e., manufacturing- and clinical-application-related handling) was confirmed. Specifically, matured constructs (i.e., about 10–50 $cm^2$) must be able to resist harvest, physical transfer and stapling to the Vaseline gauze, and transport to the clinic. Therefore, the DE-FE002-SK2 preparations displayed superiority in structural integrity retention over the CEA preparations, most likely partially due to the additional thickness/sturdiness of the complex cell sheet. Finally, as concerns the treatment of large TBSA burns, multiple DE-FE002-SK2 grafts would need to be serially manufactured and parallelly clinically applied, similarly to existing CDEA protocols. Therein, while the proposed bi-component cell-based constructs may even become available too early in the clinical pathway of severe burn patients (i.e., depending on the resuscitation and stabilization phases, with surgical wound bed preparation), their early use as temporary coverages and wound healing enhancers (i.e., first weeks of treatment) may potentially be considered. By extension, the proposed DE-FE002-SK2 constructs may also potentially be used in alternative complex and moderate cases of cutaneous affections (e.g., chronic lower limb ulcers) requiring high-quality repair interventions, taking as an example the clinical diversification already implemented in Lausanne for PBB constructs [53].

Overall, the original data reported herein have confirmed that the proposed use of allogeneic dermal progenitor fibroblasts within complex cutaneous graft manufacture addresses two critical issues of clinical relevance. Namely, the rapidity of wound coverage may be enhanced (i.e., off-the-freezer cell stock) and the structural/functional quality of cutaneous tissular repair may potentially be further optimized (i.e., early use of a dermal component and enhanced graft take). While further studies and in vivo investigative work are warranted for the proposed DE-FE002-SK2 constructs, transposition to GMP manufacturing settings and large-scale clinical translation are inherently confirmed by the locally acquired experience of the authors in cutaneous cytotherapies (i.e., CEAs, CDEAs, and PBBs). Such considerations further strengthen the rationale for working towards autologous to allogeneic clinical protocol transpositions, as the potential technical and clinical benefits are significant and quantifiable.

### 4.6. Study Limitations and Future Perspectives

Differential cell-based management approaches depend on the extent, depth, and related complications of the burn wounds. Overall, novel solutions may contribute to accelerating the recovery of burn wounds and to shortening wound healing processes, ideally with an improved quality of cutaneous scarring. Despite the technical and functional advantages of the DE-FE002-SK2 constructs, the latter remain limited by the simplicity of their cellular constituents and therefore do not optimally mimic healthy human skin. Further developments of grafts including more complex skin structures such as melanocytes, sweat glands, hair follicles, blood vessels, and lymphatic capillaries are needed, yet current approaches in this domain still lack robust clinical data [56–59]. From a transpositional viewpoint, such biomimicking applications would also require up-scaling, which will in all probability be limited by available manufacturing capabilities. Furthermore, an optimized scaffold or matrix for simplified graft preparation and delivery would be of high interest (i.e., in replacement of the Vaseline gauze). Appropriate scaffolds could potentially include thermolabile hydrogels for handling of the cell sheet or a biodegradable scaffold which could easily be removed during bandage exchanges.

From a methodological standpoint, the use of simple readouts in this study and related descriptive analyses did not enable us to characterize the mechanisms of action or the internal functional attributes of the proposed DE-FE002-SK2 constructs. Specifically, the scope of the present proof-of-concept work was built around function-oriented manufacturing process optimization, with a focus on manufacturing timeframe rationalization. Therefore, further investigation of the proposed DE-FE002-SK2 constructs at fundamental and mechanistic levels (i.e., using complementary biochemical, genomic, and proteomic methods) will allow for the optimal characterization of the proposed constructs and a tentative explanation of the mechanisms of action [60]. While the critical functional attributes of the complex grafts were confirmed (e.g., bio-adhesion capacities) in comparison to CEA or CDEA elements, the use of alternative methods for cellular activity determination (i.e., to complement the basic MTT readout) will potentially yield an enhanced understanding of key and critical functional attributes to eventually augment the quality of clinical outcomes. Therein, in addition to primary efficacy outcomes (e.g., time to complete wound closure), specific secondary outcomes related to the quality of tissular repair (e.g., biomechanical analysis of repaired skin and re-operation rates) are of prime interest for pertinent tissue engineering product efficacy benchmarking.

## 5. Conclusions

The aim of this study was to establish proofs-of-concept for a novel combinational topical tissue engineering product in view of clinical cutaneous cytotherapy workflow rationalization. Extensive local technical and clinical hindsight on the use of autologous and allogeneic skin cell sources for burn wound management was harnessed for the new manufacturing process design. It was first demonstrated that allogeneic FE002-SK2 dermal progenitor fibroblasts could be used instead of autologous fibroblasts for functional dermal template preparation, starting from a standardized cryopreserved source. Then, it was shown that DE-FE002-SK2 constructs could be manufactured in a condensed timeframe of 3 weeks, constituting a major technical advantage over the current 6–8-week-long fully autologous protocol. Ex vivo, the DE-FE002-SK2 constructs were found to be structurally equivalent to standard CDEAs and possessed enhanced bio-adhesion attributes compared to standard CEAs. Generally, the presented work constitutes a technical basis for further GMP transposition of the combinational DE-FE002-SK2 construct in view of investigative clinical work. Importantly, tangible consideration of the switch toward allogeneic cell sources for dermo-epidermal graft manufacture has been enabled by the landmark use of dermal progenitor fibroblasts (e.g., FE002-SK2 cell source) for burn wound care over the past decades in Lausanne. Overall, the rationalized manufacturing timeframes presented herein bear the potential to significantly optimize severe burn patient cytotherapeutic management workflows, potentially enabling faster wound closure and enhanced tissular healing quality.

**Supplementary Materials:** The following supporting information can be downloaded at: https://www.mdpi.com/article/10.3390/pharmaceutics15092334/s1, Figure S1: Clinical flowchart for burn patient management phases and treatments; Figure S2: Technical manufacturing workflow for CEA constructs; Figure S3: Technical manufacturing workflow for CDEA constructs; Figure S4: Technical workflow for multi-tiered primary progenitor fibroblast cell banking and PBB clinical lot preparation for use in the Lausanne Burn Center; Figure S5: Illustrated process for the ex vivo DED model preparation; Figure S6: Illustration for clinical use of CEA and CDEA constructs, with qualitative endpoints; Table S1: Comparative parameters and timeframes for manufacture of clinical batches of PBB, CEA, and CDEA constructs in the Lausanne University Hospital; Table S2: Results of statistical analyses for collagen quantification assays under vitamin C stimulation.

**Author Contributions:** Conceptualization, X.C., A.L., L.A.A. and N.H.-B.; methodology, X.C., A.L., Z.L., C.S., W.R., L.A.A. and N.H.-B.; validation, X.C., A.L., Z.L., S.J., P.A.-S., M.F., C.S., W.R., L.A.A. and N.H.-B.; formal analysis, X.C., A.L., Z.L., S.J., P.A.-S., C.S., W.R., L.A.A. and N.H.-B.; investigation, X.C., A.L., S.J., M.F., C.S., W.R., L.A.A. and N.H.-B.; resources, A.L., W.R. and L.A.A.; data curation, X.C., A.L., L.A.A. and N.H.-B.; writing—original draft preparation X.C., A.L., L.A.A. and N.H.-B.; writing—review and editing, X.C., A.L., Z.L., S.J., P.A.-S., M.F., C.S., W.R., L.A.A. and N.H.-B.; visualization, X.C., A.L., W.R., L.A.A. and N.H.-B.; supervision, W.R., L.A.A. and N.H.-B.; project administration, L.A.A. and N.H.-B.; funding acquisition, L.A.A. and N.H.-B. All authors have read and agreed to the published version of the manuscript.

**Funding:** The S.A.N.T.E and Sandoz Foundations have contributed by funding the Swiss progenitor cell transplantation program over the past fourteen years, reference numbers 27846-06 and 27866-06, respectively. The funders had no role in the design of the study; in the collection, analyses, or interpretation of data; in the writing of the manuscript; or in the decision to publish the results. This study was not supported by specific grants or institutional programs.

**Institutional Review Board Statement:** The biological starting materials used for the present study were procured according to the guidelines of the Declaration of Helsinki and approved by the appropriate Cantonal Ethics Committee [61,62]. The progenitor cell source used in the present study (i.e., FE002-SK2 primary progenitor cells) was established from the FE002 organ donation, as approved by the Vaud Cantonal Ethics Committee (University Hospital of Lausanne–CHUV, Ethics Committee Protocol N°62/07). The FE002 donation was registered under a federal cell transplantation program (i.e., Swiss progenitor cell transplantation program). Obtention and use of patient cellular materials followed the regulations of the Biobank of the CHUV Department of Musculoskeletal Medicine. Materials from adult burn patients were included in the study under the Ethics Committee Protocol N°264/12, approved by the Vaud Cantonal Ethics Committee.

**Informed Consent Statement:** Appropriate informed consent was obtained from and confirmed by starting material donors at the time of inclusion in the Swiss progenitor cell transplantation program, following specifically devised protocols and procedures which were validated by the appropriate health authorities. Informed consent (i.e., formalized in a general informed consent agreement) was obtained from all patients or from their legal representatives at the time of treatment for unrestricted use of the gathered and anonymized patient data or anonymized biological materials (i.e., donors of primary cell types).

**Data Availability Statement:** The data presented in this study are available upon written and reasonable request from the corresponding authors.

**Acknowledgments:** We would like to thank the S.A.N.T.E and Sandoz Foundations for their commitment to the Swiss progenitor cell transplantation program over the years. We would like to thank Kristina Upeski, Julianne Kocher, and Catherine Pythoud for their respective technical contributions to the presented work.

**Conflicts of Interest:** Author A.L. was employed by TEC-PHARMA SA (Bercher, Switzerland) and by LAM Biotechnologies SA (Epalinges, Switzerland) during the course of the study, within the scope of an industrial thesis. The remaining authors declare no conflict of interest.

## Abbreviations

| | |
|---|---|
| CDEA | cultured dermo-epidermal autograft |
| CEA | cultured epithelial autograft |
| CHUV | Centre Hospitalier Universitaire Vaudois |
| DED | de-epidermalized dermis |
| DE-FE002-SK2 | bioengineered skin graft based on cultured allogeneic fibroblasts and autologous keratinocytes |
| DMEM | Dulbecco's modified Eagle medium |
| DMSO | dimethyl sulfoxide |
| ECM | extracellular matrix |
| EDTA | ethylenediaminetetraacetic acid |
| EOPCB | end of production cell bank |
| FBS | fetal bovine serum |
| FE002-SK2 | clinical grade primary progenitor fibroblast cell source |
| GMP | good manufacturing practices |
| H&E | hematoxylin and eosin |
| MCB | master cell bank |
| PBB | progenitor biological bandages |
| PBS | phosphate-buffered saline |
| PCB | parental cell bank |
| TBSA | total body surface area |
| UK | United Kingdom |
| USA | United States of America |
| WCB | working cell bank |

## References


1. Greenlagh, D.G. Management of burns. *N. Engl. J. Med.* **2019**, *380*, 2349–2359. [CrossRef]
2. Schlottmann, F.; Bucan, V.; Vogt, P.M.; Krezdorn, N. A short history of skin grafting in burns: From the gold standard of autologous skin grafting to the possibilities of allogeneic skin grafting with immunomodulatory approaches. *Medicina* **2021**, *57*, 225. [CrossRef]
3. Chemali, M.; Laurent, A.; Scaletta, C.; Waselle, L.; Simon, J.-P.; Michetti, M.; Brunet, J.-F.; Flahaut, M.; Hirt-Burri, N.; Raffoul, W.; et al. Burn center organization and cellular therapy integration: Managing risks and costs. *J. Burn Care Res.* **2021**, *42*, 911–924. [CrossRef]
4. Vogt, P.M.; Busche, M.N. Evaluation of infrastructure, equipment and training of 28 burn units/burn centers in Germany, Austria and Switzerland. *Burns* **2011**, *37*, 257–264. [CrossRef]
5. Münzberg, M.; Ziegler, B.; Fischer, S.; Wölfl, C.G.; Grützner, P.A.; Kremer, T.; Kneser, U.; Hirche, C. In view of standardization: Comparison and analysis of initial management of severely burned patients in Germany, Austria and Switzerland. *Burns* **2015**, *41*, 33–38. [CrossRef]
6. Lukish, J.R.; Eichelberger, M.R.; Newman, K.D. The use of a bioactive skin substitute decreases length of stay for pediatric burn patients. *J. Pediatr. Surg.* **2001**, *36*, 1118–1121. [CrossRef]
7. Kumar, R.J.; Kimble, R.M.; Boots, R.J.; Pegg, S.P. Treatment of partial-thickness burns: A prospective, randomized trial using TransCyte®. *ANZ J. Surg.* **2004**, *74*, 622–626. [CrossRef]
8. Zaulyanov, L.; Kirsner, R.S. A review of a bi-layered living cell treatment (Apligraf®) in the treatment of venous leg ulcers and diabetic foot ulcers. *Clin. Interv. Aging* **2007**, *2*, 93–98. [CrossRef]
9. Zuliani, T.; Saiagh, S.; Knol, A.C.; Esbelin, J.; Dréno, B. Fetal fibroblasts and keratinocytes with immunosuppressive properties for allogeneic cell-based wound therapy. *PLoS ONE* **2013**, *8*, e70408. [CrossRef]
10. Debels, H.; Hamdi, M.; Abberton, K. Dermal matrices and bioengineered skin substitutes: A critical review of current options. *Plast. Reconstr. Surg. Glob. Open* **2015**, *3*, e284. [CrossRef]
11. Climov, M.; Panayi, A.C.; Borah, G.; Orgill, D.P. The life-cycles of skin replacement technologies. *PLoS ONE* **2020**, *15*, e0229455. [CrossRef]
12. Ramezankhani, R.; Torabi, S.; Minaei, N.; Madani, H.; Resaeiani, S.; Hassani, S.N.; Gee, A.P.; Dominici, M.; Silva, D.N.; Baharvand, H.; et al. Two decades of global progress in authorized Advanced Therapy Medicinal Products: An emerging revolution in therapeutic strategies. *Front. Cell Dev. Biol.* **2020**, *8*, 547653. [CrossRef] [PubMed]
13. Rheinwald, J.G.; Green, H. Serial cultivation of strains of human epidermal keratinocytes: The formation of keratinizing colonies from single cells. *Cell* **1975**, *6*, 331–343. [CrossRef] [PubMed]
14. Rheinwald, J.G.; Green, H. Epidermal growth factor and the multiplication of cultured human epidermal keratinocytes. *Nature* **1977**, *265*, 421–424. [CrossRef] [PubMed]
15. Green, H.; Kehinde, O.; Thomas, J. Growth of cultured human epidermal cells into multiple epithelia suitable for grafting. *Proc. Natl. Acad. Sci. USA* **1979**, *76*, 5665–5668. [CrossRef]
16. O'Connor, N.E.; Mulliken, J.B.; Banks-Schlegel, S.; Kehinde, O.; Green, H. Grafting of burns with cultured epithelium prepared from autologous epidermal cells. *Lancet* **1981**, *317*, 75–78. [CrossRef] [PubMed]
17. Krupp, S.; Benathan, M.; Déglise, B.; Holzer, E.; Wiesner, L.; Delacrétaz, F.; Chioléro, R. Current concepts in pediatric burn care: Management of burn wounds with cultured epidermal autografts. *Eur. J. Pediatr. Surg.* **1992**, *2*, 210–215. [CrossRef]
18. Braye, F.; Dumortier, R.; Bertin-Maghit, M.; Girbon, J.P.; Tissot, E.; Damour, O. Les cultures d'épiderme pour le traitement des grands brûlés. Etude sur deux ans (18 patients). *Ann. Chir. Plast. Esthét.* **2001**, *46*, 599–606. [CrossRef]
19. Cuono, C.B.; Langdon, R.; Birchall, N.; Barttelbort, S.; McGuire, J. Composite autologous-allogeneic skin replacement: Development and clinical application. *Plast. Reconstr. Surg.* **1987**, *80*, 626–637. [CrossRef]
20. Benathan, M.; Labidi-Ubaldi, F. Substituts épidermiques et dermo-épidermiques vivants pour le traitement des grands brûlés. *Rev. Méd. Suisse Rom.* **1998**, *118*, 149–153.
21. Brockmann, I.; Ehrenpfordt, J.; Sturmheit, T.; Brandenburger, M.; Kruse, C.; Zille, M.; Rose, D.; Boltze, J. Skin-derived stem cells for wound treatment using cultured epidermal autografts: Clinical applications and challenges. *Stem Cells Int.* **2018**, *2018*, 4623615. [CrossRef] [PubMed]
22. Atiyeh, B.S.; Costagliola, M. Cultured epithelial autograft (CEA) in burn treatment: Three decades later. *Burns* **2007**, *33*, 405–413. [CrossRef]
23. Li, Z.; Maitz, P.B. Cell therapy for severe burn wound healing. *Burn. Trauma* **2018**, *6*, 13. [CrossRef] [PubMed]
24. Gobet, R.; Raghunath, M.; Altermatt, S.; Meuli-Simmen, C.; Benathan, M.; Dietl, A.; Meuli, M. Efficacy of cultured epithelial autografts in pediatric burns and reconstructive surgery. *Surgery* **1997**, *121*, 654–661. [CrossRef]
25. Hartmann-Fritsch, F.; Marino, D.; Reichmann, E. About ATMPs, SOPs and GMP: The hurdles to produce novel skin grafts for clinical use. *Transfus. Med. Hemother.* **2016**, *43*, 344–352. [CrossRef]
26. De Wilde, S.; Veltrop-Duits, L.; Hoozemans-Strik, M.; Ras, T.; Blom-Veenman, J.; Guchelaar, H.J.; Zandvliet, M.; Meij, P. Hurdles in clinical implementation of academic Advanced Therapy Medicinal Product: A national evaluation. *Cytotherapy* **2016**, *18*, 797–805. [CrossRef]

27. Monnier, S.; Abdel-Sayed, P.; de Buys Roessingh, A.; Hirt-Burri, N.; Chemali, M.; Applegate, L.A.; Raffoul, W. Surgical management evolution between 2 massive burn cases at 17-year interval: Contribution of cell therapies in improving the surgical care. *Cell Transplant.* **2020**, *29*, 963689720973642. [CrossRef]
28. Pontiggia, L.; Klar, A.; Böttcher-Haberzeth, S.; Biedermann, T.; Meuli, M.; Reichmann, E. Optimizing in vitro culture conditions leads to a significantly shorter production time of human dermo-epidermal skin substitutes. *Pediatr. Surg. Int.* **2013**, *29*, 249–256. [CrossRef] [PubMed]
29. Meuli, M.; Hartmann-Fritsch, F.; Hüging, M.; Marino, D.; Saglini, M.; Hynes, S.; Neuhaus, K.; Manuel, E.; Middelkoop, E.; Reichmann, E.; et al. A cultured autologous dermo-epidermal skin substitute for full-thickness skin defects: A Phase I, open, prospective clinical trial in children. *Plast. Reconstr. Surg.* **2019**, *144*, 188–198. [CrossRef]
30. Moiemen, N.; Schiestl, C.; Hartmann-Fritsch, F.; Neuhaus, K.; Reichmann, E.; Löw, A.; Stenger, C.; Böttcher-Haberzeth, S.; Meuli, M. First time compassionate use of laboratory engineered autologous Zurich skin in a massively burned child. *Burns Open* **2021**, *5*, 113–117. [CrossRef]
31. Schiestl, C.; Meuli, M.; Vojvodic, M.; Pontiggia, L.; Neuhaus, D.; Brotschi, B.; Reichmann, E.; Böttcher-Haberzeth, S.; Neuhaus, K. Expanding into the future: Combining a novel dermal template with distinct variants of autologous cultured skin substitutes in massive burns. *Burns Open* **2021**, *5*, 145–153. [CrossRef]
32. Klama-Baryła, A.; Kitala, D.; Łabuś, W.; Kraut, M.; Glik, J.; Nowak, M.; Kawecki, M. Autologous and allogeneic skin cell grafts in the treatment of severely burned patients: Retrospective clinical study. *Transplant. Proc.* **2018**, *50*, 2179–2187. [CrossRef] [PubMed]
33. Coulomb, B.; Legreton, C.; Dubertret, L. Influence of human dermal fibroblasts on epidermalization. *J. Investig. Dermatol.* **1989**, *92*, 122–125. [CrossRef] [PubMed]
34. Lamme, E.N.; Van Leeuwen, R.T.J.; Brandsma, K.; Van Marle, J.; Middelkoop, E. Higher numbers of autologous fibroblasts in an artificial dermal substitute improve tissue regeneration and modulate scar tissue formation. *J. Pathol.* **2000**, *190*, 595–603. [CrossRef]
35. Hohlfeld, J.; de Buys Roessingh, A.S.; Hirt-Burri, N.; Chaubert, P.; Gerber, S.; Scaletta, C.; Hohlfeld, P.; Applegate, L.A. Tissue engineered fetal skin constructs for paediatric burns. *Lancet* **2005**, *366*, 840–842. [CrossRef] [PubMed]
36. Li, R.; Liu, K.; Huang, X.; Li, D.; Ding, J.; Liu, B.; Chen, X. Bioactive materials promote wound healing through modulation of cell behaviors. *Adv. Sci.* **2022**, *9*, e2105152. [CrossRef]
37. Al-Dourobi, K.; Laurent, A.; Deghayli, L.; Flahaut, M.; Abdel-Sayed, P.; Scaletta, C.; Michetti, M.; Waselle, L.; Simon, J.-P.; El Ezzi, O.; et al. Retrospective evaluation of Progenitor Biological Bandage use: A complementary and safe therapeutic management option for prevention of hypertrophic scarring in pediatric burn care. *Pharmaceuticals* **2021**, *14*, 201. [CrossRef]
38. Mandla, S.; Davenport Huyer, L.; Radisic, M. Review: Multimodal bioactive material approaches for wound healing. *APL Bioeng.* **2018**, *2*, 021503. [CrossRef]
39. Laurent, A.E.; Lin, P.; Scaletta, C.; Hirt-Burri, N.; Michetti, M.; De Buys Roessingh, A.S.; Raffoul, W.; She, B.-R.; Applegate, L.A. Bringing safe and standardized cell therapies to industrialized processing for burns and wounds. *Front. Bioeng. Biotechnol.* **2020**, *8*, 581. [CrossRef]
40. Hata, R.-Y.; Senoo, H. L-ascorbic acid 2-phosphate stimulates collagen accumulation, cell proliferation, and formation of a three-dimensional tissuelike substance by skin fibroblasts. *J. Cell Physiol.* **1989**, *138*, 8–16. [CrossRef]
41. MacNeil, S. Progress and opportunities for tissue-engineered skin. *Nature* **2007**, *445*, 874–880. [CrossRef] [PubMed]
42. El Ghalbzouri, A.; Jonkman, M.F.; Dijkman, R.; Ponec, M. Basement membrane reconstruction in human skin equivalents is regulated by fibroblasts and/or exogenously activated keratinocytes. *J. Investig. Dermatol.* **2005**, *124*, 79–86. [CrossRef] [PubMed]
43. Gibson, T.; Medawar, P.B. The fate of skin homografts in man. *J. Anat.* **1943**, *77*, 299–310.
44. Medawar, P.B. Immunity to homologous grafted skin; The fate of skin homografts transplanted to the brain, to subcutaneous tissue, and to the anterior chamber of the eye. *Br. J. Exp. Pathol.* **1948**, *29*, 58–69.
45. Leto Barone, A.A.; Mastroianni, M.; Farkash, E.A.; Mallard, C.; Albritton, A.; Torabi, R.; Leonard, D.A.; Kurtz, J.M.; Sachs, D.H.; Cetrulo, C.L., Jr. Genetically modified porcine split-thickness skin grafts as an alternative to allograft for provision of temporary wound coverage: Preliminary characterization. *Burns* **2015**, *41*, 565–574. [CrossRef] [PubMed]
46. Chiarini, A.; Dal Pra, I.; Armato, U. In vitro and in vivo characteristics of frozen/thawed neonatal pig split-skin strips: A novel biologically active dressing for areas of severe, acute or chronic skin loss. *Int. J. Mol. Med.* **2007**, *19*, 245–255. [CrossRef]
47. Hanna Luze, H.; Nischwitz, S.P.; Smolle, C.; Robert Zrim, R.; Kamolz, L.-P. The use of acellular fish skin grafts in burn wound management—A systematic review. *Medicina* **2022**, *58*, 912. [CrossRef]
48. Júnior, E.M.L.; Filho, M.O.D.M.; Costa, B.A.; Fechine, F.V.; Vale, M.L.; Diógenes, A.K.D.L.; Neves, K.R.T.; Uchôa, A.M.D.N.; Soares, M.F.A.D.N.; de Moraes, M.E.A. Nile Tilapia fish skin–based wound dressing improves pain and treatment-related costs of superficial partial-thickness burns: A Phase III randomized controlled trial. *Plast. Reconstr. Surg.* **2021**, *147*, 1189–1198. [CrossRef]
49. Yang, C.K.; Polanco, T.O.; Ii, J.C.L. A prospective, postmarket, compassionate clinical evaluation of a novel acellular fish-skin graft which contains Omega-3 fatty acids for the closure of hard-to-heal lower extremity chronic ulcers. *Wounds* **2016**, *28*, 112–118. [PubMed]
50. Vogt, P.M.; Thompsont, S.; Andree, C.; Liu, P.; Breuing, K.; Hatzis, D.; Brown, H.; Mulligant, R.C.; Eriksson, E.; Murray, J.E. Genetically modified keratinocytes transplanted to wounds reconstitute the epidermis. *Proc. Natl. Acad. Sci. USA* **1994**, *91*, 9307–9311. [CrossRef]

51. Sykulev, Y.; Joo, M.; Vturina, I.; Tsomides, T.J.; Eisen, H.N. Evidence that a single peptide-MHC complex on a target cell can elicit a cytolytic T cell response. *Immunity* **1996**, *4*, 565–571. [CrossRef] [PubMed]
52. Deuse, T.; Hu, X.; Gravina, A.; Wang, D.; Tediashvili, G.; De, C.; Thayer, W.O.; Wahl, A.; Garcia, J.V.; Reichenspurner, H.; et al. Hypoimmunogenic derivatives of induced pluripotent stem cells evade immune rejection in fully immunocompetent allogeneic recipients. *Nat. Biotechnol.* **2019**, *37*, 252–258. [CrossRef]
53. Laurent, A.; Rey, M.; Scaletta, C.; Abdel-Sayed, P.; Michetti, M.; Flahaut, M.; Raffoul, W.; de Buys Roessingh, A.; Hirt-Burri, N.; Applegate, L.A. Retrospectives on three decades of safe clinical experience with allogeneic dermal progenitor fibroblasts: High versatility in topical cytotherapeutic care. *Pharmaceutics* **2023**, *15*, 184. [CrossRef] [PubMed]
54. Cavalli, E.; Fisch, P.; Formica, F.A.; Gareus, R.; Linder, T.; Applegate, L.A.; Zenobi-Wong, M. A comparative study of cartilage engineered constructs in immunocompromised, humanized and immunocompetent mice. *J. Immunol. Regen. Med.* **2018**, *2*, 36–46. [CrossRef]
55. Lee, S.J.; Kim, J.; Choi, W.H.; Park, S.R.; Choi, B.H.; Min, B.H. Immunophenotype and immune-modulatory activities of human fetal cartilage-derived progenitor cells. *Cell Transplant.* **2019**, *28*, 932–942. [CrossRef]
56. Marino, D.; Luginbühl, J.; Scola, S.; Meuli, M.; Reichmann, E. Bioengineering dermo-epidermal skin grafts with blood and lymphatic capillaries. *Sci. Transl. Med.* **2014**, *6*, 221ra14. [CrossRef]
57. Klar, A.S.; Böttcher-Haberzeth, S.; Biedermann, T.; Schiestl, C.; Reichmann, E.; Meuli, M. Analysis of blood and lymph vascularization patterns in tissue-engineered human dermo-epidermal skin analogs of different pigmentation. *Pediatr. Surg. Int.* **2014**, *30*, 223–231. [CrossRef]
58. Hendrickx, B.; Verdonck, K.; Van den Berge, S.; Dickens, S.; Eriksson, E.; Vranckx, J.J.; Luttun, A. Integration of blood outgrowth endothelial cells in dermal fibroblast sheets promotes full thickness wound healing. *Stem Cell* **2010**, *28*, 1165–1177. [CrossRef]
59. Böttcher-Haberzeth, S.; Biedermann, T.; Pontiggia, L.; Braziulis, E.; Schiestl, C.; Hendriks, B.; Eichhoff, O.M.; Widmer, D.S.; Meuli-Simmen, C.; Meuli, M.; et al. Human eccrine sweat gland cells turn into melanin-uptaking keratinocytes in dermo-epidermal skin substitutes. *J. Investig. Dermatol.* **2013**, *133*, 316–324. [CrossRef]
60. Hirt-Burri, N.; Scaletta, C.; Gerber, S.; Pioletti, D.P.; Applegate, L.A. Wound-healing gene family expression differences between fetal and foreskin cells used for bioengineered skin substitutes. *Artif. Organs* **2008**, *32*, 509–518. [CrossRef]
61. World Medical Association. Declaration of Helsinki: Ethical principles for medical research involving human subjects. *JAMA* **2013**, *310*, 2191–2194. [CrossRef] [PubMed]
62. Bukovac, P.K.; Hauser, M.; Lottaz, D.; Marti, A.; Schmitt, I.; Schochat, T. The regulation of cell therapy and gene therapy products in Switzerland. *Adv. Exp. Med. Biol.* **2023**, *1430*, 41–58. [CrossRef] [PubMed]

*pharmaceutics*

MDPI

*Review*

# Cell Therapy for Retinal Degenerative Diseases: Progress and Prospects

**Kevin Y. Wu [1,*], Jaskarn K. Dhaliwal [2], Akash Sasitharan [3] and Ananda Kalevar [1]**

1 Department of Surgery, Division of Ophthalmology, University of Sherbrooke, Sherbrooke, QC J1G 2E8, Canada
2 Faculty of Health Sciences, Department of Medicine, Queen's University, Kingston, ON K7L 3N6, Canada
3 Faculty of Medicine and Health Sciences, Department of Medicine, McGill University, Montreal, QC H3A 0GA, Canada
* Correspondence: yang.wu@usherbrooke.ca

**Abstract: Background/Objectives:** Age-related macular degeneration (AMD) and retinitis pigmentosa (RP) are leading causes of vision loss, with AMD affecting older populations and RP being a rarer, genetically inherited condition. Both diseases result in progressive retinal degeneration, for which current treatments remain inadequate in advanced stages. This review aims to provide an overview of the retina's anatomy and physiology, elucidate the pathophysiology of AMD and RP, and evaluate emerging cell-based therapies for these conditions. **Methods:** A comprehensive review of the literature was conducted, focusing on cell therapy approaches, including embryonic stem cells (ESCs), induced pluripotent stem cells (iPSCs), mesenchymal stem cells (MSCs), and retinal progenitor cells. Preclinical and clinical studies were analyzed to assess therapeutic potential, with attention to mechanisms such as cell replacement, neuroprotection, and paracrine effects. Relevant challenges, including ethical concerns and clinical translation, were also explored. **Results:** Cell-based therapies demonstrate potential for restoring retinal function and slowing disease progression through mechanisms like neuroprotection and cell replacement. Preclinical trials show promising outcomes, but clinical studies face significant hurdles, including challenges in cell delivery and long-term efficacy. Combination therapies integrating gene editing and biomaterials offer potential future advancements. **Conclusions:** While cell-based therapies for AMD and RP have made significant progress, substantial barriers to clinical application remain. Further research is essential to overcome these obstacles, improve delivery methods, and ensure the safe and effective translation of these therapies into clinical practice.

**Keywords:** stem cells; mesenchymal stromal cells; cell therapy; gene therapy; retinal degenerative diseases; age-related macular degeneration; retinitis pigmentosa; embryonic stem cells; induced pluripotent stem cells; retinal progenitor cells; photoreceptor replacement; neuroprotection; paracrine effects; clinical trials

## 1. Introduction

Retinal degenerative diseases, including age-related macular degeneration (AMD) and retinitis pigmentosa (RP), are significant contributors to vision loss, affecting millions of people worldwide. AMD is particularly prevalent among older populations, while RP, though rarer, is a genetically inherited condition that progressively impairs vision. Despite advancements in ophthalmology and ocular pharmacology, effective treatments for these conditions remain limited, especially in the later stages of the disease.

Cell-based therapies have emerged as one of the potential solutions to address the complex challenges of retinal degeneration, offering the potential to replace or repair damaged retinal tissues, thereby restoring vision or at least halting further degeneration. This review provides a comprehensive examination of the anatomy and physiology of the retina, the pathophysiology of AMD, RP, glaucoma, and Stargardt disease, and the latest developments in cell therapy strategies, including the use of embryonic stem cells (ESCs), induced pluripotent stem cells (iPSCs), mesenchymal stem cells (MSCs), and progenitor cells.

A key focus of this review is on the most recent preclinical and clinical studies published within the last few years, reflecting the rapid advancements in the field. We explore the underlying mechanisms of action, such as cell replacement, neuroprotection, and paracrine effects, and discuss the challenges of translating these therapies from the laboratory to the bedside. We discuss future directions, including innovations in cell delivery techniques, combination therapies, and the ethical considerations surrounding stem cell use in retinal treatments. This review article aims to provide a clear understanding of the current state and future potential of cell therapy for retinal degenerative diseases.

## 2. Anatomy and Physiology of the Retina

### *2.1. Structure of the Retina and Choroid*

The retina is an intricate structure composed of 10 neuronal layers and 6 different cell lines (Figure 1). Layers are connected to one another via synapses and each cell line plays a role in detecting variations and movements of light [1]. These cells include photoreceptor cells, horizontal cells, bipolar cells, amacrine cells, and retinal ganglion cells.

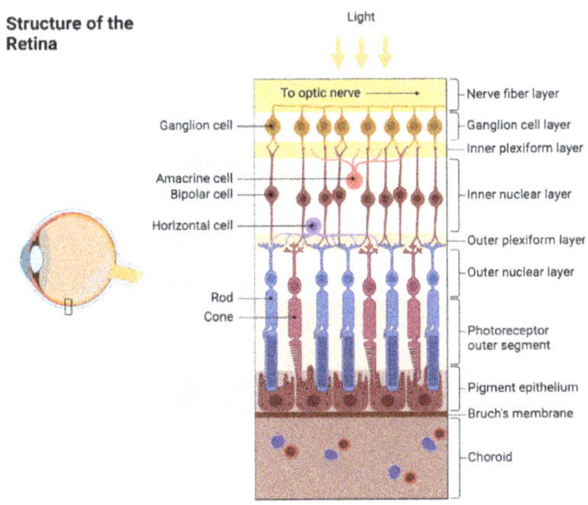


**Figure 1.** The retina consists of 10 layers: the inner limiting membrane, nerve fiber layer, ganglion cell layer, inner plexiform layer, inner nuclear layer, middle limiting membrane, outer plexiform layer, outer nuclear layer, external limiting layer, and photoreceptor layer. It also consists of 6 cell types: ganglion, amacrine, bipolar, horizontal, and photoreceptor cells. Reprinted from "Structure of the Retina", by BioRender.com (2024). Retrieved from https://app.biorender.com/biorender-templates accessed on 15 August 2024.

Photoreceptor cells include rods and cones. Rod cells comprise about 95% of photoreceptors in the retina and register low-light levels, helping to create scotopic vision [1]. Rods are concentrated in the periphery of the retina, with cone cells being concentrated in the retinal center, in the macula. Cone cells comprise about 5% of the retinal photoreceptors. Cone cells aid in processing color vision at various light levels and allow for greater spatial acuity, providing information for fine details, movement, and colors.

Horizontal cells are located between bipolar cells and photoreceptors. They provide inhibitory feedback to bipolar cells, rods, and cones and help the eyes adjust to low light and bright light [1]. Bipolar cells receive glutamatergic input from rods and cones and GABAergic inhibitory input from horizontal cells. They project their axons to retinal ganglion cells, providing glutamatergic inputs. Bipolar cells are present in the inner plexiform layer of the retina and link the outer and inner layers of the retina. Amacrine cells inhibit bipolar cells before the synapse at the inner plexiform layer. Retinal ganglion cells are photosensitive and assist with circadian rhythm, melatonin release, and regulation of pupil size.

Various retinal cells can be damaged in different ocular and retinal diseases. For example, retinitis pigmentosa (RP) primarily affects the rod cells, leading to their degeneration; glaucoma results in the destruction of retinal ganglion cells due to optic nerve damage; and in age-related macular degeneration (AMD), the compromised function of retinal pigment epithelial (RPE) cells leads to photoreceptor loss.

### 2.2. Retinal Blood Supply

The retina has a dual blood supply as it has the highest rate of oxygen consumption in the body. The dual blood supply is received by the choroid and branches of the ophthalmic artery, which arises from the internal carotid artery, giving rise to the central retinal artery and posterior ciliary arteries [1]. The central retinal artery provides blood to the inner retina. The posterior ciliary artery divides into short and long posterior ciliary arteries and provides blood flow to the outer retina. Retinal blood flow is typically low and influenced by local factors such as nitric oxide, prostaglandins, endothelin, and arterial carbon dioxide tension [2]. On the other hand, the choroid has high blood flow and low oxygen content. The choroid forms the posterior part of the uveal tract and receives blood supply from the long and short posterior ciliary arteries, nourishing the outer layers of the retina.

The blood–retina barrier is composed of the inner and outer blood–retinal barriers. The outer blood–retina barrier regulates transportation across the choriocapillaris and the retina, while the inner blood–retina barrier regulates transportation across the retinal capillaries [3]. The outer-blood retina barrier is formed at the RPE [3]. The inner is formed of very tight junctions and consists of Muller cells, which help support barrier function in the retina. An important fact of the neural retina is that it has immune privilege, proving it a suitable site for cell transplantations [4].

## 3. Retinal Degenerative Diseases

Millions of people worldwide are impacted by retinal degenerative diseases, which are a leading cause of vision loss and blindness [5]. This section provides an overview of prominent retinal degenerative disorders: age-related macular degeneration (AMD), retinitis pigmentosa (RP), glaucoma, and Stargardt disease (SD).

### 3.1. Age-Related Macular Degeneration (AMD)

Age-related macular degeneration is a leading cause of blindness globally, especially in the West [5]. It is associated with the degeneration of the macula, a region of the retina important for central vision and home to a large number of cone photoreceptors [6]. The macula also includes the fovea, which is the center of the macula. There are two types of AMD: dry AMD and wet AMD.

More than 90% of AMD patients experience dry AMD, sometimes referred to as nonexudative or non-neovascular AMD [7]. Although it usually advances gradually over decades, it can eventually lead to wet AMD. The thickening of the Bruch membrane resulting from the build-up of drusen (lipid and protein deposits) between the Bruch membrane and the retinal pigment epithelium (RPE) is a characteristic of dry AMD [8]. Retinal degeneration and atrophy are the results of this accumulation [7].

Wet AMD, or exudative/neovascular AMD, accounts for approximately 10–15% of AMD cases but is responsible for the majority of severe vision loss associated with the condition. [7]. Unlike the dry form, wet AMD progresses rapidly, often leading to significant vision loss within weeks to months. The hallmark of wet AMD is the development of choroidal neovascularization (CNV), where new, abnormal blood vessels grow from the choroid through defects in the Bruch's membrane into the subretinal space. These vessels are prone to leakage of blood, lipids, and fluids, which can cause retinal pigment epithelium (RPE) detachment and photoreceptor damage. The role of the Vascular Endothelial Growth

Factor (VEGF) is crucial in this process, as it promotes the growth and permeability of these abnormal blood vessels. The leakage from these fragile vessels leads to the accumulation of fluid and blood, resulting in rapid vision deterioration if left untreated [9].

The incidence of AMD increases after the age of 50. Risk factors for AMD include aging, blue-colored eyes, Caucasian ancestry, family history, sun exposure, smoking, alcohol intake, high blood pressure, obesity, and diabetes [10]. Clinical signs include increasing loss of central vision, trouble focusing on tasks, decreased night vision, trouble adjusting to light, fluctuating vision, and metamorphopsia [11]. Four groups can be used to categorize AMD severity (Figure 2): Group I consists of five to fifteen small lesions; early-stage AMD is characterized by more than fifteen small lesions or fewer than twenty medium-sized lesions; the intermediate stage is characterized by at least one large lesion or more than twenty medium-sized lesions or non-central geographic atrophy (GA); and the advanced stage is characterized by central geographic atrophy or wet AMD [12].

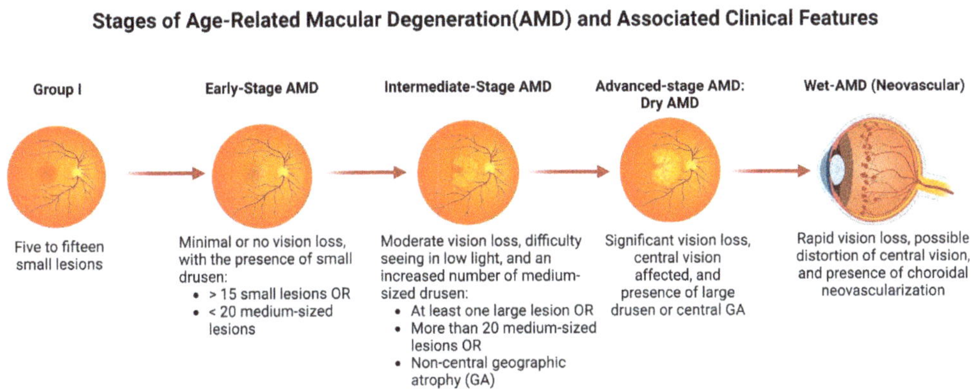


**Figure 2.** The progressive stages of age-related macular degeneration (AMD) and the associated clinical features. Adapted from the "Non-Alcoholic Fatty Liver Disease (NAFLD) Spectrum", by BioRender.com (2024). Retrieved from https://app.biorender.com/biorender-templates, accessed on 15 August 2024.

The available preventive treatment options for dry age-related macular degeneration include dietary supplements containing vitamin E, vitamin A, zinc, cupric oxide, lutein, zeaxanthin, and omega-3 fatty acids, as well as lifestyle changes like alcohol and smoking cessation [12]. Anti-VEGF therapy, which involves monthly injections of ranibizumab, bevacizumab, or aflibercept, is used to treat wet AMD [10]. Anti-VEGF therapy improves visual acuity or, at the least, it stabilizes the neo-vascularization response in a larger number of individuals [13].

### *3.2. Retinitis Pigmentosa (RP) (Disease)*

Retinitis pigmentosa (RP) is a group of genetic disorders characterized by the degeneration of photoreceptors in the retina, primarily affecting rods more than cones [14]. It is the most prevalent retinal illness that is inherited, and it can be X-linked, autosomal recessive, or autosomal dominant. In total, 1 in 5000 persons have RP, and 1 in 100 people are carriers of the disease.

Mutations cause retinal photoreceptors to undergo apoptosis, which in turn causes neighboring cells to undergo secondary apoptosis [14]. As a result, melanin deposits into perivascular regions and RPE cells separate, resulting in the formation of distinctive pigmented deposits. In spite of the term, apoptosis is the main step; inflammation is negligible. Clinical signs include flashes of light (photopsia), reduced peripheral vision leading to central vision loss, and decreased night vision (nyctalopia), which can proceed to complete night blindness.

Current therapeutic modalities for RP include supplementation with Vitamin A and E, which may slow progression in some cases [14]. The prognosis is generally poor for X-linked RP, while autosomal dominant RP has a better prognosis.

Although we have yet to develop a treatment that can restore vision for those suffering from end-stage geographic atrophy due to severe dry AMD or end-stage RP, ongoing research into cell therapy offers hope and will be discussed in detail in the next section.

### 3.3. Glaucoma

Glaucoma is a collection of eye conditions that, if untreated, frequently cause irreversible vision loss due to gradual damage to the optic nerve [15]. Elevated intraocular pressure (IOP) is the most prevalent cause; however, normal-tension glaucoma, in which optic nerve damage develops despite normal IOP levels, can also happen [16]. The trabecular meshwork's resistance to the aqueous humor's outflow usually results in a rise in intraocular pressure [17]. Retinal ganglion cell (RGC) axons, which carry visual information from the retina to the brain, are harmed by this mechanical stress on the optic nerve head caused by the elevated pressure [18]. These axons' function is disrupted by compression, gradually impairing vision [18]. Damage to the optic nerve mostly affects the optic nerve head, resulting in a distinctive pattern of loss of peripheral vision that may eventually lead to tunnel vision or total blindness [15]. RGC degeneration is believed to be facilitated by oxidative stress, neuroinflammatory processes, and mechanical injury [19]. It is well recognized that inflammatory mediators and free radicals aggravate the damage and hasten the course of glaucoma [19].

In order to halt the advancement of optic nerve damage, the main goal of current therapeutic therapies for glaucoma is to reduce IOP [20]. Medications such as carbonic anhydrase inhibitors, beta-blockers, and prostaglandin analogs, which either increase aqueous humor outflow or decrease fluid production, are commonly used as therapies [20]. A different drainage channel for the aqueous humor can also be created by surgical procedures like trabeculectomy or laser therapy [21]. Nevertheless, the damage already done to the optic nerve cannot be undone by these treatments; they can only control the illness. In addition, patients may find it difficult to follow long-term prescription regimens, and complications from surgery are a possibility. Therefore, the creation of cell-based treatments appears promising for those suffering from glaucoma. The goal of stem cell treatments is to repair or preserve injured retinal ganglion cells while regaining the function of the optic nerve. Although these treatments are still in the preliminary stages, they present a viable future option that might not only cure optic nerve damage and restore lost cells, but also halt the progression of the disease [22].

### 3.4. Stargardt Disease (SD)

The most prevalent type of inherited macular degeneration is called Stargardt disease, and it is mainly brought on by mutations in the ABCA4 gene [23]. The protein that this gene produces is in charge of removing harmful byproducts from photoreceptor cells during the visual cycle [24]. These byproducts, especially lipofuscin, accumulate in the retinal pigment epithelium (RPE) as a result of mutations in ABCA4. Both the RPE cells and the photoreceptor cells that depend on the RPE for vital metabolic support are severely damaged by the accumulation of lipofuscin [24]. Cone photoreceptors in the macula, which are in charge of central vision, gradually deteriorate as a result of lipofuscin buildup. The end outcome of this process is a progressive loss of color vision, light sensitivity, and visual acuity [23]. Lipofuscin's harmful actions exacerbate the degeneration by hindering the RPE's capacity to preserve the health of the photoreceptor cells [24]. As a result, peripheral vision usually remains intact, while central vision gradually disappears [23]. Due to the degenerative nature of Stargardt illness, many people have severe vision loss early in life, especially in youth [23].

Currently, Stargardt disease cannot be stopped from progressing further or reversed using an approved medication [23]. Supportive therapies may assist with managing symptoms but do not address the underlying pathophysiology. Examples of these therapies include the use of low-vision devices and light protection [23]. Clinical trials are still in progress for gene therapy to fix abnormalities in the ABCA4 gene [25]. The shortcomings of existing treatments highlight the possibility of cell-based therapeutics as a future modality. Damaged retinal tissue may regain its ability to function through cell replacement therapies, such as the transplanting of healthy RPE or photoreceptor cells made from stem cells. While more investigation is needed to address issues with cell survival, integration, and immune response, cell-based therapies offer patients with Stargardt illness a promising path toward retinal cell regeneration and vision preservation.

## 4. Types of Cell Therapies

With the potential to replace or repair damaged retinal cells, cell therapy holds great promise for the treatment of retinal degenerative illnesses [26]. The several kinds of cell therapies (Figure 3) that are presently being researched and developed are examined in this section.

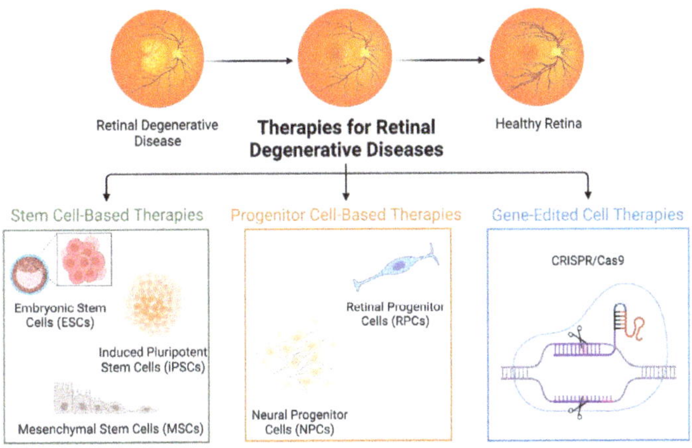


**Figure 3.** Cell-based therapies for retinal degenerative diseases. Adapted from "Immunotherapy Overview", by BioRender.com (2024). Retrieved from https://app.biorender.com/biorender-templates accessed on 15 August 2024.

### *4.1. Retinitis Pigmentosa (RP)*

#### 4.1.1. Embryonic Stem Cells

Embryonic stem cells (ESCs) are pluripotent cells derived from early-stage embryos. They have the capacity to differentiate into any cell type, including specialized retinal cells such as photoreceptors, retinal pigment epithelial (RPE) cells, and ganglion cells. This versatility makes ESCs a vital tool in regenerative medicine, notably for treating complex retinal degenerative diseases like age-related macular degeneration (AMD) and retinitis pigmentosa (RP). Although ESCs are very adaptable, transplanting them into patients carries a risk of immunological rejection and ethical issues [27]. Since ESCs are usually not produced from the patient's own cells, the transplanted cells run the risk of being recognized as foreign by the immune system, which could lead to an immunological reaction against them [27]. This may result in the transplanted cells being rejected, which would lessen the therapy's efficacy and possibly inflict further retinal tissue damage. Immunosuppressive medication carries its own risks and problems, including greater susceptibility to infections and other immune-related conditions, and may be necessary for patients in order to reduce this risk [27].

#### 4.1.2. Induced Pluripotent Stem Cells

Induced pluripotent stem cells (iPSCs) are generated by reprogramming adult somatic cells to a pluripotent state, similar to ESCs [28]. Since iPSCs can be generated from the patient's own cells, the risk of immunological rejection is reduced, and they avoid many of the ethical concerns that are related to ESCs [29]. Immunosuppressive medications, which are frequently necessary with ESC-based treatments, are not as likely to be needed when these autologous iPSCs are developed into retinal cells and transplanted back into the patient because the immune system is less likely to perceive them as alien [29]. Retinal cells can be created in vitro using iPSCs, and these cells could potentially be grafted into the injured retina to replace any missing or malfunctioning ones [29]. Furthermore, by using iPSCs to simulate retinal diseases in the lab, researchers can better understand the underlying mechanisms of these disorders and create novel treatment approaches.

#### 4.1.3. Mesenchymal Stem Cells

Mesenchymal stem cells (MSCs) are known for their immunomodulatory properties and ability to differentiate into various cell types [30]. Through immune response modulation and trophic support of injured retinal cells, MSCs have the ability to support retinal regeneration and repair [30]. The ability of MSC-derived factors, cells, and modified MSCs to repair injured retinal tissue has been the subject of numerous investigations. Preclinical models of retinal degeneration demonstrated that human dental pulp-derived MSCs (DP-MSCs) improved retinal function in a rat model of retinal degeneration through intravitreal transplantation, while rat bone-marrow-derived MSCs (BM-MSCs) restored the thickness of the outer nuclear layer (ONL) by increasing autophagy [31]. Injections of umbilical cord-derived MSCs (UC-MSCs) and their exosomes improved visual functions and decreased inflammation and retinal damage in a mouse model of intravitreal retinal injury [31].

### *4.2. Progenitor Cell-Based Therapies*

Progenitor cell-based therapies represent a promising avenue for treating retinal degenerative diseases by harnessing the regenerative potential of cells that are more differentiated than stem cells but still have the capacity to develop into specific types of retinal cells. This method focuses on replacing or repairing damaged retinal tissue with neural progenitor cells (NPCs) and retinal progenitor cells (RPCs).

#### 4.2.1. Retinal Progenitor Cells

Specialized cells called retinal progenitor cells are derived from the growing retina and have the ability to differentiate into several types of retinal cells, such as photoreceptors and retinal ganglion cells [32]. RPCs have been found to be important in regenerative therapy for retinal illnesses and to play a critical function during retinal development. RPCs are a strong contender for therapeutic intervention because of their capacity to develop into vital retinal cells and blend in with the current retinal architecture [32]. RPCs have demonstrated the ability to halt the course of disease, restore vision, and replace missing or damaged retinal cells when implanted into the retina [32]. RPC transplantation is undergoing clinical trials, and preliminary findings suggest that these cells can proliferate, migrate, and differentiate within the host retina [32].

#### 4.2.2. Neural Progenitor Cells

Neural progenitor cells (NPCs) are multipotent cells that can differentiate into various neural cell types, including neurons, astrocytes, and oligodendrocytes [33]. NPCs are particularly interesting in the context of retinal degenerative illnesses because they can replace retinal neurons while simultaneously performing vital supporting roles that keep the retina healthy [34]. NPCs have been shown to be able to adapt to the retinal environment after transplantation, and they can come from different parts of the central nervous system, such as the brain and spinal cord. Through differentiation into retinal cells and the formation of synaptic connections with pre-existing retinal neurons, NPCs have been demonstrated in preclinical investigations to restore some function of the visual system [33]. To further increase their therapeutic potential, NPCs can release neurotrophic substances that support the survival and functionality of the remaining retinal cells [33].

RPCs and NPCs in particular are progenitor cell-based therapies that provide a focused method for retinal restoration. In addition to replacing lost cells, these therapies work to foster an environment that supports the retina's long-term survival and performance.

### 4.3. Gene-Edited Cell Therapies

Gene-edited cell therapies are emerging as a revolutionary approach to treating retinal degenerative diseases by directly targeting and correcting genetic mutations responsible for these conditions. A variety of techniques for retinal gene therapy may be employed, contingent upon the kind of mutation: gene replacement or augmentation, editing or silencing the defective gene, or introducing a gene that alters the downstream or upstream pathways from the damaged gene to improve cellular function [35]. Retinal gene therapies employ several vectors and delivery systems. A plethora of gene-editing techniques have been developed, including zinc finger nucleases (ZFNs), transcription activator-like effector nucleases (TALENs), homing endonucleases or meganucleases, and CRISPR/Cas9 [35]. CRISPR/Cas9 is one of the widely used gene-editing tools in biomedical research and there are several gene therapies using this technology in clinical trials [35].

Gene therapy has long been thought to be a great fit for the retina. Advantages include a restricted, immune-privileged area protected by the blood–retina barrier [35]. Since the retina is small and does not proliferate cellularly in adults, retinal disorders can be treated with low dosages of the vector [35]. Products for ocular gene therapy might be administered by clinical protocols or established surgical methods. Nevertheless, despite these advantages, gene therapy faces a major challenge due to the enormous genetic complexity of inherited retinal illnesses, which can involve hundreds of mutations across numerous distinct genes [35]. Due to this variability, developing therapies that are one size fits all is difficult. Furthermore, a precise genetic diagnosis is necessary to pinpoint the precise mutations causing the illness, yet many patients are still without a conclusive genetic diagnosis. Without this vital information, successful gene therapy customization is difficult, which reduces the potential benefit of the treatments.

## 5. Mechanisms of Action

Cell-based therapies for retinal degenerative diseases rely on several key mechanisms of action to restore vision and prevent further damage to the retina. These mechanisms include cell replacement, neuroprotection, and paracrine effects, each contributing to the overall therapeutic potential of these advanced treatments.

### 5.1. Cell Replacement

As previously discussed, AMD and RP are characterized by the degeneration of photoreceptors and RPE cells, respectively. Consequently, the primary objective of cell-based therapy is to restore retinal function by replacing these damaged or lost cells. This approach aims to replenish the retina with healthy, functional cells that can re-establish the intricate processes of light detection and signal transmission, ultimately preserving or even restoring vision. To achieve this, stem cells or progenitor cells must be differentiated into specific retinal cells.

There exists an optimized protocol to differentiate human-induced pluripotent stem cells into retinal pigment epithelium (RPE) cells [36]. The RPE cells generated following this protocol are mature and have similar cellular and molecular properties to primary RPE cells. Furthermore, the protocol includes an enrichment step enabling large-scale GMP manufacturing, which highlights the potential for cell replacement therapies in treating AMD [36].

Human embryonic stem cells (hESC) can also serve as a stem cell source for RPE cells; however, allogeneic hESC-RPE cells can trigger immune rejection, despite the eye being considered an immune-privileged site. Petrus-Reurer et al. established that hESC-RPEs lacking HLA-I and -II, which have reduced T-cell response in vitro, do not increase NK cell cytotoxic activity, and xeno-transplanted show reduced rejection in a large-eyed animal model [37].

The potential of photoreceptor cells derived from different human iPSC sources, including blood, fibroblasts, and keratinocytes, has been investigated in numerous research studies. However, due to the challenges in developing reliable, effective, and stable techniques for the production and purification of photoreceptor cells, there is no report of the transplantation of iPSC-derived photoreceptor cells in humans for the purpose of vision restoration [38].

### 5.2. Neuroprotection and Paracrine Effects

MSCs derived from bone marrow, umbilical cords, adipose tissues, and human neural progenitor cells take on a trophic role in stem cell therapy. MSCs are known to rescue degenerating photoreceptors via paracrine factors released by the cells. These cells suppress the immune response and inflammation by releasing immunomodulatory proteins such as Th2-related cytokines, insulin-like growth factor-1, and class II major histocompatibility complex antigens. Since PRs undergo mutations that produce RP, delaying the progression of vision loss can be achieved through cell preservation techniques. However, only when sufficient PRs are present in the early stages of the disease are the preservation techniques effective. RPE produced from MSCs can also be utilized as supporting cells to give PR that are still alive trophic support [39].

## 6. Cell Therapy for Retinal Degenerative Diseases

Cell therapy for retinal degenerative diseases has been tested in multiple preclinical and clinical trials over the years. These studies have been conducted in various animal models and looked at diseases from AMD to RP, glaucoma, and retinal degeneration in general. Studies have investigated cell therapy using embryonic stem cells (ESC), induced pluripotent stem cells (iPSC), RPE stem cells, bone marrow, mesenchymal cells, and more (Figure 4). Here, we will provide a review of the preclinical (Table 1) and clinical (Table 2) studies using cell therapy for retinal diseases conducted to date.

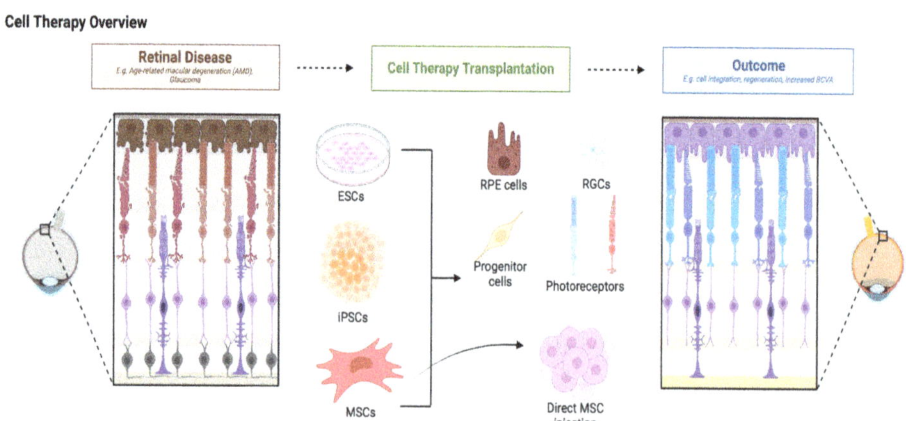


**Figure 4.** Preclinical and clinical trials to this date have utilized ESC, iPSC, MSC, and progenitor cell-derived cells to treat retinal diseases and improve functional outcomes. Adapted from "Retinal Disease and Regeneration", by BioRender.com (2024). Retrieved from https://app.biorender.com/biorender-templates accessed on 15 August 2024.

**Table 1.** Preclinical trials investigating cell therapy treatment for retinal degeneration.

| Disease Model | Animal Model | Protocol Description | Observed Effect | Reference |
|---|---|---|---|---|
| Retinal degeneration | Royal College of Surgeon (RCS) rats | Subretinal transplantation of donor RPE in host eye | RPE cells can be successfully transplanted into normal neonatal and adult rat eyes. | [40] |
| Retinal degeneration | Royal College of Surgeon (RCS) rats | Transplantation of donor RPE into subretinal space of dystrophic rat retina | Transplantation of RPE cells can prevent photoreceptor degeneration for at least 4 months. | [41] |
| Retinal degeneration | Royal College of Surgeon (RCS) rats | Subretinal transplantation of embryonic stem cells | Transplantation appeared to delay photoreceptor degeneration. | [42] |
| Retinal degeneration | Royal College of Surgeon (RCS) rats | Adult CD90 marrow stromal cells induced into cells with photoreceptor markers in vitro and then transplanted into RCS rats | MSC differentiated with autologous transplantation and integrated into the host retina with no teratoma formation. | [43] |
| AMD | Royal College of Surgeon (RCS) rats | Transplantation of RPE derived from primate ESC into subretinal space | Recovery of retinal function post-transplantation. | [44] |
| RP | C57BL/6 rho$^{-/-}$ mice at 4 week of age or C3H rd mice at 4 weeks of age | Isolated retinal progenitor cells from day 1 eGFP transgenic CH7Bl/6 mice and expanded them; then, transplanted into mice with retinal degeneration | Donor cells integrated into retina and mice who received the transplant showed improved light-mediated behavior. | [45] |
| AMD | Royal College of Surgeon (RCS) rats | RPE derived from human ESC and transplanted into subretinal space of RCS rats | Cell survived in host, photoreceptors were restored, and vision improved. | [46] |
| AMD and RP | Royal College of Surgeon (RCS) rats | hESC-derived RPE was transplanted in the subretinal space of RCS rats | Cell survived in host, photoreceptors were restored, and vision improved. | [47] |
| Retinal injury and damage | 10–12-week-old Wistar rats | Adult rat retinas underwent retinal damage via laser and then received bone marrow mesenchymal stem cell transplants | Bone marrow MSC survived in the retina and was incorporated into the outer nuclear layer, inner nuclear layer, and ganglion cell layer. Cells expressed rhodopsin and parvalbumin. | [48] |
| AMD and RP | Royal College of Surgeon (RCS) rats | RPE derived from human ESC and transplanted into subretinal space of RCS rats | Functional rescue in transplanted eyes compared to controls. | [49] |
| RP | Crx$^{-/-}$ mice (model of Leber's Congenital Amaurosis) | Retinal cells derived from human ESC were injected into mice retina using intraocular injection | Human ESC expressed markers for rod and cone photoreceptor cells once in subretinal space of mice and restored light response. | [50] |

**Table 1.** *Cont.*

| Disease Model | Animal Model | Protocol Description | Observed Effect | Reference |
| --- | --- | --- | --- | --- |
| Glaucoma | ES cell culture from mouse D3-ES cells | Embryonic stem cells were differentiated in vitro and also transplanted in vivo | Embryonic cells can be used to treat degenerative diseases as they generate RGC-like cells in vitro and also differentiate into RGC cells in vivo after transplantation. | [51] |
| Retinal degeneration | hESC and iPSC | Provide a defined method of inducing hESC and iPSC into retinal progenitors, RPE, and photoreceptors | Induced retinal progenitor cells expressed RX, MITF, PAX6, and CHX10. Hexagonal pigmented cells expressed RPE65 and CRALBP. Photoreceptors expressed recoverin, rhodopsin, and phototransduction genes. | [52] |
| Retinal degeneration | hESC and iPSC | Determine whether hESC and iPSC model retinal development upon differentiation | Demonstrated that retinal cell specification from hESC and iPSC follows a sequence and time course similar to normal retinal development. | [53] |
| Glaucoma | BALB/c mice | Trying to see if induced pluripotent stem cells can express retinal progenitor cell genes and differentiate into retinal ganglion cells. Injected iPS-derived retinal ganglion-like cells into the retina | iPS cells express Pax6, Rx, Otx2, Lhx2, and Nestin genes inherently and over expression of Math5 and DN differentiate iPS into RG-like cells. Inhibiting Hes1 increases RGC genes. iPS-derived RG-like cells survive in retina but cannot integrate post-transplant. | [54] |
| N/a | Normal retina, adult wild-type mice | Generate iPSC with *OCT4*, *SOX2*, *NANOG*, and *LIN28* to derive photoreceptors for use in cell therapy for retinal transplantation | FACS-purified iPSC-derived photoreceptors can integrate into normal mouse retina and express photoreceptor markers. | [55] |
| RP | 4–6-week-old dsRed-positive C57B1G mice were fibroblast donors and 4–6 weeks rhodopsin-null mice were transplant recipients | Adult dsRed mouse dermal fibroblast-derived iPSCs were transplanted in degenerative hosts | Cells formed teratomas. At 33 days, post-differentiation cells had markers for photoreceptors. CRX, recoverin, and rhodopsin. Increased retinol function in hosts with degenerative retina post-transplant. | [56] |
| RP | Monkey models | Determine ability of hESC-retina graft to transplant in rats and then conduct a pilot transplant in newly developed monkey models of retinal degeneration | Developed monkey models for study of retinal transplantation. Demonstrated hESC-retina graft to be effective in transplantation. | [57] |

**Table 1.** *Cont.*

| Disease Model | Animal Model | Protocol Description | Observed Effect | Reference |
|---|---|---|---|---|
| Retinal degeneration | Mouse models with mild degeneration (prom $1^{-/-}$) or severe degeneration (Cpfl1/$Rho^{-/-}$) | Derived photoreceptors from organoids and subretinal transplantation in wild-type hosts | Retinal organoids had high photoreceptors and survived in the subretinal space of all mice. In mild degeneration cells integrated and had mature morphology. In the severe degeneration model, transplants remained in subretinal space and had rod-specific markers but no mature morphology. | [58] |
| Glaucoma | 1–3-month Sprague Dawley rats | Transplanted GFP-labeled retinal ganglion cells into normal rat retinas by intravitreal injection | Cells integrated into the retina of adult rats (1–3 months) and made synapses post-transplantation. | [59] |
| Retinal degeneration | Female mice of inbred strain BALB/c age 7–9 weeks | Cultured MSCs to see growth factor expression, anti-inflammatory effects, and differentiation | Mesenchymal cells can differentiate into cells that show retinal markers, produce neuroprotective factors for retinal regeneration, and inhibit production of pro-inflammatory cytokines. | [60] |
| Retinal degeneration | 4-week albino Royal College of Surgeon (RCS) rats | Isolated rat embryonic stem cells and induced them into retinal progenitor cells in vitro; transplanted into RCS rat retina | Visual function was restored in RCS rats. Potential clinical application of ESC cell therapy. | [61] |
| Retinal degeneration | Mice and pigs | Oncogene mutation-free iPSC was taken from AMD patients and differentiated into iPSC retinal pigment epithelium patches | Protocol was robust and efficient in generating RPE cells and rescuing degenerating retina in mice and pigs. | [62] |
| Retinal degeneration | Rhodopsin mutant SD-Foxn1 Tg (S334ter)3LacRrrc nude rats and 2 monkeys | Transplanted human iPSC retinas into animal models | Mature photoreceptors survived in the host retina for 5 months (rat) and 2 years (monkey). Some light responses detected in grafted areas in rats (4 of 7) and monkeys. | [63] |
| Retinal degeneration | BALB/c-mu mice | Transplanted human retinal progenitor cells via intravitreal injection into BALB/c-mu mice | Differentiated hRPCs had high retinal markers, no teratoma was formed, and retinal function improved. Slowed retinal degeneration. However, hRPCs were no longer effective 12 weeks post-transplant. | [64] |
| Retinal degeneration | Royal College of Surgeon (RCS) rats | Compared combined hiPSC-derived RPE and retinal precursor cell (RPCs) transplantation to either alone; in vivo monitoring conducted | Combined transplantation of hiPSC-derived RPE and RPC may be better than either transplant alone in retinal degeneration. Better visual response and conservation of outer nuclear layer. | [65] |

**Table 1.** *Cont.*

| Disease Model | Animal Model | Protocol Description | Observed Effect | Reference |
| --- | --- | --- | --- | --- |
| RP | Royal College of Surgeon (RCS) rats | hiPSC-derived retinal cells and photoreceptor progenitor (PRP) cells transplanted in vivo via trans-scleral subretinal injection | Strong efficacy and safety for hiPSC-derived RPE and PRP cells in animals. No animal had teratoma formation and there was graft survival and integration. RPE transplant rescued vision function and there was functional photoreceptor activity. | [66] |
| AMD—geographic atrophy | Swine | Subretinal transplantation of hiPSC-derived RPE into healthy and degenerative retina areas | In vitro analysis showed the hiPSC-RPE cells to be differentiated, have typical epithelial morphology, and RPE-related gene expression. In the healthy retina, they engrafted and formed mature epithelium, but were patchy in atrophic areas. | [67] |
| Retinal degeneration | Royal College of Surgeon (RCS) rats | Transplanted retinal progenitor cells derived from mouse ESC-derived retinal organoids into RCS rats | The transplanted cells migrated to the inner retina and differentiated into photoreceptors, interneurons, and ganglion cells. The grafted cells elicited robust responses to light stimuli and integrated with the host retina. | [68] |
| RP | Royal College of Surgeon (RCS) rats | Derived umbilical cord mesenchymal stem cells (UCMSC) and then intravenously infused into RCS rats | Small UCMSC became stuck in lungs less and left quicker than UCMSC. Inflammation was inhibited and neurotrophic factors upregulated in retina and serum after transplantation. May be a potential therapeutic approach and delay degeneration in rats. | [69] |
| RP | *rd10* mice | Intravitreal injection of MSCs into mouse retina | Increase in survival rate of photoreceptors and visual function enhancement was observed through optomotor and electroretinogram responses. | [70] |
| RP | *rd12* mouse models with retinal degeneration | Intravitreal injection of adult MSC-derived RPCs into mouse retina | Transplanted RPCs led to improved vision and function. Observed anti-inflammation, retinal protection, and increased expression of genes involved in neurogenesis. | [71] |

**Table 1.** *Cont.*

| Disease Model | Animal Model | Protocol Description | Observed Effect | Reference |
|---|---|---|---|---|
| RP | Two animal models: RCS and P23H-1 rats | Utilized either intravitreal or subretinal injections of bone marrow mononuclear stem cell transplantations | Both forms of injections increased cell survival, as seen through mitigation of photoreceptor degeneration. No enhanced retinal function observed. | [72] |
| RP and AMD | Sodium iodate-induced retinal injury rat model | Transplantation of human adipose-derived MSCs | Transplantation facilitated photoreceptor regeneration and restoration of retinal function. | [73] |
| Retinal degeneration | 3-week-old RCS rats | Compared subretinal transplant of stem cells, human adipose-derived stem cells, amniotic fluid stem cells, bone marrow stem cells, dental pulp stem cells, induced pluripotent stem cells, and hiPSC-derived RPE | Rats transplanted with any stem cell other than hiPSC had better visual function 4 weeks post-injection. Rats with hiPSC maintained visual function 8 weeks post-injection. | [74] |

**Table 2.** Clinical trials investigating cell therapy treatment for retinal degeneration.

| Trial Stage | Type of Cell Used | Disease | Sample Size | Approach | Country | Identifier |
|---|---|---|---|---|---|---|
| Phase I/II | hESC-derived RPE (MA09-hRPE) | SMD | 13 | Subretinal injection of 50,000–200,000 cells | USA | NCT01345006 |
| Phase I and II—completed | hESC-derived RPE (MA09-hRPE) | Dry AMD | 13 | Subretinal injection of 50,000–150,000 cells in 5 cohorts | USA | NCT01344993 |
| Terminated | hESC-derived RPE (MA09-hRPE) | Advanced Dry AMD | 10 | Transplantation of MA09-hRPE | Republic of Korea | NCT01674829 |
| Phase I/II—completed | hESC-derived RPE (MA09-hRPE) | SMD | 12 | 5 cohorts with 50,000–200,000 cell injections | UK | NCT01469832 |
| Phase I—completed | hESC-derived RPE (MA09-hRPE) | Stargardt Macular Dystrophy | 3 | Subretinal transplantation of MA09-hRPE cells | Republic of Korea | NCT01625559 |
| Phase I/II—unknown status | hESC-derived RPE | AMD and Stargardt | 15 | Subretinal transplantation | China | NCT02749734 |
| Phase I/II—enrolling | hESC-RPE | AMD | 36 | Evaluating occurrence of late-onset adverse effects after hESC-RPE subretinal transplant | UK, USA | NCT03167203 |

**Table 2.** *Cont.*

| Trial Stage | Type of Cell Used | Disease | Sample Size | Approach | Country | Identifier |
|---|---|---|---|---|---|---|
| Phase 1 | hESC-derived RPE | RP | 10 | Transplant into subretinal space | China | NCT03944239 |
| Phase 1—recruiting | PF-05206388—hESC-derived RPE | Wet AMD | 10 | Implantation of PF-05206388 | UK | NCT01691261 |
| Phase I and II—active | hESC-derived RPE | RP | 12 | Implantation of monolayer therapeutical patch into eye with worse acuity | France | NCT03963154 |
| Phase I/II—completed | hESC-derived RPE | Dry AMD, wet AMD, and Stargardt disease | 15 | Compare the safety of surgical implantation of hESC-RPE monolayer on s polymeric scaffold versus hESC-RPE injections into subretinal space | Brazil | NCT02903576 |
| Phase I/II—unknown status | hESC-derived RPE on parylene membrane (CPCB-RPE1) | Advanced dry AMD patients with geographic atrophy and central fovea involvement | 16 | Subretinal implantation of 100,000 differentiated RPE cells attached to a small parylene membrane | USA | NCT02590692 |
| Phase I/IIa—active, not recruiting | OpRegen hESC-derived RPE | Dry AMD | 24 | Subretinal transplantation of 50,000–200,000 cells; see how cells engraft, survive, and moderate disease progression | Israel | NCT02286089 |
| Phase I/II—enrolling | Retinal stem and progenitor cells | AMD | 20 | Cultured retinal stem and progenitor cells are injected subretinally | Belarus | NCT05187104 |
| Phase I/II—unknown status | hESC-derived RPE | Dry AMD | 10 | Transplant into subretinal space | China | NCT03046407 |
| Phase I/II—recruiting | RPESC-RPE-4W (allogeneic RPE stem-cell-derived RPE cells isolated from human cadaver) | Dry AMD | 18 | Patients will receive 50,000, 150,000, or 250,000 RPESC-RPE-4W cells in the macula of the eye. | USA | NCT04627428 |
| Phase 1 | Autologous iPSC-derived RPE | AMD | 6 | Determine safety of transplanting iPSC-derived RPE sheets | Japan | UMIN000011929 |
| Phases I/IIa—recruiting | Autologous iPSC-derived RPE | Dry AMD | 20 | Subretinal transplantation of autologous iPSC-derived RPE in one eye | USA | NCT04339764 |

**Table 2.** *Cont.*

| Trial Stage | Type of Cell Used | Disease | Sample Size | Approach | Country | Identifier |
|---|---|---|---|---|---|---|
| Phase I/IIa—recruiting | hiPSC-derived Eyecyte-RPE | Geographic atrophy secondary to dry AMD | 54 | Single-dose subretinal injection at varying doses: 100,000, 200,000, and 300,000 | India | NCT06394232 |
| Phase I—recruiting | Induced pluripotent stem cell (iPSC) | AMD | 10 | Autologous transplantation of iPSC-derived retinal pigment epithelium (RPE) into subretinal pace | Beijing | NCT05445063 |
| Phase I | $CD34^+$ stem cells from bone marrow | Irreversibly blind patients due to various retinal conditions | 15 | $CD34^+$ bone marrow stem cells intravitreal | USA | NCT01736059 (pilot) |
| Phase I—completed | Autologous $CD34^+$ stem cells harvested from bone marrow | RP | 4 | Intravitreal injection into 1 eye and followed for 6 months | USA | NCT04925687 |
| Phase 1—completed | Autologous bone marrow stem cells | RP | 5 | Single intravitreal injection | Brazil | NCT01068561 |
| Phase II—completed | Autologous bone marrow stem cells | RP | 50 | Single intravitreal injection | Brazil | NCT01560715 |
| Phase I | Adult human bone-marrow-derived MSC | RP | 14 | Intravitreal injection | Thailand | NCT01531348 |
| Phase I/II—completed | Autologous bone marrow stem cell | AMD or Stargardt with best-corrected ETDRS visual acuity <20/200 | 20 | Intravitreal injection | Brazil | NCT01518127 |
| Not noted | Autologous bone-marrow-derived stem cells | AMD, RP, Stargardt | 500 | Injection of autologous bone-marrow-derived stem cells | USA, United Arab Emirates | NCT03011541 |
| Phase 3—completed | Umbilical cord Wahrton's jelly-derived mesenchymal stem cells | RP | 32 | Cells implanted in sub-tenon space | Turkey | NCT04224207 |
| Phase I—recruiting | Allogeneic adult umbilical cord-derived mesenchymal stem cells (UC-MSCs) | RP | 20 | Intravenous and sub-tenon delivery of 100 million UC-MSCs | Antigua and Barbuda, Argentia, Mexico | NCT05147701 |

## 6.1. Preclinical Studies

### 6.1.1. Preclinical Studies Using ESCs

Some of the initial studies showing promise for the use of cell therapy in retinal disorders showed rescue and prevention of photoreceptor degeneration by transplanting retinal pigment epithelium (RPE) in Royal College of Surgeon (RCS) rats [40,41,75]. Limitations of these methods included the need for healthy RPE. Later, Schraermeyer and colleagues [42] transplanted ESC and found it to delay photoreceptor degeneration in RCS rats, making ESC a potential source for cell transplantation in retinal diseases.

While there was promise for the use of mouse ESCs, there had been no reports showing the use of primate ESC until Haruta and colleagues [44] investigated the generation of epithelial cells from primate embryonic cells. Embryonic cells were obtained from cynomolgus monkeys, differentiated into embryonic stem-cell-derived pigment epithelial cells (ESPE), and transplanted into the subretinal space of RCS rats, resulting in photoreceptor death and vision loss [44]. After transplantation, the RCS rats were observed to have recovery and retinal function, providing evidence for the use of ESPEs for cell-replacement therapy for retinal degenerative diseases [44]. An advantage of using ESCs for degenerative diseases is that they have the capacity to indefinitely differentiate into any cell type.

Further studies investigated the use of human ESCs (hESCs) for retinal diseases and found hESC-derived RPE to exhibit morphology, marker expression, and function of authentic RPE, rescuing retinal function in animal models of retinal degeneration [46,47,49]. In RCS rats, an improvement in visual performance was observed compared to untreated controls, after hESC-derived RPE transplantation [46]. Idelson and colleagues [49] confirmed that retinal rescue was not a nonspecific effect by also transplanting human fibroblasts into the subretinal space. Transplantation of fibroblasts did not result in protection of the photoreceptor layer and delay in degradation [49]. Similarly, in $Crx^{-/-}$ mice (a model of Leber's Congenital Amaurosis), hESC-derived retinal cells differentiated into functional rod and cone photoreceptors and restored light responses in the animals [50].

Additional studies found ESC to also possess the potential to differentiate into cells similar to retinal ganglion cells (RGC). In this study, neural progenitors (NP) were first derived from FGF2-induced ESC cells, which then differentiated into RGC-like cells, expressing RGC regulators and markers, such as Ath5, Brn3b, RPF-1, Thy-1, and Islet-1, in vitro [51]. The ESC-NP cells were then exposed to FGF2, which, upon transplantation, integrated and differentiated into RGCs in vivo [51]. This research provided a method for differentiating ESC into RGC and showed efficacy in vivo. Other research has successfully induced rat ESCs into RPEs and photoreceptors, restoring visual function in RCS rats after retinal transplantation [61].

Comparison of subretinal transplantation of mouse ESC-derived rod photoreceptors in mild retinal degeneration and severe retinal degeneration mice showed differences between the two models. The mice ESCs integrated into the mild retinal degeneration models and acquired mature morphology expressing photoreceptor markers, whereas, in severe retinal degeneration models, the transplanted cells survived but did not have mature morphologic features [58]. This may have been due to severely degenerated retinas creating a hostile environment and activated microglia resulting in immune responses and rejection [58]. This study highlights a primary concern of using ESCs, as they are not autologous and may induce immune reactions and rejection upon transplantation in the degenerated host retina.

### 6.1.2. Preclinical Studies Using iPSCs

While ESC-based replacement therapy is valuable for retinal regeneration, it is complicated due to immune rejection, tumor formation, and ethical concerns. Therefore, several researchers investigated the use of induced pluripotent stem cells (iPSCs) for retinal cell-replacement therapy. Results demonstrated that iPSCs express various retinal progenitor cell-related proteins, such as *Pax6*, *Rx*, *Otx2*, *Lhx2*, and *Nestin* [52–54]. Direct differentiation of iPSCs into retinal ganglion (RG)-like cells was achieved with overexpression of *Math5* and the addition of DN and DAPT, with the cells surviving in the mice retina post-transplantation, but not integrating into the retina [54].

However, Venugopalan and colleagues [59] transplanted primary mouse RGC into uninjured mature rats' retina in vivo by intravitreal injection and found results similar to using human iPSC and mesenchymal stem cells. The transplanted RGCs survived, migrated to the ganglion cell layer, and made functional synaptic connections in the host retina, responding to light stimulation [59]. The synaptic integration shows promise for allogeneic stem-cell-derived transplants as mice RGCs were successfully transplanted into rat retina [59]. Additionally, another study found that greater differentiation of iPSC-derived photoreceptors and purifying using fluorescence-activated cell sorting (FACS) allowed the cells to integrate into the outer nuclear layer and express photoreceptor markers after transplantation to the subretinal space of normal adult mice [55]—providing hope for autologous transplantation as a treatment for retinal degeneration.

Subretinal transplantation of iPSCs into retinal degenerative mice has resulted in iPSCs successfully integrating into the retinal outer nuclear layer and increased retinal function in hosts, as seen through electroretinographic analysis and functional anatomy [56]. The studies mentioned above have demonstrated the feasibility of photoreceptor replacement therapy using ESCs and iPSCs; however, transplant success based on disease stage remained unclear.

As mentioned before, a concern with cell transplants is immune rejection. To address this concern and oncogenic mutations, Sharma and colleagues [62] developed an oncogene mutation-free clinical-grade iPSC from AMD patients and differentiated them into RPE patches on biodegradable scaffolds. This allowed the cells to integrate into both rat and porcine models with AMD-like eye conditions [62]. On the other hand, another study of swine models mimicking end-stage AMD subretinal transplantation of hiPSC-derived RPE cells did not graft well in atrophic areas compared to healthy areas [67]. However, several engrafted RPE cells showed possible interaction with host photoreceptors as seen by the expression of immunolabeled phagosomes, suggesting a delay of the loss of visual function by decreasing GA progression [67]. A comparison of these two studies suggests that methods using scaffolds may provide more benefit and feasibility for autologous clinical-grade-induced RPE cell transplantation.

Human iPSCs-derived cells have also been shown to be effective in the long term post-transplantation. Human iPSC-retina grafts have been shown to survive up to 5 months in rats and up to 2 years in monkey models [57,63]. However, while some transplanted RGCs showed light responses in these models, it was not clear whether these responses were residual from the host retina or due to cell transplantation [63].

Another study reported that a combination of hiPSC-derived RPE cells and retinal precursor cells preserved endogenous photoreceptors and visual function, more than transplantation of either cell alone in early- and late-stage disease degeneration [65]. Further work is needed to investigate the benefit of a combination transplant and which cell combinations provide the most benefit.

#### 6.1.3. Preclinical Studies Using MSCs

One method to support autologous cell transplant and reduce immune rejection is through the use of mesenchymal stem cells (MSCs). Mesenchymal cells may be obtained from the bone marrow or adipose tissue of a particular patient and used as autologous cells for cell-replacement therapy. It has been shown that MSCs have anti-inflammatory properties, produce growth factors, and contribute to tissue regeneration, making them suitable for retinal degenerative cell therapy [60]. Additionally, MSCs can differentiate into RPE, photoreceptor-like, bipolar, and amacrine cells [43,48,69]. Recent studies have shown intravitreal injections of MSCs to have protective effects on the retina and enhance vision function [70,71]. On the other hand, a study using intravitreal or subretinal injections of bone marrow mononuclear stem cells reported increased cell survival, but no enhancement of retinal function in RCS and P23H-1 rats [72]. This calls for the need for further studies looking at various animal models. Another study observed photoreceptor regeneration and restoration of retinal function, following human adipose-derived MSCs in sodium iodate-induced retinal injury mice models, showing promise for MSC therapy in RP and AMD [73]. In addition to bone marrow and adipose-derived MSCs, they can also be derived from the umbilical cord. Notably, intravenously delivered small umbilical cord mesenchymal stem cells (average diameter $8.636 \pm 2.256$ μm) are safer and may protect visual function in RCS rats [69].

#### 6.1.4. Preclinical Studies Using Progenitor Cells

Preclinical studies using progenitor cells have shown them to restore some visual function in mice models. Klassen and colleagues [45] report successful engraftment of retinal progenitor cells in the degenerating retina of mature mice, with some cells maturing into neurons such as photoreceptors and expressing recoverin, rhodopsin, or cone opsin. Mice who received the transplant showed improved light-mediated behavior compared to controls [45]. Recently, He and colleagues [68] transplanted retinal progenitor cells from mouse ESC-derived retinal organoids and reported successful differentiation of transplanted cells, along with responses to light stimuli and integration with the host retina. While this study shows promising results, long-term effects and results need to be further investigated.

Moreover, while many studies before have used two methodologies to generate various retinal cells, one study created RPE and photoreceptor progenitor cells (PRP) cells using a single methodology. This unified protocol was created to generate RPE and PRP cells simultaneously from the same source of iPSCs, with cells surviving and integrating into rodent models of retinal degeneration post-transplant and improved vision [66]. This method provides an efficient and effective way to generate cells for combined transplantation. Further, intravitreal injection of human retinal progenitor cells (RPC) is shown to preserve retinal morphology but is only effective up to 12 weeks post-transplantation [64].

As there is a variety of stem cells that may be utilized in cell therapy for retinal degeneration, a study investigated which may be the most effective. It was reported that hiPSC-RPE cells have the best protective effect for retinal degeneration, transplanting better and longer than human adipose-derived stem cells, amniotic stem cells, bone marrow stem cells, dental pulp stem cells, and hiPSCs [74]. However, this finding must be further investigated, as there are differences between diseases, such as RP being genetic and AMD being related to older age, and studies with disease-specific animal models should be conducted. Preclinical studies have provided insight that stem cell therapy has the potential to stabilize or reverse progressive vision loss in both non-primates and primates, paving the way for clinical studies.

### 6.2. *Clinical Trials*

Most current clinical trials are currently in the early phases, focusing on initial responses and the safety of cell therapy (see Table 2). Current human trials are focusing on confirming that transplanted cells do not form teratomas, do not migrate into other organs, do not lead to immune rejection, and do not have other unintended adverse effects.

#### 6.2.1. Clinical Trials Using hESCs

Schwartz and colleagues conducted the first study investigating hESC-derived subretinal cell transplantation in human patients with Stargardt macular dystrophy and dry AMD (NCT01345006 and NCT01344993). Preliminary reports of two patients at 4 months post-transplant of hESC-derived RPE show that there were no signs of hyperproliferation, tumor formation, or transplant rejection [76]. A subsequent follow-up involving 18 patients, 9 with Stargardt and 9 with AMD, for a median 22-month period was reported. In this report, there were 10 eyes with an improvement in the Best Corrected Visual Acuity (BCVA) score, 7 eyes with a stable score, and 1 eye with a 10-letter decrease [77]. In addition, complications included cataracts in four eyes and the development of endophthalmitis in one patient [77]. These complications were reported to be attributed to pars plana vitrectomy surgery and the use of immunosuppressive treatment, not specifically with the hESC transplant [77].

While the participants in Schwartz and colleagues' study were primarily white and black, W.K. Song and colleagues [78] investigated the safety and efficacy of hESC-derived RPE transplantation in four Asian patients: two with AMD and two with Stargardt disease (NCT01674829). Preliminary results were similar to Schwartz and colleagues [77], with some visual acuity improvement in three patients and stable acuity in one patient one year post-transplant [78]. There was no reported adverse proliferation, tumor formation, or serious safety issues [78]. While there were some adverse reactions following immunosuppression, these stopped after cessation of the immunosuppression [78]. This study provided greater promise for the use of hESC-derived RPE transplantation in patients of various ethnicities.

Mehat and colleagues [79] found subretinal transplantation of hESC-derived RPE cells in 12 Stargardt patients to be safe and to result in no inflammatory reaction or uncontrolled proliferation (NCT01469832). There was evidence of subretinal hyperpigmentation in all 12 patients, suggesting survival and engraftment of the transplanted hESC-derived RPE cells [79]. However, they did not report any significant improvement or decline in retinal function by electroretinography post-transplant in any patient and only borderline BCVA improvements in four patients [79]. This was hypothesized to be due to the advanced stage of the disease at the start of the study and the slow rate of progression in Stargardt, suggesting protection against further deterioration may only be seen in a longer follow-up period.

A recent study in Korea has investigated the long-term safety of hESC-derived RPE transplantation in three Asian patients with Stargardt disease (NCT01625559). Sung and colleagues [80] found no serious adverse events to be present during a 3-year follow-up period, with improvement of BCVA in one patient and stable BCVA in the other two patients. Favorable function and anatomical results were reported, compared to the natural progression of Stargardt disease. Further, Li and colleagues [81] reported no adverse reactions in a longitudinal 5-year study investigating hESC-derived RPE subretinal transplantation in seven Stargardt patients (NCT02749734). While these studies show promise for the long-term safety and efficacy of subretinal hESC-derived RPE transplantation, further multicenter studies with a larger number of patients are needed. A study that is currently in progress aims to follow 36 patients for up to 10 years after an hESC-derived RPE cell subretinal transplantation (NCT03167203). A study in China is also investigating the treatment of dry AMD using hESC-derived RPE (NCT03046407); however, the results of this study and its progress are currently unknown.

Further work by da Cruz and colleagues [82] (NCT01691261) aimed to determine the feasibility and safety of using subretinal transplantation using a biocompatible hESC-RPE monolayer on a synthetic basement membrane (a 'patch'), rather than a suspension, in patients with wet AMD. Results from two patients show the stability of the hESC-RPE patch and improved BCVA and reading speed over 12 months [82]. As there were no control patients, the results of this study must be critically analyzed, but do suggest that an RPE patch transplant may be a beneficial form of treatment for retinal degeneration.

Preliminary safety results of a study (NCT03963154) investigating the use of a patch created using a novel tissue-engineered product consisting of hESC-derived RPE cells report successful integration in the retina, with no local inflammation or retinal deterioration observed in seven patients [83]. A recent study in Brazil is comparing whether surgical implantations of hESC-RPE monolayer on a polymeric scaffold or hESC-RPE injections into subretinal space are safer in AMD and Stargardt patients (NCT02903576).

Moreover, a five-year follow-up of a phase 1/2a clinical trial (NCT02590692) assessing scaffold-based hESC-derived RPE transplantation in 16 legally blind patients with GA reported the implant to be safe and tolerated [84]. The primary endpoint of the study was a safety assessment at 1-year post-transplant, which reported four patients in cohort 1 to have serious adverse events, including retinal hemorrhage, edema, retinal detachment, or RPE detachment [85]. However, these adverse events were mitigated in cohort 2 by using hemostasis during surgery. Patients were followed for a median of 3 years and reported a higher likelihood of BCVA improvements than worsening [84]. Patients who experienced worsening in BCVA had experienced the adverse events mentioned before during post-transplantation [84]. This study shows that scaffold-based transplants are successful and tolerated in patients with GA, suggesting this method as a possible treatment.

Recently, primary 24-month results from the currently active OpRegen hESC-derived RPE cell therapy trial (NCT02286089) suggest that subretinal transplantation of OpRegen is successful and safe. The data suggest that OpRegen counteracts RPE dysfunction and loss in GA [86]. Results report sustained BCVA gains at 24 months and greater improvement in retinal structure observed in patients with extensive coverage of GA with OpRegen and less advanced GA [86].

A study of unknown status in China is investigating the safety and efficacy of hESC-derived RPE cell subretinal transplantation in patients with RP (NCT03944239). An ongoing trial is also investigating the safety, tolerability, feasibility, and efficacy of retinal pigment epithelium stem cell (RPEESC)-derived RPE transplantation in patients with dry AMD (NCT04627428). The RPEESC is obtained from eyes donated to eye banks and the study aims to enroll 18 participants.

#### 6.2.2. Clinical Trials Using hiPSCs

While hESC-derived cell transplantations have proven to be safe and effective, there remains the concern of immune rejection. Hence, clinical trials are starting to be conducted utilizing hiPSC-derived cells, offering an autologous approach to cell transplantation.

Mandai and colleagues [87] reported iPSC-derived RPE sheets to be intact one-year after transplantation in one patient with AMD, but with no improvements in BCVA (UMIN000011929). Notably, the patient did not receive any immunosuppressants and there was no transplant rejection [87]. This same patient was then followed for a period of 4 years, showing survival of the RPE sheet and no adverse reactions [88]. This clinical trial showed promise for the use of autologous iPSC-derived transplantation for patients with retinal degeneration. However, there remains a need for larger study sizes and a variety of disease states to be investigated. The first of these trials in the United States is currently underway, investigating autologous transplantation of iPSC-derived RPE in AMD patients with GA (NCT04339764).

In India, investigators are evaluating the safety and efficacy of a novel hiPSC-derived formulation, Eyecyte-RPE, in patients with GA due to dry AMD (NCT06394232). This formulation is speculated to replace damaged RPE and potentially enable tissue regeneration.

A study in China is currently recruiting patients for autologous transplantation of hiPSC-derived RPE in AMD patients (NCT05445063).

#### 6.2.3. Clinical Trials Using MSCs

As mentioned before, MSCs provide paracrine effects and contribute to tissue regeneration, making them suitable for retinal degeneration cell therapy. Park and colleagues explored the safety and feasibility of intravitreal autologous $CD34^+$ bone marrow cell injection in patients with AMD or RP (NCT01736059; NCT04925687). Preliminary findings of the pilot study conducted in six participants reported a single intravitreal injection to be well tolerated with no intraocular inflammation and no worsening of BCVA after 6 months [89]. These promising results led to a follow-up study conducted in RP patients to determine the number of $CD34^+$ cells isolated for injection and adverse events (NCT04925687). Seven patients were enrolled in this study and a mean of $3.26 \pm 0.66$ million viable $CD34^+$ cells were intravitreally injected in each eye [90]. While patients tolerated the injection 6 months post-injection, four patients had an extended follow-up and three of these four patients had progressive vision loss in both eyes [90]. Park and colleagues [90] note that it is unknown if repeat intravitreal injection of CD34$^+$ would result in a greater therapeutic effect and larger studies are needed.

Another study investigated the safety of a single intravitreal injection of autologous bone-marrow-derived cells in patients with RP and the vision-related quality of life of these patients after the injection (NCT01068561; NCT01560715). Phase 1 (NCT01068561) results reported no adverse events associated with the injection over a period of 10 months [91]. Phase 2 (NCT01560715) results found there to be an initial improvement in the vision-related quality of life of these patients, but no difference from baseline at 12 months post-injection [92].

Tuekprakhon and colleagues [93] also investigated intravitreal autologous bone-marrow-derived MSC (BM-MSC) injection in 14 patients with advanced RP (NCT01531348). Their findings found improvements in BCVA initially, but BCVA returned to baseline at 12 months [93]. Researchers observed several patients with discomfort, such as mild pain, pressure, redness, and irritation, and mild adverse events, such as localized posterior synechiae, cystoid macular edema, and localized choroidal detachment, in their 12-month follow-up period [93]. One patient experienced a serious adverse event (diffuse vitreous hemorrhage) 3 years post-injection and required surgery, after which, vision was restored for the patient [93]. The adverse reactions and little improvement in visual function results warrant further investigation of BM-MSC injections in patients with RP.

On the other hand, Siqueira and colleagues [94] investigated intravitreal autologous bone-marrow-derived stem cell injection in patients with dry AMD (NCT01518127). Data reported intravitreal injections to be safe in patients with dry AMD and showed that there were slight increases in BCVA three months after injection [94]. We wonder if a longer-term follow-up period would result in findings similar to Tuekprakhon and colleagues [93], with BCVA returning to baseline.

The Stem Cell Ophthalmology Treatment Study (SCOTS and SCOTS2) is a multicenter trial investigating autologous BM-MSC treatment for the treatment of retinal disease and optic nerve damage (NCT03011541). This study aims to recruit 500 participants and follow them for a 12-month period. Weiss and Levy have reported findings of Stargardt disease, AMD, and RP patients. In the study, 34 eyes with Stargardt disease received autologous bone marrow injections using retrobulbar, sub-tenons, intravitreal or subretinal, and intravenous injection [95]. Over one year, statistically significant results ($p = 0.0004$) showed 21 (61.8%) eyes to improve, 8 (23.5%) to remain stable, and 5 (14.7%) to continue to have disease progression [95]. Visual acuity improvement was also seen in some patients [95]. Similarly, there were significant clinical improvements in visual acuity and a delay in vision loss seen in 32 patients with AMD [96]. In the 33 patients with RP, there were also improvements in visual acuity and stability of disease progression seen over a follow-up period of at least 6 months [97].

A phase 3 clinical trial investigated the management of RP using Wharton's jelly-derived MSCS (WJ-MSC) (NCT04224207). It was found that sub-tenon transplantation of WJ-MSCs was effective and safe during a 1-year follow-up period, in both autosomal dominant and autosomal recessive inheritance of RP [98].

Another clinical trial is currently enrolling participants for a study investigating the safety and efficacy of intravenous and sub-tenon delivery of allogeneic adult umbilical cord-derived MSC cells for the treatment of RP (NCT05147701). Adverse effects will be monitored for a four-year follow-up period.

#### 6.2.4. Clinical Trials Using Progenitor Cells

We did not come across many clinical trials investigating the use of progenitor cells. A clinical trial is currently enrolling participants in a study investigating retinal stem and progenitor cell therapy for the treatment of AMD (NCT05187104).

## 7. Future Directions

There have been numerous advances in the utilization of cell therapy for retinal degenerative diseases. Progress continues to be made in this field with new advances in cell therapy techniques and combinations of therapies. However, there remain challenges in translating research findings to clinical populations and ethical sourcing of stem cells. In this section, we will highlight progress made and outline some challenges that need to be addressed.

### *7.1. Advances in Cell Therapy Techniques*

The method of delivering cells into the ocular region is critical to ensure cell survival and transplantation success. Currently, there are three methods that are commonly used to deliver cells into the ocular region: subretinal, intravitreal, and suprachoroidal injections. While subretinal injections enable direct effects on cells and tissue in the subretinal space, there can be complications such as retinal detachment [99]. On the other hand, although an intravitreal injection can be quite invasive, the vitreous is an immune-privileged site and shows promise for being a site of stem cell delivery. Wang and colleagues [64] found intravitreal injections to be safe to inject human retinal progenitor cells in RCS rats with no teratoma formation following injection and a delay in retinal degeneration, showing promise for clinical models. Another method of cell delivery has been the suprachoroidal injection. This method is less invasive and has high bioavailability, as it targets the choroid, retinal pigment epithelium, and neuroretina [100].

### *7.2. Combination Therapies*

Integration of gene therapy and biomaterials shows promising advances in cell transplantation and retinal degeneration treatment. Gene therapy, specifically CRISPR-Cas9, enhances hESC survival by reducing cell immunogenicity and eliminating the need for immunosuppression [101]. The integration with gene therapy has also shown the success of autologous transplantation in Stargardt patients. CRISPR-Cas9 was used to correct the ABCA4 variant in hiPSCs of these patients and autologous transplantation was performed without any adverse effects [102]. This research shows that gene therapy in combination with cell therapy allows for in vitro gene editing and differentiation of retinal cells for autologous transplantation treatment of retinal dystrophy [102].

Additionally, biomaterials and scaffolds have been combined with cell therapy to optimize its results. The use of scaffold technology plays two major roles in cell therapy. One role is providing a platform to deliver a layer of cells and the other role is the delivery of drugs, promoting cell survival and integration, and immunosuppression [103]. For example, sometimes the transplanted RPE does not adhere well to Bruch's membrane, resulting in the need for a scaffold to help the transplanted RPE adhere and differentiate [103]. Ideal scaffolds are biocompatible, biodegradable, and injectable [104]. Historically, gelatin substrate was used during photoreceptor transplantation to maintain the photoreceptor layer, as it dissolves at room temperature and is not neurotoxic [105]. Today, scaffolds are typically made of biomaterials such as parylene C, polyethylene, terephthalate, or poly (lactic-co-glycolic acid), and deliver cells in a more structured way, allowing for a better understanding of cell survival and differentiation [103]. Aside from scaffolds, biomaterial such as bone marrow has its own advantages in cell therapy. Bone marrow stromal cells migrate to sites of injury and can differentiate into various cells, including retinal cells, and produce neurotrophic factors to help with cell survival [27]. Bone marrow stromal cells can be used in autologous transplantation, reducing concerns of immune rejection [27].

Moreover, 3D bioprinting technology is being utilized to study retinal degeneration, and 3D-bioprinted eye tissue has been created using patient stem cells [106]. This bioprinted tissue will allow scientists to better understand AMD and its progression to wet AMD and allow for modeling of the disease process in vitro. The future of 3D bioprinting and its possibility to be used for therapeutic development provides an exciting area to develop further.

### 7.3. Barrier to Clinical Translation

Although the eye and subretinal space provide a unique immunological environment with immune privilege, there remain barriers to clinical translation. One of these barriers is the risk and occurrence of immunogenicity. As some cell therapy methods utilize allogeneic stem cells and embryonic cells, there is the possibility of host-mediated immune responses and allogeneic graft rejection post-transplant [39]. After a cell transplant, there is an innate immune response that mediates tissue stress and inflammation; sometimes, with this response, natural killer cells become activated and play a role in allogeneic cell rejection [39]. Some have attempted to use systemic immunosuppression to overcome graft rejection; however, this leads to the issue of increased infection. Recent advances are utilizing gene editing, such as CRISPR-Cas9 to reduce immunogenicity, but there remains a need to ensure the safety of using gene-edited cells in clinical settings [101].

As mentioned before, a method to overcome the issue of graft rejection and promote cell survival and integration is to use iPSCs. Takahashi and colleagues [107] demonstrated the creation of induced pluripotent cells from adult human fibroblasts, providing evidence of the creation of patient-specific iPSCs. The use of iPSCs provides an autologous method for cell transplantation, decreases the risk of immune rejection, and eliminates the need for systemic immunosuppression [107]. However, the promise of iPSC in cell therapy is not without concerns as reprogramming of the cells raises concerns of genetic instability [108]. It has been stated that iPSC cells may have epigenetic memory and continue to proliferate, causing an increased risk of teratomas [39,109]. The unlimited differentiation possibility can also cause concern for the creation of human clones [110]. It is necessary that the use of stem cells for therapies be safety checked to ensure that there are benefits for the patients post-transplantation.

The clinical translation of cell therapy for retinal diseases faces several other challenges. Ensuring transplanted cells survive, integrate into the retinal tissue, and restore function is also critical, as is mitigating off-target effects that could lead to unintended complications [109]. Demonstrating meaningful functional recovery in vision and proving the long-term efficacy of these therapies are essential steps for clinical success. Scalability and standardization present additional barriers, as developing cost-effective, reproducible manufacturing processes that maintain consistent product quality is complex. Furthermore, cost remains a significant obstacle, with high therapy expenses limiting accessibility; ensuring broad patient access will require strategic efforts in cost reduction and healthcare reimbursement [29]. Finally, adequate and optimal delivery methods must be identified through clinical studies to ensure the correct and effective placement of cells within the retina [109].

### 7.4. Ethical Issues

The source of stem cells, in particular the derivation of pluripotent stem cells from human embryos and oocytes, has been a controversial topic amongst the clinical and public community since its utilization in medicine. However, iPSCs, which are reprogrammed from somatic cells, avoid ethical controversies as they do not use embryos or oocytes and are more commonly used today for cell therapy. While autologous stem cell transplantation minimizes ethical concerns and the risk of immune reaction, they raise concerns of genetic anomalies being present, a concern as retinal degenerative diseases have genetic origins [31]. As mentioned before, iPSCs do have complications of their own; therefore, it is important to optimize iPSC differentiation protocols to ensure that ethical concerns are mitigated.

## 8. Conclusions

This review has highlighted the promising potential of cell-based therapies in treating retinal degenerative diseases such as age-related macular degeneration (AMD) and retinitis pigmentosa (RP). We explored the anatomy and physiology of the retina, the pathophysiology of these diseases, and the various cell therapy approaches being developed, including embryonic stem cells (ESCs), induced pluripotent stem cells (iPSCs), mesenchymal stem cells (MSCs), and progenitor cells. Our focus on the most recent preclinical and clinical studies underscores the rapid advancements in this field.

Despite the progress, several barriers remain in translating these therapies into clinical practice. Challenges such as immune rejection, ensuring long-term survival and integration of transplanted cells, and the need for scalable and standardized manufacturing processes are critical areas that must be addressed.

For future research, we recommend a focused effort on overcoming these barriers to clinical translation. This includes developing strategies to enhance cell survival and integration, refining delivery methods, and addressing the immune responses that may arise from allogeneic transplants. Additionally, further exploration into the combination of gene therapy and biomaterials with cell therapy could provide a more comprehensive approach to treating retinal degenerative diseases. By addressing these challenges, the field of ocular cell therapy can advance toward developing clinically viable and widely accessible treatments, ultimately offering new therapeutic options for patients suffering from vision loss.

**Author Contributions:** Conceptualization, K.Y.W.; writing—original draft preparation, K.Y.W., J.K.D. and A.S.; writing—review and editing, K.Y.W., J.K.D. and A.S; supervision, K.Y.W. and A.K. All authors have read and agreed to the published version of the manuscript.

**Funding:** This research received no external funding.

**Institutional Review Board Statement:** Not applicable.

**Informed Consent Statement:** Not applicable.

**Data Availability Statement:** Not applicable.

**Acknowledgments:** The authors acknowledge Nada Barakat for help with references and formatting.

**Conflicts of Interest:** The authors declare no conflicts of interest.

## References


1. Mahabadi, N.; Al Khalili, Y. Neuroanatomy, Retina. In *StatPearls*; StatPearls Publishing: Treasure Island, FL, USA, 2024.
2. Delaey, C.; van de Voorde, J. Regulatory Mechanisms in the Retinal and Choroidal Circulation. *Ophthalmic Res.* **2000**, *32*, 249–256. [CrossRef] [PubMed]
3. Vinores, S.A. Breakdown of the Blood–Retinal Barrier. *Encycl. Eye* **2010**, *5*, 216–222. [CrossRef]
4. Forrester, J.V.; McMenamin, P.G.; Dando, S.J. CNS Infection and Immune Privilege. *Nat. Rev. Neurosci.* **2018**, *19*, 655–671. [CrossRef] [PubMed]
5. Ellis, R.R. Age-Related Macular Degeneration (AMD): An Overview. Available online: https://www.webmd.com/eye-health/macular-degeneration/age-related-macular-degeneration-overview (accessed on 16 August 2024).
6. Hageman, G.S.; Gehrs, K.; Johnson, L.V.; Anderson, D. Age-Related Macular Degeneration (AMD). In *Webvision: The Organization of the Retina and Visual System*; Kolb, H., Fernandez, E., Nelson, R., Eds.; University of Utah Health Sciences Center: Salt Lake City, UT, USA, 1995.
7. Fernandes, A.R.; Zielińska, A.; Sanchez-Lopez, E.; dos Santos, T.; Garcia, M.L.; Silva, A.M.; Karczewski, J.; Souto, E.B. Exudative versus Nonexudative Age-Related Macular Degeneration: Physiopathology and Treatment Options. *Int. J. Mol. Sci.* **2022**, *23*, 2592. [CrossRef] [PubMed]
8. Somasundaran, S.; Constable, I.J.; Mellough, C.B.; Carvalho, L.S. Retinal Pigment Epithelium and Age-Related Macular Degeneration: A Review of Major Disease Mechanisms. *Clin. Exp. Ophthalmol.* **2020**, *48*, 1043–1056. [CrossRef]
9. Ruan, Y.; Jiang, S.; Gericke, A. Age-Related Macular Degeneration: Role of Oxidative Stress and Blood Vessels. *Int. J. Mol. Sci.* **2021**, *22*, 1296. [CrossRef]
10. Pugazhendhi, A.; Hubbell, M.; Jairam, P.; Ambati, B. Neovascular Macular Degeneration: A Review of Etiology, Risk Factors, and Recent Advances in Research and Therapy. *Int. J. Mol. Sci.* **2021**, *22*, 1170. [CrossRef]
11. Dry Macular Degeneration—Symptoms and Causes—Mayo Clinic. Available online: https://www.mayoclinic.org/diseases-conditions/dry-macular-degeneration/symptoms-causes/syc-20350375 (accessed on 16 August 2024).
12. Ruia, S.; Kaufman, E.J. Macular Degeneration. In *StatPearls*; StatPearls Publishing: Treasure Island, FL, USA, 2024.
13. Cunningham ET Jr, Adamis AP, Altaweel M, Aiello LP, Bressler NM, D'Amico DJ, Goldbaum M, Guyer DR, Katz B, Patel M, Schwartz SD; Macugen Diabetic Retinopathy Study Group. A Phase II Randomized Double-Masked Trial of Pegaptanib, an Anti–Vascular Endothelial Growth Factor Aptamer, for Diabetic Macular Edema. *Ophthalmology* **2005**, *112*, 1747–1757. [CrossRef]
14. O'Neal, T.B.; Luther, E.E. Retinitis Pigmentosa. In *StatPearls*; StatPearls Publishing: Treasure Island, FL, USA, 2024.

15. Glaucoma | National Eye Institute. Available online: https://www.nei.nih.gov/learn-about-eye-health/eye-conditions-and-diseases/glaucoma (accessed on 28 September 2024).
16. Types of Glaucoma | National Eye Institute. Available online: https://www.nei.nih.gov/learn-about-eye-health/eye-conditions-and-diseases/glaucoma/types-glaucoma (accessed on 28 September 2024).
17. Carreon, T.; van der Merwe, E.; Fellman, R.L.; Johnstone, M.; Bhattacharya, S.K. Aqueous Outflow—A Continuum from Trabecular Meshwork to Episcleral Veins. *Prog. Retin. Eye Res.* **2017**, *57*, 108–133. [CrossRef]
18. Glaucoma and Eye Pressure | National Eye Institute. Available online: https://www.nei.nih.gov/learn-about-eye-health/eye-conditions-and-diseases/glaucoma/glaucoma-and-eye-pressure (accessed on 28 September 2024).
19. Vernazza, S.; Tirendi, S.; Bassi, A.M.; Traverso, C.E.; Saccà, S.C. Neuroinflammation in Primary Open-Angle Glaucoma. *J. Clin. Med.* **2020**, *9*, 3172. [CrossRef]
20. Glaucoma Medicines | National Eye Institute. Available online: https://www.nei.nih.gov/Glaucoma/glaucoma-medicines (accessed on 28 September 2024).
21. Laser Treatment for Glaucoma | National Eye Institute. Available online: https://www.nei.nih.gov/learn-about-eye-health/eye-conditions-and-diseases/glaucoma/treatment (accessed on 28 September 2024).
22. Hu, B.-Y.; Xin, M.; Chen, M.; Yu, P.; Zeng, L.-Z. Mesenchymal Stem Cells for Repairing Glaucomatous Optic Nerve. *Int. J. Ophthalmol.* **2024**, *17*, 748–760. [CrossRef] [PubMed]
23. Stargardt Disease | National Eye Institute. Available online: https://www.nei.nih.gov/learn-about-eye-health/eye-conditions-and-diseases/stargardt-disease (accessed on 28 September 2024).
24. Ghenciu, L.A.; Hațegan, O.A.; Stoicescu, E.R.; Iacob, R.; Șișu, A.M. Emerging Therapeutic Approaches and Genetic Insights in Stargardt Disease: A Comprehensive Review. *Int. J. Mol. Sci.* **2024**, *25*, 8859. [CrossRef] [PubMed]
25. Auricchio, A.; Trapani, I.; Allikmets, R. Gene Therapy of ABCA4-Associated Diseases. *Cold Spring Harb. Perspect. Med.* **2015**, *5*, a017301. [CrossRef] [PubMed]
26. Yalla, G.R.; Kuriyan, A.E. Cell Therapy for Retinal Disease. *Curr. Opin. Ophthalmol.* **2024**, *35*, 178–184. [CrossRef]
27. Radu, M.; Brănișteanu, D.C.; Pirvulescu, R.A.; Dumitrescu, O.M.; Ionescu, M.A.; Zemba, M. Exploring Stem-Cell-Based Therapies for Retinal Regeneration. *Life* **2024**, *14*, 668. [CrossRef]
28. Cerneckis, J.; Cai, H.; Shi, Y. Induced Pluripotent Stem Cells (iPSCs): Molecular Mechanisms of Induction and Applications. *Signal Transduct. Target. Ther.* **2024**, *9*, 112. [CrossRef]
29. Voisin, A.; Pénaguin, A.; Gaillard, A.; Leveziel, N. Stem Cell Therapy in Retinal Diseases. *Neural Regen. Res.* **2022**, *18*, 1478–1485. [CrossRef]
30. Adak, S.; Magdalene, D.; Deshmukh, S.; Das, D.; Jaganathan, B.G. A Review on Mesenchymal Stem Cells for Treatment of Retinal Diseases. *Stem Cell Rev. Rep.* **2021**, *17*, 1154–1173. [CrossRef]
31. Sharma, A.; Jaganathan, B.G. Stem Cell Therapy for Retinal Degeneration: The Evidence to Date. *BTT* **2021**, *15*, 299–306. [CrossRef]
32. German, O.L.; Vallese-Maurizi, H.; Soto, T.B.; Rotstein, N.P.; Politi, L.E. Retina Stem Cells, Hopes and Obstacles. *World J. Stem Cells* **2021**, *13*, 1446–1479. [CrossRef]
33. Shahin, S.; Tan, P.; Chetsawang, J.; Lu, B.; Svendsen, S.; Ramirez, S.; Conniff, T.; Alfaro, J.S.; Fernandez, M.; Fulton, A.; et al. Human Neural Progenitors Expressing GDNF Enhance Retinal Protection in a Rodent Model of Retinal Degeneration. *Stem Cells Transl. Med.* **2023**, *12*, 727–744. [CrossRef] [PubMed]
34. Nair, D.S.R.; Thomas, B.B. Stem Cell-Based Treatment Strategies for Degenerative Diseases of the Retina. *Curr. Stem Cell Res. Ther.* **2022**, *17*, 214–225. [CrossRef] [PubMed]
35. Drag, S.; Dotiwala, F.; Upadhyay, A.K. Gene Therapy for Retinal Degenerative Diseases: Progress, Challenges, and Future Directions. *Investig. Ophthalmol. Vis. Sci.* **2023**, *64*, 39. [CrossRef] [PubMed]
36. Surendran, H.; Soundararajan, L.; Reddy, V.B.K.; Subramani, J.; Stoddard, J.; Reynaga, R.; Tschetter, W.; Ryals, R.C.; Pal, R. An Improved Protocol for Generation and Characterization of Human-Induced Pluripotent Stem Cell-Derived Retinal Pigment Epithelium Cells. *STAR Protoc.* **2022**, *3*, 101803. [CrossRef]
37. Petrus-Reurer, S.; Winblad, N.; Kumar, P.; Gorchs, L.; Chrobok, M.; Wagner, A.K.; Bartuma, H.; Lardner, E.; Aronsson, M.; Plaza Reyes, Á.; et al. Generation of Retinal Pigment Epithelial Cells Derived from Human Embryonic Stem Cells Lacking Human Leukocyte Antigen Class I and II. *Stem Cell Rep.* **2020**, *14*, 648–662. [CrossRef]
38. Shrestha, R.; Wen, Y.-T.; Tsai, R.-K. Induced Pluripotent Stem Cells and Derivative Photoreceptor Precursors as Therapeutic Cells for Retinal Degenerations. *Tzu Chi Med. J.* **2019**, *32*, 101–112. [CrossRef]
39. Wu, K.Y.; Kulbay, M.; Toameh, D.; Xu, A.Q.; Kalevar, A.; Tran, S.D. Retinitis Pigmentosa: Novel Therapeutic Targets and Drug Development. *Pharmaceutics* **2023**, *15*, 685. [CrossRef]
40. Li, L.; Turner, J.E. Inherited Retinal Dystrophy in the RCS Rat: Prevention of Photoreceptor Degeneration by Pigment Epithelial Cell Transplantation. *Exp. Eye Res.* **1988**, *47*, 911–917. [CrossRef]
41. Gouras, P.; Kjeldbye, H.; Sullivan, B.; Reppucci, V.; Britfis, M.; Wapner, F.; Goluboff, E. Transplanted Retinal Pigment Epithelium Modifies the Retinal Degeneration in the RC5 Rat. *Investig. Ophthalmol.* **1989**, *30*, 586–588.
42. Schraermeyer, U.; Thumann, G.; Luther, T.; Kociok, N.; Arnhold, S.; Kruttwig, K.; Andressen, C.; Addicks, K.; Bartz-Schmidt, K.U. Subretinally Transplanted Embryonic Stem Cells Rescue Photoreceptor Cells from Degeneration in the RCS Rats. *Cell Transplant.* **2001**, *10*, 673–680. [CrossRef]

43. Kicic, A.; Shen, W.-Y.; Wilson, A.S.; Constable, I.J.; Robertson, T.; Rakoczy, P.E. Differentiation of Marrow Stromal Cells into Photoreceptors in the Rat Eye. *J. Neurosci.* **2003**, *23*, 7742–7749. [CrossRef]
44. Haruta, M.; Sasai, Y.; Kawasaki, H.; Amemiya, K.; Ooto, S.; Kitada, M.; Suemori, H.; Nakatsuji, N.; Ide, C.; Honda, Y.; et al. In Vitro and In Vivo Characterization of Pigment Epithelial Cells Differentiated from Primate Embryonic Stem Cells. *Investig. Ophthalmol. Vis. Sci.* **2004**, *45*, 1020–1025. [CrossRef]
45. Klassen, H.J.; Ng, T.F.; Kurimoto, Y.; Kirov, I.; Shatos, M.; Coffey, P.; Young, M.J. Multipotent Retinal Progenitors Express Developmental Markers, Differentiate into Retinal Neurons, and Preserve Light-Mediated Behavior. *Investig. Ophthalmol. Vis. Sci.* **2004**, *45*, 4167–4173. [CrossRef] [PubMed]
46. Lund, R.D.; Wang, S.; Klimanskaya, I.; Holmes, T.; Ramos-Kelsey, R.; Lu, B.; Girman, S.; Bischoff, N.; Sauvé, Y.; Lanza, R. Human Embryonic Stem Cell–Derived Cells Rescue Visual Function in Dystrophic RCS Rats. *Cloning Stem Cells* **2006**, *8*, 189–199. [CrossRef] [PubMed]
47. Vugler, A.; Carr, A.-J.; Lawrence, J.; Chen, L.L.; Burrell, K.; Wright, A.; Lundh, P.; Semo, M.; Ahmado, A.; Gias, C.; et al. Elucidating the Phenomenon of HESC-Derived RPE: Anatomy of Cell Genesis, Expansion and Retinal Transplantation. *Exp. Neurol.* **2008**, *214*, 347–361. [CrossRef]
48. Castanheira, P.; Torquetti, L.; Nehemy, M.B.; Goes, A.M. Retinal Incorporation and Differentiation of Mesenchymal Stem Cells Intravitreally Injected in the Injured Retina of Rats. *Arq. Bras. Oftalmol.* **2008**, *71*, 644–650. [CrossRef] [PubMed]
49. Idelson, M.; Alper, R.; Obolensky, A.; Ben-Shushan, E.; Hemo, I.; Yachimovich-Cohen, N.; Khaner, H.; Smith, Y.; Wiser, O.; Gropp, M.; et al. Directed Differentiation of Human Embryonic Stem Cells into Functional Retinal Pigment Epithelium Cells. *Cell Stem Cell* **2009**, *5*, 396–408. [CrossRef] [PubMed]
50. Lamba, D.A.; Gust, J.; Reh, T.A. Transplantation of Human Embryonic Stem Cell-Derived Photoreceptors Restores Some Visual Function in Crx-Deficient Mice. *Cell Stem Cell* **2009**, *4*, 73–79. [CrossRef] [PubMed]
51. Jagatha, B.; Divya, M.S.; Sanalkumar, R.; Indulekha, C.L.; Vidyanand, S.; Divya, T.S.; Das, A.V.; James, J. In Vitro Differentiation of Retinal Ganglion-like Cells from Embryonic Stem Cell Derived Neural Progenitors. *Biochem. Biophys. Res. Commun.* **2009**, *380*, 230–235. [CrossRef]
52. Osakada, F.; Jin, Z.-B.; Hirami, Y.; Ikeda, H.; Danjyo, T.; Watanabe, K.; Sasai, Y.; Takahashi, M. In Vitro Differentiation of Retinal Cells from Human Pluripotent Stem Cells by Small-Molecule Induction. *J. Cell Sci.* **2009**, *122*, 3169–3179. [CrossRef]
53. Meyer, J.S.; Shearer, R.L.; Capowski, E.E.; Wright, L.S.; Wallace, K.A.; McMillan, E.L.; Zhang, S.-C.; Gamm, D.M. Modeling Early Retinal Development with Human Embryonic and Induced Pluripotent Stem Cells. *Proc. Natl. Acad. Sci. USA* **2009**, *106*, 16698–16703. [CrossRef] [PubMed]
54. Chen, M.; Chen, Q.; Sun, X.; Shen, W.; Liu, B.; Zhong, X.; Leng, Y.; Li, C.; Zhang, W.; Chai, F.; et al. Generation of Retinal Ganglion–like Cells from Reprogrammed Mouse Fibroblasts. *Investig. Ophthalmol. Vis. Sci.* **2010**, *51*, 5970–5978. [CrossRef] [PubMed]
55. Lamba, D.A.; McUsic, A.; Hirata, R.K.; Wang, P.-R.; Russell, D.; Reh, T.A. Generation, Purification and Transplantation of Photoreceptors Derived from Human Induced Pluripotent Stem Cells. *PLoS ONE* **2010**, *5*, e8763. [CrossRef] [PubMed]
56. Tucker, B.A.; Park, I.-H.; Qi, S.D.; Klassen, H.J.; Jiang, C.; Yao, J.; Redenti, S.; Daley, G.Q.; Young, M.J. Transplantation of Adult Mouse iPS Cell-Derived Photoreceptor Precursors Restores Retinal Structure and Function in Degenerative Mice. *PLoS ONE* **2011**, *6*, e18992. [CrossRef] [PubMed]
57. Shirai, H.; Mandai, M.; Matsushita, K.; Kuwahara, A.; Yonemura, S.; Nakano, T.; Assawachananont, J.; Kimura, T.; Saito, K.; Terasaki, H.; et al. Transplantation of Human Embryonic Stem Cell-Derived Retinal Tissue in Two Primate Models of Retinal Degeneration. *Proc. Natl. Acad. Sci. USA* **2016**, *113*, E81–E90. [CrossRef]
58. Santos-Ferreira, T.; Völkner, M.; Borsch, O.; Haas, J.; Cimalla, P.; Vasudevan, P.; Carmeliet, P.; Corbeil, D.; Michalakis, S.; Koch, E.; et al. Stem Cell–Derived Photoreceptor Transplants Differentially Integrate Into Mouse Models of Cone-Rod Dystrophy. *Investig. Ophthalmol. Vis. Sci.* **2016**, *57*, 3509–3520. [CrossRef]
59. Venugopalan, P.; Wang, Y.; Nguyen, T.; Huang, A.; Muller, K.J.; Goldberg, J.L. Transplanted Neurons Integrate into Adult Retinas and Respond to Light. *Nat. Commun.* **2016**, *7*, 10472. [CrossRef]
60. Holan, V.; Hermankova, B.; Kossl, J. Perspectives of Stem Cell–Based Therapy for Age-Related Retinal Degenerative Diseases. *Cell Transplant.* **2017**, *26*, 1538–1541. [CrossRef]
61. Wu, H.; Li, J.; Mao, X.; Li, G.; Xie, L.; You, Z. Transplantation of Rat Embryonic Stem Cell-Derived Retinal Cells Restores Visual Function in the Royal College of Surgeons Rats. *Doc. Ophthalmol.* **2018**, *137*, 71–78. [CrossRef]
62. Sharma, R.; Khristov, V.; Rising, A.; Jha, B.S.; Dejene, R.; Hotaling, N.; Li, Y.; Stoddard, J.; Stankewicz, C.; Wan, Q.; et al. Clinical-Grade Stem Cell-Derived Retinal Pigment Epithelium Patch Rescues Retinal Degeneration in Rodents and Pigs. *Sci. Transl. Med.* **2019**, *11*, eaat5580. [CrossRef]
63. Tu, H.-Y.; Watanabe, T.; Shirai, H.; Yamasaki, S.; Kinoshita, M.; Matsushita, K.; Hashiguchi, T.; Onoe, H.; Matsuyama, T.; Kuwahara, A.; et al. Medium- to Long-Term Survival and Functional Examination of Human iPSC-Derived Retinas in Rat and Primate Models of Retinal Degeneration. *EBioMedicine* **2019**, *39*, 562–574. [CrossRef] [PubMed]
64. Wang, Z.; Gao, F.; Zhang, M.; Zheng, Y.; Zhang, F.; Xu, L.; Cao, L.; He, W. Intravitreal Injection of Human Retinal Progenitor Cells for Treatment of Retinal Degeneration. *Med. Sci. Monit.* **2020**, *26*, e921184-1–e921184-10. [CrossRef] [PubMed]

65. Salas, A.; Duarri, A.; Fontrodona, L.; Ramírez, D.M.; Badia, A.; Isla-Magrané, H.; Ferreira-de-Souza, B.; Zapata, M.Á.; Raya, Á.; Veiga, A.; et al. Cell Therapy with hiPSC-Derived RPE Cells and RPCs Prevents Visual Function Loss in a Rat Model of Retinal Degeneration. *Mol. Ther. Methods Clin. Dev.* **2021**, *20*, 688–702. [CrossRef] [PubMed]
66. Surendran, H.; Nandakumar, S.; Reddy, V.B.K.; Stoddard, J.; Mohan, K.V.; Upadhyay, P.K.; McGill, T.J.; Pal, R. Transplantation of Retinal Pigment Epithelium and Photoreceptors Generated Concomitantly via Small Molecule-Mediated Differentiation Rescues Visual Function in Rodent Models of Retinal Degeneration. *Stem Cell Res. Ther.* **2021**, *12*, 70. [CrossRef] [PubMed]
67. Duarri, A.; Rodríguez-Bocanegra, E.; Martínez-Navarrete, G.; Biarnés, M.; García, M.; Ferraro, L.L.; Kuebler, B.; Aran, B.; Izquierdo, E.; Aguilera-Xiol, E.; et al. Transplantation of Human Induced Pluripotent Stem Cell-Derived Retinal Pigment Epithelium in a Swine Model of Geographic Atrophy. *Int. J. Mol. Sci.* **2021**, *22*, 10497. [CrossRef]
68. He, X.-Y.; Zhao, C.-J.; Xu, H.; Chen, K.; Bian, B.-S.-J.; Gong, Y.; Weng, C.-H.; Zeng, Y.-X.; Fu, Y.; Liu, Y.; et al. Synaptic Repair and Vision Restoration in Advanced Degenerating Eyes by Transplantation of Retinal Progenitor Cells. *Stem Cell Rep.* **2021**, *16*, 1805–1817. [CrossRef]
69. Liang, Q.; Li, Q.; Ren, B.; Yin, Z.Q. Intravenous Infusion of Small Umbilical Cord Mesenchymal Stem Cells Could Enhance Safety and Delay Retinal Degeneration in RCS Rats. *BMC Ophthalmol.* **2022**, *22*, 67. [CrossRef]
70. Zhang, J.; Li, P.; Zhao, G.; He, S.; Xu, D.; Jiang, W.; Peng, Q.; Li, Z.; Xie, Z.; Zhang, H.; et al. Mesenchymal Stem Cell-Derived Extracellular Vesicles Protect Retina in a Mouse Model of Retinitis Pigmentosa by Anti-Inflammation through miR-146a-Nr4a3 Axis. *Stem Cell Res. Ther.* **2022**, *13*, 394. [CrossRef]
71. Brown, C.; Agosta, P.; McKee, C.; Walker, K.; Mazzella, M.; Alamri, A.; Svinarich, D.; Chaudhry, G.R. Human Primitive Mesenchymal Stem Cell-Derived Retinal Progenitor Cells Improved Neuroprotection, Neurogenesis, and Vision in Rd12 Mouse Model of Retinitis Pigmentosa. *Stem Cell Res. Ther.* **2022**, *13*, 148. [CrossRef]
72. Di Pierdomenico, J.; Gallego-Ortega, A.; Martínez-Vacas, A.; García-Bernal, D.; Vidal-Sanz, M.; Villegas-Pérez, M.P.; García-Ayuso, D. Intravitreal and Subretinal Syngeneic Bone Marrow Mononuclear Stem Cell Transplantation Improves Photoreceptor Survival but Does Not Ameliorate Retinal Function in Two Rat Models of Retinal Degeneration. *Acta Ophthalmol.* **2022**, *100*, e1313–e1331. [CrossRef]
73. Dezfuly, A.R.; Safaee, A.; Amirpour, N.; Kazemi, M.; Ramezani, A.; Jafarinia, M.; Dehghani, A.; Salehi, H. Therapeutic Effects of Human Adipose Mesenchymal Stem Cells and Their Paracrine Agents on Sodium Iodate Induced Retinal Degeneration in Rats. *Life Sci.* **2022**, *300*, 120570. [CrossRef] [PubMed]
74. Liu, Q.; Liu, J.; Guo, M.; Sung, T.-C.; Wang, T.; Yu, T.; Tian, Z.; Fan, G.; Wu, W.; Higuchi, A. Comparison of Retinal Degeneration Treatment with Four Types of Different Mesenchymal Stem Cells, Human Induced Pluripotent Stem Cells and RPE Cells in a Rat Retinal Degeneration Model. *J. Transl. Med.* **2023**, *21*, 910. [CrossRef] [PubMed]
75. Sheedlo, H.J.; Li, L.; Gaur, V.P.; Young, R.W.; Seaton, A.D.; Stovall, S.V.; Jaynes, C.D.; Turner, J.E. Photoreceptor Rescue in the Dystrophic Retina by Transplantation of Retinal Pigment Epithelium. In *International Review of Cytology*; Jeon, K.W., Friedlander, M., Eds.; Academic Press: Cambridge, MA, USA, 1992; Volume 138, pp. 1–49.
76. Schwartz, S.D.; Hubschman, J.-P.; Heilwell, G.; Franco-Cardenas, V.; Pan, C.K.; Ostrick, R.M.; Mickunas, E.; Gay, R.; Klimanskaya, I.; Lanza, R. Embryonic Stem Cell Trials for Macular Degeneration: A Preliminary Report. *Lancet* **2012**, *379*, 713–720. [CrossRef] [PubMed]
77. Schwartz, S.D.; Regillo, C.D.; Lam, B.L.; Eliott, D.; Rosenfeld, P.J.; Gregori, N.Z.; Hubschman, J.-P.; Davis, J.L.; Heilwell, G.; Spirn, M.; et al. Human Embryonic Stem Cell-Derived Retinal Pigment Epithelium in Patients with Age-Related Macular Degeneration and Stargardt's Macular Dystrophy: Follow-up of Two Open-Label Phase 1/2 Studies. *Lancet* **2015**, *385*, 509–516. [CrossRef]
78. Song, W.K.; Park, K.-M.; Kim, H.-J.; Lee, J.H.; Choi, J.; Chong, S.Y.; Shim, S.H.; Del Priore, L.V.; Lanza, R. Treatment of Macular Degeneration Using Embryonic Stem Cell-Derived Retinal Pigment Epithelium: Preliminary Results in Asian Patients. *Stem Cell Rep.* **2015**, *4*, 860–872. [CrossRef]
79. Mehat, M.S.; Sundaram, V.; Ripamonti, C.; Robson, A.G.; Smith, A.J.; Borooah, S.; Robinson, M.; Rosenthal, A.N.; Innes, W.; Weleber, R.G.; et al. Transplantation of Human Embryonic Stem Cell-Derived Retinal Pigment Epithelial Cells in Macular Degeneration. *Ophthalmology* **2018**, *125*, 1765–1775. [CrossRef]
80. Sung, Y.; Lee, M.J.; Choi, J.; Jung, S.Y.; Chong, S.Y.; Sung, J.H.; Shim, S.H.; Song, W.K. Long-Term Safety and Tolerability of Subretinal Transplantation of Embryonic Stem Cell-Derived Retinal Pigment Epithelium in Asian Stargardt Disease Patients. *Br. J. Ophthalmol.* **2021**, *105*, 829–837. [CrossRef]
81. Li, S.; Liu, Y.; Wang, L.; Wang, F.; Zhao, T.; Li, Q.; Xu, H.; Meng, X.; Hao, J.; Zhou, Q.; et al. A Phase I Clinical Trial of Human Embryonic Stem Cell-derived Retinal Pigment Epithelial Cells for Early-stage Stargardt Macular Degeneration: 5-years' Follow-up. *Cell Prolif.* **2021**, *54*, e13100. [CrossRef]
82. da Cruz, L.; Fynes, K.; Georgiadis, O.; Kerby, J.; Luo, Y.H.; Ahmado, A.; Vernon, A.; Daniels, J.T.; Nommiste, B.; Hasan, S.M.; et al. Phase 1 Clinical Study of an Embryonic Stem Cell–Derived Retinal Pigment Epithelium Patch in Age-Related Macular Degeneration. *Nat. Biotechnol.* **2018**, *36*, 328–337. [CrossRef]
83. Monville, C.; Bertin, S.; Devisme, C.; Brazhnikova, E.; Jaillard, C.; Walter, H.; Plancheron, A.; Jarraya, M.; Bejanariu, A.; Abbas, S.; et al. Phase I/II Open-Label Study of Implantation into One Eye of hESC-Derived RPE in Patients with Retinitis Pigmentosa Due to Monogenic Mutation: First Safety Results. *Investig. Ophthalmol. Vis. Sci.* **2023**, *64*, 3829.

84. Humayun, M.S.; Clegg, D.O.; Dayan, M.S.; Kashani, A.H.; Rahhal, F.M.; Avery, R.L.; Salehi-Had, H.; Chen, S.; Chan, C.; Palejwala, N.; et al. Long-Term Follow-up of a Phase 1/2a Clinical Trial of a Stem Cell-Derived Bioengineered Retinal Pigment Epithelium Implant for Geographic Atrophy. *Ophthalmology* **2024**, *131*, 682–691. [CrossRef] [PubMed]
85. Kashani, A.H.; Lebkowski, J.S.; Rahhal, F.M.; Avery, R.L.; Salehi-Had, H.; Chen, S.; Chan, C.; Palejwala, N.; Ingram, A.; Dang, W.; et al. One-Year Follow-Up in a Phase 1/2a Clinical Trial of an Allogeneic RPE Cell Bioengineered Implant for Advanced Dry Age-Related Macular Degeneration. *Trans. Vis. Sci. Technol.* **2021**, *10*, 13. [CrossRef]
86. Telander, D. OpRegen® Retinal Pigment Epithelium (RPE) Cell Therapy for Patients with Geographic Atrophy (GA): Month 24 Results from the Phase 1/2a Trial. 2024.
87. Mandai, M.; Watanabe, A.; Kurimoto, Y.; Hirami, Y.; Morinaga, C.; Daimon, T.; Fujihara, M.; Akimaru, H.; Sakai, N.; Shibata, Y.; et al. Autologous Induced Stem-Cell–Derived Retinal Cells for Macular Degeneration. *N. Engl. J. Med.* **2017**, *376*, 1038–1046. [CrossRef] [PubMed]
88. Takagi, S.; Mandai, M.; Gocho, K.; Hirami, Y.; Yamamoto, M.; Fujihara, M.; Sugita, S.; Kurimoto, Y.; Takahashi, M. Evaluation of Transplanted Autologous Induced Pluripotent Stem Cell-Derived Retinal Pigment Epithelium in Exudative Age-Related Macular Degeneration. *Ophthalmol. Retin.* **2019**, *3*, 850–859. [CrossRef] [PubMed]
89. Park, S.S.; Bauer, G.; Abedi, M.; Pontow, S.; Panorgias, A.; Jonnal, R.; Zawadzki, R.J.; Werner, J.S.; Nolta, J. Intravitreal Autologous Bone Marrow CD34+ Cell Therapy for Ischemic and Degenerative Retinal Disorders: Preliminary Phase 1 Clinical Trial Findings. *Investig. Ophthalmol. Vis. Sci.* **2015**, *56*, 81–89. [CrossRef]
90. Park, S.S.; Bauer, G.; Fury, B.; Abedi, M.; Perotti, N.; Coleal-Gergum, D.; Nolta, J.A. Phase I Study of Intravitreal Injection of Autologous CD34+ Stem Cells from Bone Marrow in Eyes with Vision Loss from Retinitis Pigmentosa (AAO Meeting Paper). *Ophthalmol. Sci.* **2024**, *5*, 100589. [CrossRef]
91. Siqueira, R.C.; Messias, A.; Voltarelli, J.C.; Scott, I.U.; Jorge, R. Intravitreal Injection of Autologous Bone Marrow–Derived Mononuclear Cells for Hereditary Retinal Dystrophy: A Phase I Trial. *Retina* **2011**, *31*, 1207–1214. [CrossRef]
92. Siqueira, R.C.; Messias, A.; Messias, K.; Arcieri, R.S.; Ruiz, M.A.; Souza, N.F.; Martins, L.C.; Jorge, R. Quality of Life in Patients with Retinitis Pigmentosa Submitted to Intravitreal Use of Bone Marrow-Derived Stem Cells (Reticell-Clinical Trial). *Stem Cell Res. Ther.* **2015**, *6*, 29. [CrossRef]
93. Tuekprakhon, A.; Sangkitporn, S.; Trinavarat, A.; Pawestri, A.R.; Vamvanij, V.; Ruangchainikom, M.; Luksanapruksa, P.; Pongpaksupasin, P.; Khorchai, A.; Dambua, A.; et al. Intravitreal Autologous Mesenchymal Stem Cell Transplantation: A Non-Randomized Phase I Clinical Trial in Patients with Retinitis Pigmentosa. *Stem Cell Res. Ther.* **2021**, *12*, 52. [CrossRef]
94. Siqueira, R.C.; Costa Cotrim, C.; Messias, A.; Sousa, M.V.d.; Toscano, L.; Jorge, R. Intravitreal Autologous Bone Marrow Derived Stem Cells in Dry Age-Related Macular Degeneration. *Investig. Ophthalmol. Vis. Sci.* **2016**, *57*, 3704.
95. Weiss, J.N.; Levy, S. Stem Cell Ophthalmology Treatment Study (SCOTS): Bone Marrow-Derived Stem Cells in the Treatment of Stargardt Disease. *Medicines* **2021**, *8*, 10. [CrossRef] [PubMed]
96. Weiss, J.N.; Levy, S. Stem Cell Ophthalmology Treatment Study (SCOTS): Bone Marrow-Derived Stem Cells in the Treatment of Age-Related Macular Degeneration. *Medicines* **2020**, *7*, 16. [CrossRef] [PubMed]
97. Weiss, J.N.; Levy, S. Stem Cell Ophthalmology Treatment Study: Bone Marrow Derived Stem Cells in the Treatment of Retinitis Pigmentosa. *Stem Cell Investig.* **2018**, *5*, 18. [CrossRef] [PubMed]
98. Özmert, E.; Arslan, U. Management of Retinitis Pigmentosa by Wharton's Jelly Derived Mesenchymal Stem Cells: Preliminary Clinical Results. *Stem Cell Res. Ther.* **2020**, *11*, 25. [CrossRef] [PubMed]
99. Peng, Y.; Tang, L.; Zhou, Y. Subretinal Injection: A Review on the Novel Route of Therapeutic Delivery for Vitreoretinal Diseases. *Ophthalmic Res.* **2017**, *58*, 217–226. [CrossRef]
100. Chiang, B.; Jung, J.H.; Prausnitz, M.R. The Suprachoroidal Space as a Route of Administration to the Posterior Segment of the Eye. *Adv. Drug Deliv. Rev.* **2018**, *126*, 58–66. [CrossRef]
101. Lotfi, M.; Morshedi Rad, D.; Mashhadi, S.S.; Ashouri, A.; Mojarrad, M.; Mozaffari-Jovin, S.; Farrokhi, S.; Hashemi, M.; Lotfi, M.; Ebrahimi Warkiani, M.; et al. Recent Advances in CRISPR/Cas9 Delivery Approaches for Therapeutic Gene Editing of Stem Cells. *Stem Cell Rev. Rep.* **2023**, *19*, 2576–2596. [CrossRef]
102. Siles, L.; Ruiz-Nogales, S.; Navinés-Ferrer, A.; Méndez-Vendrell, P.; Pomares, E. Efficient Correction of ABCA4 Variants by CRISPR-Cas9 in hiPSCs Derived from Stargardt Disease Patients. *Mol. Ther. Nucleic Acids* **2023**, *32*, 64–79. [CrossRef]
103. Klymenko, V.; González Martínez, O.G.; Zarbin, M. Recent Progress in Retinal Pigment Epithelium Cell-Based Therapy for Retinal Disease. *Stem Cells Transl. Med.* **2024**, *13*, 317–331. [CrossRef]
104. Ballios, B.G.; Cooke, M.J.; van der Kooy, D.; Shoichet, M.S. A Hydrogel-Based Stem Cell Delivery System to Treat Retinal Degenerative Diseases. *Biomaterials* **2010**, *31*, 2555–2564. [CrossRef]
105. Silverman, M.S.; Hughes, S.E. Transplantation of Photoreceptors to Light-Damaged Retina. *Investig. Ophthalmol. Vis. Sci.* **1989**, *30*, 1684–1690.
106. Song, M.J.; Quinn, R.; Nguyen, E.; Hampton, C.; Sharma, R.; Park, T.S.; Koster, C.; Voss, T.; Tristan, C.; Weber, C.; et al. Bioprinted 3D Outer Retina Barrier Uncovers RPE-Dependent Choroidal Phenotype in Advanced Macular Degeneration. *Nat. Methods* **2023**, *20*, 149–161. [CrossRef] [PubMed]
107. Takahashi, K.; Tanabe, K.; Ohnuki, M.; Narita, M.; Ichisaka, T.; Tomoda, K.; Yamanaka, S. Induction of Pluripotent Stem Cells from Adult Human Fibroblasts by Defined Factors. *Cell* **2007**, *131*, 861–872. [CrossRef] [PubMed]

108. Jin, Z.-B.; Okamoto, S.; Osakada, F.; Homma, K.; Assawachananont, J.; Hirami, Y.; Iwata, T.; Takahashi, M. Modeling Retinal Degeneration Using Patient-Specific Induced Pluripotent Stem Cells. *PLoS ONE* **2011**, *6*, e17084. [CrossRef] [PubMed]
109. Rohowetz, L.J.; Koulen, P. Stem Cell-Derived Retinal Pigment Epithelium Cell Therapy: Past and Future Directions. *Front. Cell Dev. Biol.* **2023**, *11*, 1098406. [CrossRef]
110. Zheng, Y.L. Some Ethical Concerns About Human Induced Pluripotent Stem Cells. *Sci. Eng. Ethics* **2016**, *22*, 1277–1284. [CrossRef]

*pharmaceutics*

MDPI

*Review*

# Immunotherapies Targeting Tumor-Associated Macrophages (TAMs) in Cancer

**Mei-Ye Li [1], Wei Ye [1] and Ke-Wang Luo [1,2,*]**

1 School of Pharmaceutical Sciences, Southern Medical University, Guangzhou 510515, China; meiyeli2023@gmail.com (M.-Y.L.); yeyewei2023@gmail.com (W.Y.)

2 People's Hospital of Longhua, The affiliated hospital of Southern Medical University, Shenzhen 518109, China

* Correspondence: kewangluo@126.com or kewangluo@smu.edu.cn

**Abstract:** Tumor-associated macrophages (TAMs) are one of the most plentiful immune compositions in the tumor microenvironment, which are further divided into anti-tumor M1 subtype and pro-tumor M2 subtype. Recent findings found that TAMs play a vital function in the regulation and progression of tumorigenesis. Moreover, TAMs promote tumor vascularization, and support the survival of tumor cells, causing an impact on tumor growth and patient prognosis. Numerous studies show that reducing the density of TAMs, or modulating the polarization of TAMs, can inhibit tumor growth, indicating that TAMs are a promising target for tumor immunotherapy. Recently, clinical trials have found that treatments targeting TAMs have achieved encouraging results, and the U.S. Food and Drug Administration has approved a number of drugs for use in cancer treatment. In this review, we summarize the origin, polarization, and function of TAMs, and emphasize the therapeutic strategies targeting TAMs in cancer treatment in clinical studies and scientific research, which demonstrate a broad prospect of TAMs-targeted therapies in tumor immunotherapy.

**Keywords:** TAMs; polarization; therapies; clinical application

## 1. Introduction

Cancer is a significant health problem and a major cause of death in the world. In the process of cancer development, tumor microenvironment (TME) is widely recognized as dynamically regulating cancer progression and influencing therapeutic efficacy, and it is a complex multicellular environment which includes a variety of immune cells, endothelial cells (ECs), cancer-associated fibroblasts (CAFs), pericytes, and other cell types [1]. Among the TME, immune cells, especially macrophages, have recently become an attractive target for cancer therapy, and achieve desirable results in treatment.

Macrophages indeed play a crucial role in maintaining tissue homeostasis and host defense [2]. Three main functions of these cells are phagocytosis, exogenous antigen presentation, and immunomodulation through the secretion of cytokines and growth factors [3]. Mature macrophages are differentiated from circulating bone marrow-derived monocytes [4]. Within the TME, macrophages are a significant stromal component and are often referred to as TAMs. TAMs can be found in various types of tumor, and are proven to play a complex function in tumor progression and immune response against cancer. In general, TAMs are classified into two types: classical M1 macrophages and alternative M2 macrophages; M1 macrophages are engaged in mechanistic responses, pathogen removal, and anti-tumor immunity. On the contrary, M2 macrophages have a connection with anti-inflammatory responses, wound healing, and the properties of tumorigenicity. TAMs have received widespread attention over the past decades due to their effects on leukocytes, cytokines, and inflammatory mediators. Currently, drugs targeting TAMs include pexidartinib, which produces promising therapeutic outcomes in the treatment of patients with solid tumors. Lee et al. indicated that patients with advanced solid tumors, and treated with 600 mg/day of pexidartinib, experienced an objective remission and prolonged survival, with one third of participants experiencing at least a 30% reduction in the sum diameter of the target lesions, and a 66.7% disease-control rate [5]. Furthermore, the US Food and Drug Administration (FDA) declared their approval of pexidartinib for the treatment of adult patients with giant cell tumor of the tendon sheath on 2 August 2019. Based on the good results demonstrated by TAMs in tumor therapy, we address the origins, polarization, and targeted therapies of TAMs, and also summarize recent advances in immunotherapy for the tumor-targeted treatment of TAMs in recent years.

## 2. Tumor-Associated Macrophages (TAMs)

TAMs are a specific category of macrophages that exist in the TME. It is believed that TAMs are predominantly derived from circulating monocytes. When stimulated by varying factors, these macrophages show variable phenotypes and functions, which are also known as the polarization of TAMs. The plasticity of TAMs allows them to dynamically respond to changes in the TME and adopt different activation states. In the present section, we will concentrate on the origin and polarization of TAMs.

### 2.1. TAMs' Origins

It has been proposed for a considerable time that TAMs originated from circulating monocytes, and are attracted to tumors through chemotactic signals emitted by the tumor, such as C-C motif chemokine ligand 2, CCL2) [6]. This single origin of macrophages was not questioned until the discovery of the embryonic origin of tissue-resident macrophages [7]. Increasing evidence suggests that, in addition to circulating monocytes, embryo-derived TAMs are a non-negligible source of TAMs in TME. Although it is suggested that monocyte-derived macrophages could support the growth of TAMs in the inflammatory environment of a tumor, the potentially different contributions of monocyte- and embryo-derived TAMs to tumorigenesis remain a fascinating question.

Circulating monocytes originate from hematopoietic stem cells in bone marrow, such as intestinal macrophages [8]. Yolk sac macrophages and fetal liver could localize to specific tissues and then evolve into functional tissue-resident macrophages [9]. The latest available evidence demonstrates that the recruitment of circulating monocytes is critical for the accumulation of TAMs [10–12]. Chemokines, cytokines, and products of the complement cascade [13] are major determinants of macrophage recruitment and positioning in tumors [12]. Also, complement components, especially C5a, are linked to the recruitment and functional polarization of TAMs [14]. The coexistence of circulating monocytes and tissue-resident macrophages has been confirmed in tumor types such as breast tumors [11], brain tumors [15], lung cancer [8], and hepatocellular carcinoma [16]. In lung, brain, and pancreas tumors, TAMs from hematopoietic stem cells express antigen–presenting–related genes, and exhibit extensive immunosuppression, while embryonic–origin–TAMs–expressed genes are closely related to tissue remodeling and wound healing, suggesting that macrophages from different sources produce different physiological effects, even in the same tissue [17,18]. Different sources of TAMs are one of the important causes of the complexity of TME.

### 2.2. TAMs Polarization

TAMs polarization is the process of macrophages exhibiting characteristic phenotypic and functional responses to microenvironmental stimuli and signals encountered by each particular tissue. In this section, we will concentrate on the polarization of TAMs.

Macrophages are classified into two groups according to their function: classical M1-type macrophages and alternative M2-type macrophages (Figure 1). M1 macrophages are typically activated by lipopolysac charides, viral products, IFN-$\gamma$, or granulocyte-macrophage colony-stimulating factor (GM-CSF). M1 produces nitric oxide (NO) and reactive oxygen species (ROS), and also expresses a variety of pro-inflammatory cytokines, for example IL-1, IL-6, IL-12, TNF-$\alpha$, IL23, and CCL2. M1 also has phagocytosis and could kill target cells. For this reason, M1 macrophages represent a critical cellular component participating in the inflammatory response and anti-tumor immunity. Conversely, M2 macrophages are activated by macrophage colony-stimulating factor (M-CSF), IL-10, IL-4, IL-13, or glucocorticoids [19]. M2 expresses TGF-β, IL-1b, IL-4, IL-12, INF-γ, matrix metalloprotein (MMP), and vascular endothelial growth factor (VEGF) [20], thus it has the ability to repair damaged tissues, stimulate angiogenesis, and promote tumorigenesis and progression [21]. Furthermore, M2 macrophages can be categorized into at least four phenotypes, including M2a, which is induced by IL4 and IL13; M2b, which is induced by immune complexes or LPS; M2c, which is induced by IL10, TGF-β, or glucocorticoids; and M2d, which is the immune-suppressing type of M2 macrophages [22,23].

The main signaling pathways related to M1/M2 polarization are the JAK/STAT signaling pathway, the IRF signaling pathway, the Notch signaling pathway, the PI3K/AKT signaling pathway, and the TLR4 signaling pathway. STAT1 and STAT3/STAT6 are members of the STAT family and play a key role in signal transduction and transcriptional activation. Up-regulation of the suppressor of cytokine signaling (SOCS)1 expression activates the JAK1/STAT1 pathway, which promotes macrophages polarization to the M1 type, leading to an inflammatory response of cytotoxicity and tissue damage [24]. However, activation of STAT3 [25] and STAT6 [26] can polarize macrophages to M2, resulting in immunosuppressive effects. An LPS-induced TLR4 pathway activates JAK2/STAT1, thereby promoting M1 macrophage polarization [27]. M2 TAMs trigger IL-6 production in normal oxytumor cells, which promotes tumorigenesis by regulating JAK-STAT3 [28]. It has been found that the interaction between PPAR γ and the IL-4-STAT6 axis controls the M2 phenotypic transition [29]. In addition, the IRF-signaling pathway has a critical role in the progression of macrophages polarization. Mammals have nine IRFs, and they have significant differences in gene expression and regulation. Related studies have found that IRF-4 specifically regulates M2 cell polarization with the help of histone demethylase Jmjd3 in response to chitin [30]. IRF5 has been shown to be necessary for IL12 and pro-inflammatory cytokine expression [31]. In another study, the expression of IL12 and pro-inflammatory factors in GM-CSF-polarized macrophages was found to be increased along with the up-regulation of IRF5, which in turn activated T cells to stimulate M1 macrophages formation [32]. IRF6 participates in the negative regulation of M2 polarization of mouse bone marrow-derived macrophages by inhibiting PPARγ. In addition, the Notch pathway has an indispensable function in the activation of macrophages polarization. A study found that miR-148a-3p enhanced macrophage M1 polarization and inhibited M2 polarization when activated by Notch [33]. Activation of signal regulatory protein α (SIRPα) can promote macrophage M2 polarization. Notch activation may inhibit the expression of SIRPα through Hes family co-inhibitors, thereby promoting M1 polarization [34]. Apart from that, the PI3/AKT signaling pathway has a critical effect in macrophages polarization. The PI3K/Akt signaling pathway can be affected by TLR4, cytokine chemokines, and the Fc receptor. Activated PI3K I phosphatidylinositol 4,5-bisphosphate (PIP2) produces phosphatidylinositol 3,4,5-triphosphate (PIP3) at the membrane, and the PIP3 further triggers the activation of akt. Activated akt phosphorylates and inactivates the negative regulator of the mechanistic target of rapamycin complex (mTORC)1, thereby activating mTORC1. Consequently, Akt-mTORC1 signaling in macrophages contributes to increased histone acetylation, and generates M2 phenotypes [35]. Ship is a negative modulator of PI3K/Akt signaling; lacking ship results in a polarized M2 phenotype and reduces the production of inflammatory cytokines. Pten is another negative regulator of PI3K signaling, and its absence significantly enhances akt signaling and induces the formation of M2 macrophages [36]. TLR4 is a pathogen-pattern-recognition receptor [37]. TLR4 complex binds to adapter molecules (e.g., LPS) via myeloid differentiation factor 88 (Myd88), thereby enhancing the induction of inflammatory factor expression and inducing macrophages polarization [38]. In addition to the above pathway, it is found that the polarization of TAMs can be induced by the change in a nanocarrier's surface physical properties [39].

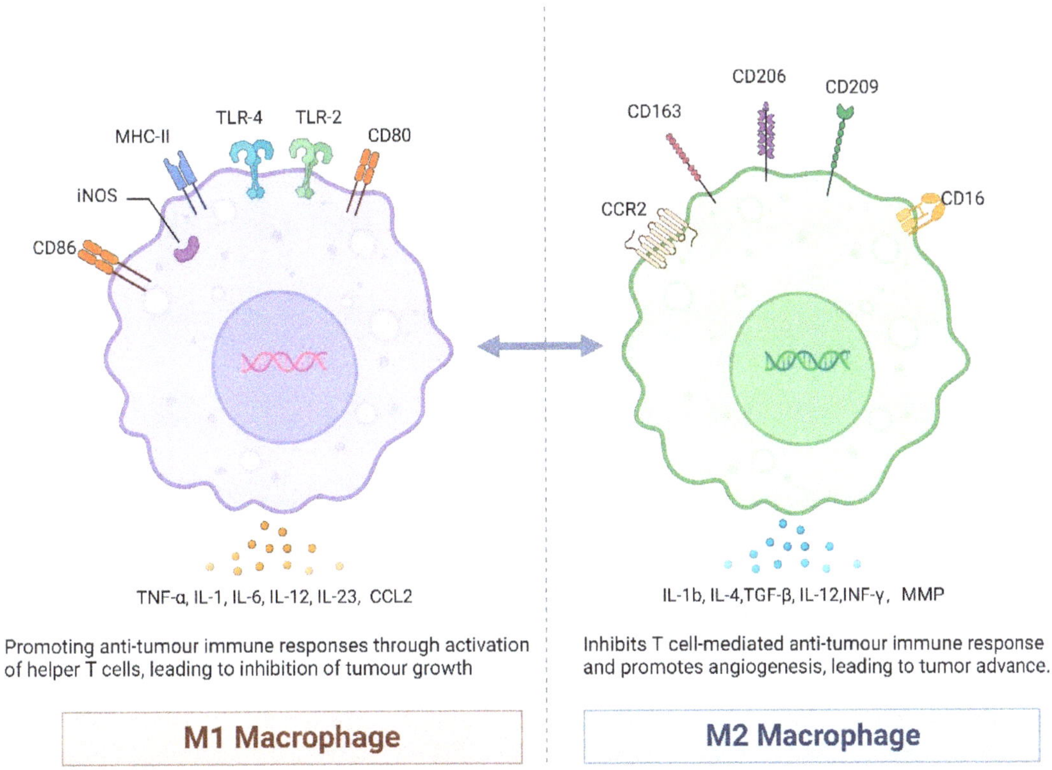


**Figure 1.** Two major subtypes of TAMs. TAMs are a type of immune cell that infiltrates the tumor microenvironment and plays a significant role in tumor development and progression. TAMs can exhibit different functional phenotypes, often referred to as M1 and M2 polarizations. M1-TAMs are typically associated with an anti-tumor response, and express certain surface markers, such as CD80 and CD86. M1-TAMs produce pro-inflammatory cytokines, such as IL-12, TNF-α. These cytokines contribute to the activation of natural killer cells, cytotoxic T cells, and other immune cells, thereby promoting an anti-tumor immune response. M1-TAMs also produce chemokines like CCL2, which recruit and activate T cells, further enhancing the anti-tumor immune response. On the other hand, M2-TAMs are associated with a pro-tumorigenic function, and express different surface markers, such as CD163 and CD206. M2-TAMs secrete anti-inflammatory cytokines, including TGF-β and IFN-γ, which can suppress immune responses and promote tumor growth. M2-TAMs also produce factors such as MMPs that facilitate tissue remodeling and angiogenesis, supporting tumor invasion and metastasis. It is important to note that the phenotypes and functions of TAMs can be influenced by various factors in the tumor microenvironment, including cytokines, chemokines, and signals from cancer cells themselves. This plasticity allows TAMs to adapt their functions based on the specific conditions within the tumor.

### *2.3. Functions of TAMs*

TAMs are an important pro-tumorigenic cell population in the TME, and they play multiple critical roles in tumor development. In this section, we will briefly outline the functions of TAMs in promoting tumor angiogenesis and in affecting metabolism and immunosuppression.

The formation of new blood vessels is essential to provide nutrients and oxygen for further tumor growth. It is known that TAMs are accumulated in hypoxic areas of tumor tissue, and that they secrete various pro-angiogenic molecules including TNF-α, matrix metalloproteinase (MMP), and vascular endothelial growth factor (VEGF) to promote blood vessel formation in tumors [40]. In addition, STAT3 activation in TAMs upregulates the production of angiogenic factors such as VEGF and basic fibroblast growth factor (bFGF), which in turn activates STAT3 signaling in endothelial cells and induces angiogenesis [41]. In addition, TIE2-expressing macrophages are characterized by elevating pro-angiogenic activity and attenuating pro-inflammatory phenotype, which is a receptor for angiostatin and plays an essential function in angiogenesis [42,43]. TAMs promote tumor angiogenesis, cell invasion, and metastasis. During epithelial mesenchymal transition (EMT), tumor cells lose intercellular junctions and apical-basal polarity due to the inhibition of E-cadherin, and consequently acquire the ability to invade [44]. TAMs-derived TGF-β triggers the activation of the β-catenin pathway in the tumor, thereby inducing EMT and accelerating tumor invasion [45]. The extracellular matrix (ECM) provides structural and biochemical support for tumor growth. TAMs provide a variety of ECM regulators, such as MMP and histone proteases, to facilitate tumor cell escape [46].

Tumors arise under hypoxic conditions, and tumor cells mainly use aerobic glycolysis to produce energy. TAMs are closely associated with tumor cell metabolism. Studies have reported that TAMs increase glycolysis in NSCLC cells through TNF-α secretion and promote hypoxia through AMP-activated protein kinase and PGC-1α activation, which in turn sustains tumor development [47]. In addition, TAMs have been found to be effective in enhancing aerobic glycolysis and inducing apoptosis resistance in breast cancer cells by transmitting myeloid-specific, HIF-1α-stable, long, non-coding RNA through extracellular vesicles [48]. Furthermore, some secreted molecules of TAMs can shape their immune phenotype. One study showed that ovarian cancer cells promote membrane cholesterol efflux from TAMs. On the one hand, the cholesterol derived from TAMs promotes tumorigenesis, on the other hand, high cholesterol efflux destroys lipid rafts in TAMs, leading to the reprogramming of TAMs to M2 type. The immune response of T-cells is also affected by the metabolites of TAMs. Studies have reported that arginine depletion via Arginase, a marker of M2-like TAMs, inhibits T-cell receptor expression and T-cell cytotoxicity [49].

Tumor immunosuppression is a well-established mechanism for regulating tumor growth. In the early stages of tumorigenesis, M1 macrophages maintain themselves by secreting large amounts of the pro-inflammatory cytokines IFNγ and IL12, which demonstrate anti-tumor activity, and induce the infiltration and activation of cytotoxic T-cells at the tumor site [50]. M1 macrophages can be captured by the tumor, and then transformed to an M2-like state by secreting immunosuppressive cytokines. M2 macrophages inhibit the secretion of IL10 by cytotoxic T cells, while IL10 supports the expression of immunosuppressive regulatory T-cells (Treg) [51]. However, in most types of cancer, TAMs show a higher degree of similarity to anti-inflammatory macrophages and biases toward a pro-tumor state [52]. Numerous studies have shown that TAMs secrete cytokines, such as TGF-β, IL-10, and arginase 1 (Arg 1), which directly inhibit the effector functions of CD4 + and CD8 + T cells, and enhance the expression of Treg cells, thus contributing to the formation of an immunosuppressive microenvironment [53]. TGF-β promotes the polarization of TAMs into M2 phenotypes in the innate immune response, which further promotes TGF-β production and deepens immunosuppression [54]. In the adaptive immune response, TGF-β regulates the production of a variety of cytolytic genes including granzyme A, granzyme B, IFNγ, and FAS ligands, which impair the anti-tumor activity of CD8 + T cells, ultimately leading to pro-tumor TME [55,56]. IL-10 is an important cytokine in the TME, and TAMs-derived IL-10 plays a role in inhibiting IL-12 expression in the autocrine circuit [57]. IL-10 inhibits the release of the cytotoxic cytokine IFN-γ, which is a major stimulus for the differentiation of naïve T-cells, thereby promoting immune evasion [58]. It has been demonstrated that Arg1 metabolizes L-arginine mainly to polyamines and proline, which leads to the dysregulation of T-cell receptor (TCR) signaling, and subsequently induces CD8 + T-cell unresponsiveness [59,60]. Furthermore, a variety of chemokines produced by TAMs have been implicated in immunosuppression. For example, TAM-derived CCL17/CCL22 significantly contributes to the entry of Tregs into the TME via the chemokine receptor CCR4 [61]. CCL18 produced by TAMs attracts naïve T-cells to the tumor site, leading to T-cell unresponsiveness [62].

## 2.4. Therapeutic Strategies Targeting TAMs

Numerous investigations have demonstrated that TAMs represent the most plentiful immune cells infiltrating the TME. TAMs mainly exert M2-like pro-cancer effects in TME, and regulate a variety of malignant effects including angiogenesis, immunosuppression, and metastasis of tumors. Currently, many drugs targeting TAMs have entered the clinical research stage. Therapeutic strategies targeting TAMs include: (1) inhibiting recruitment of TAMs, (2) killing TAMs, (3) regulating the polarization of TAMs [63]. In addition, therapies such as exosomes and CAR-M have also achieved good results in actual treatment. At this stage, drug development for TAMs mainly focuses on the following targets (Figure 2).

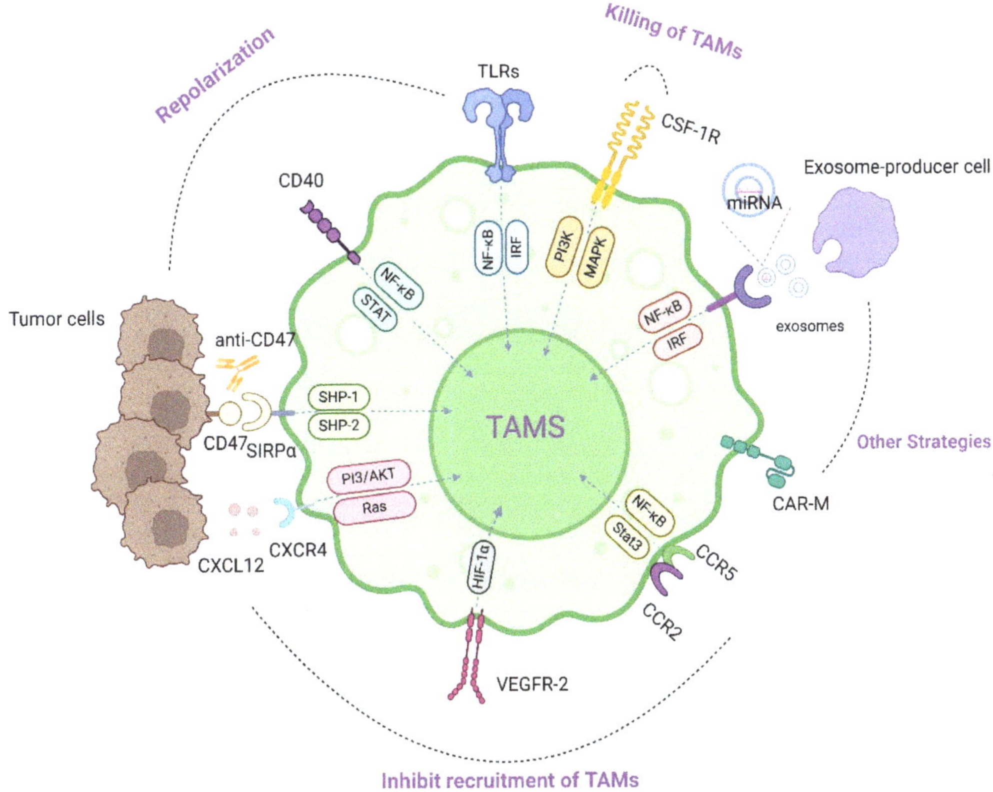


**Figure 2.** Immunotherapies targeting TAMs. Immunotherapies targeting TAMs have emerged as a potential strategy to enhance anti-tumor immune responses. There are three main categories involved in targeting TAMs: (1) Inhibition of macrophage recruitment: aims to prevent the recruitment of TAMs into the tumor microenvironment. It involves suppressing the production of chemokines like CCL2, CCL5, CXCL12, and their corresponding receptors such as CXCR4. Additionally, inhibition of VEGF formation can also prevent TAMs recruitment by reducing tumor angiogenesis; (2) Killing of TAMs: focuses on directly eliminating TAMs. One way to achieve this is by inhibiting the CSF1-R,

which is vital for the survival and proliferation of TAMs. Blocking CSF1-R can lead to the depletion of TAMs within the tumor. The mechanism of action may be related to the activation of the PI3K-dependent pathway and the Ras/mediator-activated protein kinase-dependent pathway; (3) Reprogramming of TAMs into anti-tumor macrophages: aims to convert TAMs from a pro-tumor phenotype into an anti-tumor phenotype. It involves activating specific receptors on TAMs, such as CD40 and TLRs. The mechanism of CD40 can be related to NF-κB and the transcriptional activator STAT. The mechanism of TLR can be related to NF-κB and IRF signaling. Moreover, the binding of CD47 to SIRP-α leads to activation and phosphorylation of the SIRP-α ITIM matrix and recruitment of the SHP-1 and SHP-2 phosphatases, which inhibit the phagocytosis of tumor cells by preventing myosin IIA from aggregating at phagocytic synapses. Interfering with the SIRP-α-CD47 axis has been investigated as a way to restore the recognition and phagocytosis of tumor cells by TAMs. In addition, exosomes and CAR-M have also been studied recently. Exosomes are small vesicles that can be used to deliver therapeutic agents directly to TAMs, allowing targeted modulation of their functions. The mechanism of miRNA can be related to NF-κB and IRF signaling. CAR-M refers to genetically modified macrophages expressing chimeric antigen receptors, enabling them to recognize and eliminate tumor cells more effectively.

#### 2.4.1. Inhibiting Recruitment of TAMs

A strategy aimed at TAMs is to block their recruitment or prevent monocytes/macrophages penetrating into the tumor. The recruitment of TAMs in tumors is typically driven by monocyte recruitment via the C-C motif chemokine ligand (CCL)-2-C-chemokine receptor (CCR)-2 axis. Alternative pathways engaged in the recruitment of TAMs are C-X-C ligand (CXCL)-12-C-X-C receptor (CXCR)-4 axis and the VEGF receptor pathway. Targeting all of these pathways is effective at inhibiting TAMs recruitment, as described in more detail below.

Chemokines are small molecular proteins, which perform their function by binding to G protein-coupled chemokine receptors (GPCRs) expressed on the cell surface [64]. The CCL2, also known as monocyte chemotactic protein-1 (MCP-1), was the first CC chemokine discovered and investigated for its inhibition of TAMs recruitment, and it prefers to bind to its receptor, CCR2 [65]. CCL2 is released by tumor cells, stromal cells, and monocytes in TME. Mechanistically, the expression of CCL2 is regulated by the NF-κB signaling pathway. Various stimulatory factors released by tumor cells, such as TNF-α, IL-1β, etc., can activate the NF-κB signaling pathway, thus promoting the expression of CCL2. Inhibition of the NF-κB signaling pathway can reduce the expression of CCL2, thereby reducing the recruitment of TAMs [66]. In addition, it has been reported that STAT3 increases the expression of CCL2, which in turn promotes the infiltration of TAMs [67]. Its receptor, CCR2, has a major part in recruiting bone marrow monocytes into solid tumors, and progression towards TAMs [68]. It has been found that inhibition of the CCL2/CCR2 signaling pathway with anti-CCL2 antibodies can block the recruitment of TAMs, and delay the progression of breast cancer [6]. A clinical trial (NCT01413022) observed that the combination of a CCR2 inhibitor (PF-04136309) with chemotherapy for the treatment of regional pancreatic cancer was safe and well-tolerated—[69]. When compared to chemotherapy on its own, the combination of the CCR2 antagonist CCX827-B (NCT02345408) and the chemotherapeutic agent FOLFIRINOX enhanced overall survival in patients [70]. These studies indicate that blocking the CCL2/CCR2 axis is a potent way to suppress macrophages recruitment. However, it is noteworthy that discontinuation of anti-CCL-2 therapy can lead to rebound, increasing the liberation of monocytes formerly lodged inside the bone marrow, and thus expediting breast cancer metastasis through the promotion of angiogenesis [71]. Therefore, caution should be taken when using anti-CCL2 antibodies for future clinical trials. Apart from CCL2, it is noteworthy that another C motif chemokine ligand, CCL5, also promotes the recruitment of TAMs and contributes to tumor metastasis and recurrence, which can be restricted by the CCL5 receptor antagonist maraviroc and the Raf kinase inhibitory protein [72].

The C-X-C ligand (CXCL)12CXC receptor (CXCR)4 axis and the vascular endothelial growth factor receptor pathway can also inhibit the recruitment of TAMs. Matrix cell-derived CXCL-12 could promote macrophages' migratory movement across the inner-endothelial barrier and contribute to the aggregation and survival of TAMs in hypoxic areas of the tumor [73]. Targeting CXCR-4 can dramatically lower overall tumor load and metastasis in multiple models of preclinical cancer, including ovarian, prostate, and breast cancers. CXCL12 binding to CXCR4 activates various signaling pathways and promotes cell proliferation and survival. PI3 kinase, Ras, and AKT are all downstream effectors of the CXCL12/CXCR4 axis, and activation of them promotes tumor cell growth, spread, and migration [74,75]. Therefore, inhibiting CXCL-12-CXCR-4 signaling is an active tool for regulating macrophages infiltration and preventing metastasis. A stage I clinical trial (NCT02737072) in advanced refractory solid tumors showed that the combination of the CXCR4 antagonist LY2510924 with durvalumab resulted in a safe and controlled response, with a good overall response of stable condition in four out of nine patients (44.4%) after treatment [76]. VEGF is also involved in the function of recruiting macrophages into the tumor, which requires macrophage-expressed VEGF receptor 2. Huang et al. alleviated the hypoxic environment by using anti-VEGFR2 antibodies. They also reported that low-dose anti-vascular endothelial growth factor receptor 2 inhibited the HIF-1$\alpha$ pathway, improved vascular perfusion, and subsequently repolarized TAMs to the M1 phenotype [77]. Further research found that selective inhibition of VEGF receptor 2 reduces the infiltration of macrophages and reduces angiogenesis in models of breast and pancreatic cancer [78].

#### 2.4.2. Killing of TAMs

TAMs exhibit a variety of tumor-promoting effects, and are negatively associated with the prognosis of patients with malignant tumors [79]. Therefore, elimination of existing TAMs is an appealing cancer treatment approach. A strategy has been explored to block colony-stimulating factor 1 (CSF1)-mediated signaling in TAMs. CSF-1, a predominant growth and differentiation factor, widely expresses in cancer cells that cooperate with colony-stimulating factor receptors (CSF-1R) [80]. CSF-1R is a kind of tyrosine kinase receptor expression on monocytes, which could dimerize and transmit signals upon binding to CSF-1 or IL-34 [17]. CSF-1 triggers the dimerization of CSF-1R, and the subsequent autophosphorylation of specific tyrosine residues (e.g., Tyr723) in the intracellular structural domain of CSF-1R [81]. Phosphotyrosine residues in the CSF-1R cytoplasmic domain induce intracellular signaling molecule translocations and activate signaling cascades through SH2 interactions, thereby activating PI3K-dependent and Ras/mitogen-activated protein kinase-dependent pathways [82], ultimately promoting M2-TAMs proliferation, migration, and survival. In addition, blocking the CSF1/CSF-1R axis can reduce the differentiation and recruitment of monocytes to tumor sites, thus further hampering the viability of existing TAMs [83]. Compound D2923 (2-oxo-3,4-dihydropyrimido[4,5-d]pyrimidine derivative) is derived from a series of organic synthesis studies. It is a novel CSF1R-selective inhibitor with potent anti-tumor activity in vitro and in vivo, capable of removing M2-like TAMs from tumors [84]. Apart from that, monoclonal antibodies against CSF1, lacnotuzumab, showed improved patient responses in combination therapy with advanced triple-negative breast cancer in a recent randomized phase II clinical trial (NCT02435680) [85]. Similarly, LY3022855 (NCT01346358) was demonstrated to be useful in reducing levels of TAMs in intractable solid tumors [86]. Besides, a phase 1b/2 study of CSF-1R (ARRY-382), in combination with the PD-1 antibody pembrolizumab for the treatment of individuals with advanced solid tumors (NCT02880371), demonstrated that the combination was effective, with a partial response in 2 patients (10.5%) with pancreatic ductal adenocarcinoma and ovarian carcinoma, who lasted 29.2 months and 3.1 months, respectively. This indicated a great potential of CSF-1R inhibitors in immunotherapy [87].

Apart from that, recent studies have proven that osteoporosis bisphosphonates can remove TAMs by inducing macrophages to produce extraosseous myelin cytotoxicity. In preclinical breast cancer models, bisphosphonates effectively decrease breast tumor growth by reducing the tumor invasion of TAMs [88]. Moreover, it has been found that the anti-tumor drug trabectedin could induce apoptosis of TAMs through receptors of TNF-associated apoptosis-inducing ligand (TRAIL), thereby selectively depleting monocytes or macrophages in blood and tumors [89]. In pancreatic ductal adenocarcinoma, trabectedin effectively depletes monocytes, and changes the TME by reducing IL10 production and inducing CD8 T cell activation, leading to favorable clinical outcomes [90]. Excessive macrophages depletion may disrupt immune homeostasis, as well as increase the incidence of infections and autoimmune diseases. To address the above side effects, we can take measures such as implementing rigorous immune monitoring, promptly detecting immune toxic reactions, and adjusting treatment plans based on the specific situation of the patient. Additionally, combining immunotherapy with other treatment methods, such as chemotherapy or radiotherapy, can better regulate the immune system's response and reduce immune toxicity; more clinical practice is needed to facilitate the maturation of this therapeutic strategy.

#### 2.4.3. Regulating the Polarization of TAMs

Altering TAMs phenotype is a new potential therapeutic approach to activate anti-tumor immunity. A large number studies have shown that macrophage phenotypes are highly plastic and can be easily regulated by the external microenvironment. This provides an opportunity for TAMs to repolarize into M1-type macrophages, which can effectively fight tumors and activate other immune cells [91]. Recent studies have found that affecting CD40, CD47, TLR, etc., can change macrophages polarization.

CD40 belongs to the TNF receptor superfamily with extensive expression in antigen-presenting cells, including macrophages, dendritic cells, and B cells, through interaction with its ligand CD40 (CD40L). Moreover, the combination of CD40 and CD40L would activate the expression of major histocompatibility complex (MHC) molecules and then release pro-inflammatory cytokines, including IL-12, to promote the activation of T-cells [92]. The most common transcription factors activated by CD40 signaling are NF-κB and activator of transcription STAT [93]. Researchers elucidated that CD40 activation triggered glutamine metabolism and fatty acid oxidation (FAO) to promote ATP citrate lyase-dependent epigenetic reprogramming of pro-inflammatory genes and anti-tumorigenic phenotypes in macrophages [94]. Recently, three cloned CD40 monoclonal antibodies have displayed good anti-tumor effects [95–97]: SGN-40, CHIR12.12, and CP-870,893. For example, CP-870,893, a humanized CD40 monoclonal antibody developed by Roche, showed promising efficacy in combination with chemotherapeutic agents, such as paclitaxel. In a phase I clinical trial (NCT00607048), advanced solid tumor patients were treated with CP-870,893 and chemotherapy, resulting in four melanoma patients (27% of patients with melanoma) getting an objective partial response at restaging (day 43) [98]. What is more, Wiehgen et al. found that dual-targeting TAMs blocked by CD40 agonists and CSF-1 transformed TAMs into pro-inflammatory phenotypes [99].

TLR is an innate immune–pattern–recognition receptor that can be activated by invading bacterial particles or viral nucleic acids, leading to macrophages polarization towards the M1 type [100]. TLR agonists (mainly TLR4, TLR7, and TLR9 agonists) are reported to be available for cancer therapy to stimulate polarization of TAMs to a pro-inflammatory phenotype [101]. TLR4 agonists stimulate activator protein 1 and interferon regulatory factor (IRF) 3 signaling, leading to widespread activation of M1-related genes [102]. Studies indicate that cationic polymers for clinical nucleic acid drug therapy can promote therapeutic anti-tumor immunity in a mouse sarcoma model by activating TLR4 signaling to cause the repolarization of TAMs [103]. Currently, TLR7 activation is another attractive target for the repolarization of TAMs as it activates NF-κB and IRF7 signaling in macrophages [102]. TLR7 agonists convert myeloid-derived suppressor cells into tumor-killing M1 macrophages, thereby effectively reversing oxaliplatin resistance in colorectal cancer patients [104]. In addition, TLR9 activation with synthetic unmethylated cytosine-guanine oligodeoxynucleotides (CpG-ODN) leads to the activation of the interleukin 1 receptor-associated kinase

1 (IRAK)/TNF receptor-associated factor (TRAF) pathway, which in turn activates the NF-κB [105]. The TLR9 agonist IMO-2125 can cause anti-tumor macrophages proliferation and tumor regression in mouse models, as assessed in the clinical study of metastatic melanoma [106].

Normal human cells can interact with SIRPα expressed on the surface of macrophages by expressing CD47, and transmit the signal "do not eat me" to macrophages to avoid accidental injury by macrophages [107]. However, tumor cells can evade the killing of macrophages with anti-tumor activity through high expression of CD47. The binding of tumor cell CD47 to macrophage SIRP-α leads to the activation and phosphorylation of the SIRP-α ITIM motif, and recruitment of SHP-1 and SHP-2 phosphatases, which inhibit tumor cell phagocytosis by preventing the accumulation of myosin IIA at phagocytic synapses [108]. Thus, by disrupting with the SIRP-α-CD47 axis (e.g., by using antibodies against SIRPα and CD47), it is possible to restore recognition and phagocytosis of tumor cells by TAMs, and to activate anti-tumor immune responses [107,109]. Anti-CD47 monoclonal antibody Hu5F9-G4 can activate the phagocytosis and other killing effects of macrophages on tumor cells [110]. Clinical trials of its association with rituximab in the treatment of patients with non-Hodgkin's lymphoma are being conducted in phase 1b/2 (NCT02953509), providing a new approach for tumor immunotherapy [111]. Although blocking CD47-SIRRP alpha is a promising therapeutic strategy, and the monoclonal, double-clonal, and fusion proteins of this target have been extensively studied, off-target toxicity is still a limitation of this strategy.

#### 2.4.4. Other Targeting Strategies

In recent years, treatment strategies for cancer that target TAMs have been rapidly evolving, with numerous relevant research findings. As a new type of drug carrier, exosomes are used for drug delivery as natural nanoscale vesicles with a structure similar to the cell membrane, which can penetrate the biofilm to enter the receptor cell and secrete the drug through biofilm fusion (including endocytosis, cytotoxicity, and phagocytosis). In addition, they have good biocompatibility, targetability, and low immunogenicity [112]. Exosomes do not act directly on tumors, but affect them by releasing internal substances and they contain various substances inside them, such as proteins and miRNAs [113]. MicroRNA, a 19-24 nucleotide non-coding RNA, is a key transcriptional regulator of gene expression in organisms [114]. Mature miRNAs are processed from hairpin-like precursor miRNAs by the RNAse III enzyme double-stranded RNA (dsRNA)-specific endonuclease (DICER) [115]. Deletion of DICER in macrophages induces M1-like TAMs reprogramming, which is characterized by promoting the recruitment of activated CTLs into tumors [116]. MiRNAs are strongly associated with macrophage polarization. Thulin et al. indicated that miRNA-9 in monocytes activated PPARδ, which in turn enhanced M1 macrophages polarization [117]. Furthermore, overexpression of miRNA-125b in macrophages was found to be effective in enhancing macrophage responses to M1-inducing factor IFN-γ by targeting IRF4. Thus, knockdown of IRF4 enhanced M1 activation and pro-inflammatory responses in macrophages [118]. The hypoxic glioma-derived exosome miRNA-1246 promotes glioma proliferation, migration, and invasion in vitro and in vivo by inhibiting the NF-κB signaling pathway, activating the STAT3 signaling pathway and inducing M2 macrophages polarization [119]. The lung cancer exosome miRNA-19b-3p targets PTPRD-mediated dephosphorylation of STAT3 in macrophages, activates STAT3, and causes M2 polarization in macrophages [120]. Exosomes secreted by tumor cells with cell-of-origin-related genetic information can be used as a means of tumor immunotherapy. For example, the presence of miRNA-155 and miRNA-125b in exosomes secreted by pancreatic cancer cells induces a tumor-killing M1 phenotype in macrophages [121]. Similarly, the secretion of miRNA-125b-transfected exosomes from colon cancer mediates macrophage repolarization towards the M1 phenotype [122]. Given the critical role of exosomal miRNAs in macrophage polarization, we believe that exosomes have great potential in clinical therapeutics. Moreover, miRNA vaccines are currently in the developmental stage and offer a promising approach to targeting TAMs and enhancing anti-tumor immunity.

During the past decade, a hot topic of research in immunotherapies has been the chimeric antigen receptor (CAR). It is a single-chain changeable fragment antibody attached to specific proteins in tumor cells. Depending on the intracellular structural domains, CAR has been developed into its fourth generation and has achieved good therapeutic results in hematological tumors. Similar cell therapies such as CAR-M and CAR-NK are inspired by the genetically engineered CAR-T [123]. A central component of CAR-M contains an extracellular structural domain in which a single-chain variable fragment (scFv) offers specific recognition, a hinge structural domain, a membrane-spanning structural domain, and an intracellular structural domain providing outstream signaling [124]. CAR-M expresses pro-inflammatory cytokines and chemokines, promotes the transgenesis from M2 macrophages to M1, recruits antigens and presents them to T cells, and also resists the effects of immunosuppressive cytokines. In addition, it is found that CAR-M is further proven to induce pro-inflammatory TME and to augment anti-tumor T-cell activity in humanized mouse models [125]. CAR-M technology continues to develop, and studies have shown that MPEI/pCAR-IFN-$\gamma$ could indulge CAR-M1 macrophages to produce potent anti-tumor immunity in vivo. This approach could improve the poor response of CAR-T cell therapy to tumor treatment [126]. A clinical trial (NCT03608618) involved the construction of CAR immune cells (including CAR-M) by transfecting peripheral blood mononuclear cells with mRNA for patients with recurrent/refractory ovarian cancer and peritoneal mesothelioma, but unfortunately the study was discontinued without any results [127]. The CAR family of cellular therapeutics, despite challenges such as off-target toxicity, neurotoxicity, and inflammatory factor storms, also points to a new direction for anti-tumor therapy (Figure 2).

## 3. Clinical Application and Scientific Research in TAMs

Clinical studies targeting TAMs have indeed gained significant attention in the field of tumor therapy. Therapeutic strategies aimed at TAMs include approaches to block their origin and aggregation, as well as to modulate their polarization. These strategies recognize the importance of TAMs in TME, and seek to manipulate their function to enhance anti-tumor immune responses. Clinical research is being conducted to explore novel therapeutic agents and immunotherapies specifically targeting TAMs. Promising results have been observed in liver, breast, lung, and colorectal cancers. This section focuses on clinical studies of TAMs in different types of cancer (Table 1).

### 3.1. Liver Cancer

Hepatocellular carcinoma (HCC) is a highly prevalent malignant tumor of the gastrointestinal system. TAMs are crucial immunological cells present within TME of HCC. It has been demonstrated that TAMs could increase the cell proliferation, invasion, and migration ability of HCC by secreting various cytokines, inducing the occurrence of epithelial–mesenchymal transition, and then accelerating the progression of HCC [128]. In addition, Bao et al. found that DNA stress caused by mitochondrial fission accelerated the infiltration of TAMs in the microenvironment of HCC, and enhanced the growth and metastasis of HCC [129]. Researchers are investigating various approaches to modulate TAMs in HCC to shift their polarization from the immunosuppressive M2 macrophages to pro-inflammatory M1 macrophages, killing or inhibiting the recruitment of TAMs. By doing so, the anti-tumor immune reaction can be enhanced, potentially leading to improved therapy outcomes. Currently, the major drugs for HCC treatment targeting TAMs in clinical or scientific trials are SNDX-6352, BMS-813160, and Sorafenib.

SNDX-6352, a CSFR-1 inhibitor, could affect the proliferation, differentiation, and survival of TAMs by binding to CSF-1R. In a clinical trial (NCT04301778), the combination of SNDX-6352 (CSFR-1 inhibitor) and Durvalumab (MEDI4736) was superior to Durvalumab alone in treating patients with intrahepatic cholangiocarcinoma who had received chemotherapy or radiation therapy. Durvalumab combined with CSF-1R inhibitor SNDX-6352 improved overall survival (OS) in previously treated intrahepatic cholangiocarcinoma patients without causing any serious adverse effects, indicating the great potential of the CSF-1R inhibitor immunotherapy [130].

BMS-813160 is identified as a potent and selective dual CCR2/5 antagonist. Studies have confirmed its ability to inhibit the migration of inflammatory monocytes and macrophages [131]. A clinical study (NCT04123379) of nabulizumab and a CCR2/5 inhibitor (BMS-813160) given before and after surgery to HCC patients is underway, to investigate whether the drug BMS-813160 can boost long-term survival in cancer patients [132].

Sorafenib, a multi-targeted kinase inhibitor that inhibited VEGF2 to reduce the density of TAMs [133], is currently the most effective drug for treating patients with advanced HCC [134]. Numerous preclinical investigations have indicated that sorafenib significantly suppresses tumor growth and lung metastasis [135]. A clinical trial (NCT02971696) to assess the efficacy of sorafenib versus optimal supportive therapy in two cohorts of patients with advanced HCC showed sorafenib (VEGF2 inhibitor) improved overall survival compared with optimal treatment [136]. In addition, a phase II study (NCT01259193) was designed to assess the safety, overall survival, and time to progression of sorafenib in combination with zoledronic acid in advanced HCC. Unfortunately, this clinical trial has been terminated [137].

Recent studies have found that levatinib can regulate cancer immunity in TME by decreasing TAMs, especially exhibiting enhanced anti-tumor activity in the IFN signaling pathway when combined with PD-1 blockers [138]. It is reported that the natural compound baicalin directly induces reprogramming of TAMs into M1-like macrophages via activation of the autophagy-related reticuloendotheliosis virus oncogene homologue B (RelB)/p52. This study demonstrated that the tumor-suppressive effect of baicalin is dependent on the conversion of macrophages for the treatment of HCC from M2-like phenotype to M1-like phenotype [139].

Clinical trials of CAR-M therapies have opened up a new frontier in the use of macrophages to treat solid tumors. An open-label, single-arm, phase I clinical trial (NCT04660929) is underway to assess the tolerability and safety of CT-0508 in terms of the frequency and severity of adverse events in subjects [140]. However, because of the heterogeneity of liver cancer, it remains challenging to discover hepatic tumor cell-specific targets and the effect of engineered macrophages in hepatic TME. Whether CAR-M enhances tumor suppression in combination with CAR-T, multi-targeted kinase inhibitors, and ICIs remains to be further investigated.

### 3.2. Breast Cancer

Breast cancer ranks 2nd in global cancer mortality among females [141]. Abundant laboratory studies have provided evidence of the role of M2-polarized macrophages in breast cancer. These macrophages with an M2-like phenotype have been shown to promote tumor-cell proliferation, interfere with immunosuppression, and promote angiogenesis (the formation of new blood vessels) [12]. The high density of cells expressing macrophage-associated labels in primary breast cancer is usually related to a poorer prognosis for the patient; CD68 and CD163 have been widely used as human pan-macrophage markers [142]. Recently, clinical drugs for TAMs, such as PLX3397, Selicrelumab, Imiquimod, 852A, etc., have been used in clinical trials and have gained good prospects.

Pexidartinib (PLX3397), a CSF1/CSF1R-signaling inhibitor, could induce a reduction in the number of TAMs and lead to a remarkable delay in tumor recurrence [143]. A clinical trial (NCT01596751) assessing the safety and efficacy of eribulin in combination with CSF1 inhibitor PLX3397 in patients with metastatic breast cancer showed that 5 participants in phase II obtained an objective response [144]. Furthermore, a phase 1b study evaluating the safety of PLX3397(NCT01525602) and paclitaxel in advanced solid tumor patients (includes breast cancer) has been completed. The results were promising and without any serious adverse effects in patients receiving PLX3397 1600 mg/day, with 1 in 20 (5%) receiving complete remission, 2 in 20 (10%) obtaining partial remission, and 6 in 20 (30%) with a stable disease [145].

Selicrelumab (also known as RO7009789) is a wholly human IgG2 antibody with strong agonistic activity and low binding affinity for human FcγR. To date, selicrelumab is the most widely evaluated agonist CD40 antibody in clinical research [146]. Apart from being tested as a single therapy, it has been assessed in combination with other therapies. An open-label, multicentre, dose-escalation phase Ib clinical trial (NCT02760797) was designed to evaluate the safety, pharmacokinetics, pharmacodynamics, and therapeutic activity of emactuzumab (CSF-1R) combined with selicrelumab (CD40 Antibody) in patients with advanced solid tumors (including breast cancer) [147]. The results revealed a manageable safety profile and evidence of progressive disease activity of emactuzumab in combination with selicrelumab, but did not translate into objective clinical responses [148].

Imiquimod is an immune response modifier that can induce the immune-mediated rejection of primary cutaneous malignancies when applied locally. It was evaluated in a phase II study (NCT00899574) in patients with cutaneous breast cancer metastases; 10 patients participated and completed the study [149]. The results indicated that patients tolerated the imiquimod treatment well, with only grade 1 to 2 transient topical and systemic adverse effects, consistent with the immunomodulatory effects of imiquimod. Interestingly, the results revealed that topical imiquimod was an active and well-tolerated treatment for skin/chest wall metastases of breast cancer [150].

Molecule 852A, TLR 7 agonist, is a novel immune response modulator. In a phase II trial (NCT00319748), molecule 852A was administered subcutaneously in patients with recurrent ovarian cancer ($n$ = 10), breast cancer ($n$ = 3), and cervical cancer ($n$ = 2) who had been treated with strict therapy [151]. The optimal response was the stabilization of all patients. Unexpected toxicities such as myocardial infarction and infection also occurred [152] (Table 1).

In addition, Li et al. found that Andrographolide suppressed breast cancer progression by regulating TAMs towards M1 polarization via the Wnt/β-catenin pathway [153]. It was found that Cordyceps sinensis extract could inhibit the progression of triple-negative breast cancer by enhancing the polarization of TAMs towards M1-type via activation of the NF-κB pathway [154]. Research found that dendrosomal curcumin exerted a protective effect on metastatic breast cancer in mice by increasing macrophage M1 levels in TME [155]. Immunotherapies targeting TAMs for the treatment of breast cancer have achieved promising results in both clinical research and scientific studies, however there is still a long way to go to bring individualized treatment options to patients.

### 3.3. Lung Cancer

Lung cancer represents one of the most common malignant tumors in the world and its incidence is increasing year by year [141]. Although the treatment of lung cancer has been highly successful, the 5-year survival rate of patients is still less than 15% [156]. Recently, immunotherapy targeting TAMs has received widespread attention. Casanova-Acebes et al. found that early in the course of human and mouse non-small cell lung cancer (NSCLC), tissue-resident macrophages congregated around lung cancer cells and contributed to cancer cell aggression, resulting in an increased number of regulatory T-cells and the promotion of tumor-immune escape. Thus, the removal of tissue-resident macrophages could reduce the quantity of regulatory T-cells, facilitate the accumulation of CD8 + T cells, and inhibit tumor growth [157]. TAMs are critical for the survival of circulating lung cancer cells, and the removal of TAMs by genetic approaches could significantly inhibit cancer cell survival in lung capillaries and lead to lung metastasis [158]. In addition, Lu et al. found that octamer-binding transcription factor 4 (Oct4) expressed by lung cancer cells promoted macrophages' polarization towards M2-type TAMs through upregulation of M-CSF, leading to tumor growth and the progression of metastasis. These findings indicate that TAMs play indispensable functions in the process of lung cancer proliferation and metastasis, and drugs-targeted TAMs may gain promising results in lung cancer.

Emactuzumab is a CSFR-1inhibitor. It was used in a clinical trial (NCT02323191) combination with PD-L1 (atezolizumab) inhibitor therapy to assess the safety, pharmacokinetics, and activity for participants with advanced solid tumor [159]. The findings indicated that the confirmed objective response rate (ORR) was 12.5% for immune checkpoint blockers (ICB)-experienced NSCLC, and emactuzumab in combination with atezolizumab demonstrated a manageable safety profile, which suggested that the combination of CSFR-1 inhibitors with PD-L1 inhibitors has great promise.

Tazemetostat, is a small molecule enhancer of the zeste homolog 2 (EZH2) inhibitor. It has been found that EZH2 could promote lung cancer metastasis and macrophages infiltration through the up-regulation of CCL5, therefore inhibition of EZH2 could suppress lung cancer progression [160]. An open-label, single-arm, phase Ib/II clinical study (NCT05467748) is currently underway, in which pembrolizumab is being used in conjunction with tazemetostat in the treatment of patients with advanced NSCLC who experienced disease progression from front- or second-line treatment [161].

Eganelisib (IPI-549) is a first-in-class, innovative, oral PI3K-$\gamma$ inhibitor [162]. Preclinical research revealed that PI3K-$\gamma$ had an essential role in sustaining the immunosuppressive condition of TAMs in TME. Eganelisib targeting PI3K-$\gamma$ could reprogram key immunosuppressive macrophages (M2) to anti-tumor macrophages (M1) within TME, thereby downregulating immunosuppression, increasing immunoreactivity, and eventually leading to the mobilization and multiplication of killer T-cells [163]. A period 1/1b dose-escalation trial (NCT02637531), designed to investigate the safety, tolerability, pharmacokinetics, and pharmacodynamics of IPI-549 single-agent treatment in combination with nivolumab for the treatment of subjects with NSCLC, is in the enrolment phase [164] (Table 1).

Furthermore, scientific studies have found that shuangshen granules could inhibit the growth and formation of lung cancer. The mechanism may be related to the regulation of TAMs [165]. Astragaloside IV blocks macrophage M2 polarization via the AMPK signaling pathway, reducing lung tumor growth, infiltration, migration, and angiogenesis, which might play an active part in inhibiting lung cancer metastasis [166]. Targeting TAMs might be an outstanding strategy for lung cancer treatment, as shown in clinical trials and scientific studies. However, the clinical use of current strategies for treating lung cancer, such as surgery and chemotherapy, is still very limited and we still have a long way to go.

### 3.4. Colorectal Cancer

TAMs play an indispensable role in the pathogenesis of colorectal cancer (CRC). Increasing evidence suggests that TAMs are associated with the prognosis of CRC patients. CD68, as a surface marker of pan-TAMs, is found to be associated positively with overall survival in CRC tissues [167]. From a study of 159 primary CRC, Algars et al. discovered that the count of peritumoral M2 macrophages was positively correlated with survival in earlier-stage CRC, but negatively correlated with survival in stage IV CRC [168]. Furthermore, TAMs in colon cancer secrete TNF-$\alpha$, IL-1$\beta$, and stimulate the NF-$\kappa$B pathway in the vessel endothelium to generate VEGF, which in turn boosts angiogenesis and alters the TME [169]. Indeed, the findings suggest that TAMs might be a prospective target for new anti-colorectal cancer therapeutic strategies.

Maglumab (Hu5F9-G4), a humanized IgG4 monoclonal antibody, shows high affinity for human CD47. Hu5F9-G4 is designed to disrupt the identification of CD47 by the SIRP$\alpha$ receptor on macrophages, thereby preventing cancer cells from using the "do not eat me" message to avoid macrophage phagocytosis [110]. In preclinical in vivo models, Hu5F9-G4 is active against a variety of solid tumors, including breast, ovarian, colon, liver, brain, and other organ cancers [170–172]. A phase 1b/2 clinical trial (NCT02953782) has revealed that 2 in 30 CRC patients confirmed partial remission for 7.0 and 12.5 months, with an objective remission rate of 6.7%, in which Hu5F9-G4 in conjunction with cetuximab were treated for patients suffering from advanced CRC [173]. Moreover, patients with CRC treated with Hu5F9-G4 in combination with cetuximab did not experience any serious adverse effects, and therefore Hu5F9-G4 has a favorable safety and tolerability profile.

Tumor-associated macrophage kinase (TAMK) commonly expresses on tumor cells in the process of malignant transformation. Suppression of TAMK family members AXL and MERTK could lower the threshold of immune activation and enhance anti-tumor immunity. PF-07265807 is a small molecule inhibitor of MERTK and AXL [174]. A clinical trial (NCT04458259) is underway to test the safety, pharmacokinetics, and tolerability of PF-07265807 in participants with advanced CRC, which is still in the recruitment phase [175].

A phase I dose-escalation clinical trial (NCT02777710) was designed to estimate the clinical efficacy and safety of the combination of pexidartinib (anti-CSF1R antibody) and durvalumab (PD-L1 agonist) in individuals diagnosed with advanced/metastatic CRC, and results demonstrated that toxicity was consistent with the expected profile of the individual agents, and no unexpected events were identified with this combination [176] (Table 1).

In addition, scientific studies have found that the nutrient β-carotene is effective at inhibiting M2 macrophages polarization and fibroblast activation, which in turn could suppress the growth and metastasis of CRC [177]. In summary, targeted TAMs therapy has potential efficacy in the cure of CRC, with the deepening of research and continuous technological advancement. It is believed that TAMs therapy will become an important means of CRC treatment. Future clinical studies and clinical applications will further validate its efficacy and safety, bringing more treatment options and hope to CRC patients.

### 3.5. Other Types of Cancer

Other than the cancer types mentioned above, the investigation of TAMs in other kinds of cancer is rapidly evolving, with varying results in patients, and it has attracted widespread attention.

A phase Ib/II trial (NCT02807844) assessed the safety and efficacy of lacnotuzumab (MCS110) versus spartalizumab (PDR001) for patients with pancreatic cancer, endometrial cancer, and advanced melanoma. Common adverse events (AEs) suspected to be drug-related were oedema around the eyes (30%), elevated aspartate aminotransferase (24%), and elevated blood creatine phosphokinase (24%), with the most common grade $\geq$3 AEs suspected to be related to the drug (6%). Out of 30 patients suffering from pancreatic cancer, 1 achieved a partial response (346 days into the study) and 2 had durable stable disease (328 and 319 days into the study, respectively). The results showed that MCS110, combined with PDR001, was generally well tolerated [178].

In addition, a clinical trial (NCT01676831) found a favorable safety profile with the topical use of raquinimod (TLR7/8 agonist) in treating early-stage cutaneous T-cell lymphoma [179]. However, due to the small number of subjects, further in-depth studies are needed. What is more, a clinical trial [180] (NCT00537368) evaluated the safety, efficacy, and pharmacokinetics of CNTO888(CCL2 antibody) alone or in combination with other commonly used chemotherapeutic agents for the therapy of solid tumors such as ovarian and prostate cancers. Durable disease stabilization of 5–15.7 months was observed in 4 patients. Moreover, two of these patients with ovarian and prostate cancer experienced sustained reductions in cancer antigen 125 and prostate-specific antigen of more than 50% at 10 and 5 months, respectively [181]. In addition, a clinical study (NCT00992186) designed to determine the efficacy and safety of carlumab in patients with metastatic refractory prostate cancer demonstrated that carlumab was well tolerated but failed to show single-agent anti-tumor activity [182]. For individuals with a recurrent or refractory primary malignant central nervous system tumor or freshly diagnosed diffuse endogenous pontine gliomas, a phase I clinical trial (NCT03389802) is currently underway, assessing the site-specific tolerability and safety of a monoclonal antibody to CD40 agonist (APX005M) in patients [183]. Furthermore, histone deacetylase inhibitors were found to be effective in modulating the polarization of TAMs towards the M1-type, and thus exerting anti-tumor effects [184]. A phase II clinical trial (NCT00134043) was conducted to estimate the objective response to a histone deacetylase inhibitor (vorinostat) in 19 participants with progressive thyroid cancer. The results showed that there were no patients achieved partial or complete remission [185] (Table 1).

**Table 1.** Relevant clinical trials of immunotherapies targeting TAMs in different types of cancer.

| Clinical Trials.gov Identifier | Target | Drug | Study Design | Type | Patients | Outcomes | Status | References |
|---|---|---|---|---|---|---|---|---|
| NCT01413022 | CCR2 | PF-04136309 | Oxaliplatin + Irinotecan + Leucovorin + Fluorouracil vs. Oxaliplatin + Irinotecan + Leucovorin + Fluorouracil + PF-04136309 | Pancreatic Neoplasms | 44 | TCR↑ | Completed | [69] |
| NCT02345408 | CR2 | CCX872-B | CCX872-B | Pancreatic Cancer | 54 | PFS↑ | Completed | [70] |
| NCT02737072 | CXCL-12-CXCR-4 | LY2510924 | LY2510924 + Durvalumab | Solid Tumor | 9 | Safe | Completed | [76] |
| NCT02435680 | CSF1 | Lacnotuzumab | Lacnotuzumab + Larboplatin + Gemcitabine vs.Carboplatin + Gemcitabine | Advanced Triple Negative Breast Cancer | 50 | PFS↑ | Completed | [85] |
| NCT01346358 | CSF-1R | LY3022855 | LY3022855 | Neoplasms | 72 | Well Tolerated | Terminated Has Results | [86] |
| NCT02880371 | CSF-1R | ARRY-382 | ARRY-382 + Pembrolizumab | Advanced Solid Tumors | 82 | ORR↑ | Completed | [87] |
| NCT00607048 | CD40 | CP-870,893 | Paclitaxel + Carboplatin + CP-870,893 | Solid Tumor | 34 | Safe | Completed | [98] |
| NCT02953509 | CD47 | Magrolimab | Magrolimab + Rituximab vs.Magrolimab + Rituximab + Gemcitabine + Oxaliplatin | Non Hodgkin Lymphoma | 178 | ongoing | Active, not recruiting | [111] |
| NCT03608618 | CAR-M | MCY-M11 | MCY-M11 + Cyclophosphamide | Advanced Ovarian Cancer and Peritoneal Mesothelioma | 14 | unknow | Terminated | [127] |
| NCT04301778 | CSF-1R | SNDX-6352 | Durvalumab vs. SNDX-6352 | Intrahepatic Cholangiocarcinoma | 5 | OS↑ | Completed | [130] |
| NCT04123379 | CCR2 | BMS-813160 | Nivolumab vs.BMS-813160 | Hepatocellular Carcinoma | 36 | Ongoing | Active, not recruiting | [132] |
| NCT02971696 | VEGF2 | Sorafenib | Sorafenib vs. Best Supportive Care | Hepatocellular Carcinoma | 55 | OS↑ | complete | [136] |
| NCT01259193 | VEGF2 | Sorafenib + Zoledronic Acid | Sorafenib + Zoledronic Acid | Hepatocellular Carcinoma | 50 | Unknow | Terminated | [137] |
| NCT04660929 | CAR-M | CT-0508 | CT-0508 vs.CT-0508 + Pembrolizumab | Hepatocellular Carcinoma | 48 | Ongoing | Recruiting | [140] |
| NCT01596751 | CSF1 | PLX3397 | PLX3397 vs. Eribulin | Metastatic Breast Cancer | 67 | PFS↑ | Completed | [144] |
| NCT01525602 | CSF1 | PLX3397 | PLX3397 + Paclitaxel | Breast Cancer | 74 | Relief Degree↑ | Completed | [145] |
| NCT02760797 | CD40 | RO7009789 | Emactuzumab + RO7009789 | Metastatic Triple-Negative Breast Cancer | 38 | PFS↑ | Completed | [147] |
| NCT00899574 | TLR7 | Imiquimod | Imiquimod | Breast Cancer | 10 | Relief Degree↑ | Completed | [149] |
| NCT00319748 | TLR7 | 852A | 852A | Breast Cancer | 15 | Relief Degree↑ | Completed | [151] |
| NCT02323191 | CSF-1R | Emactuzumab | Atezolizumab vs. Emactuzumab | Lung Cancer | 221 | Relief Degree↑ | Completed | [159] |
| NCT05467748 | CCL5 | Tazemetostat | Tazemetostat | Nonsmall Cell Lung Cancer | 66 | Ongoing | Not yet recruiting | [161] |
| NCT02637531 | PI3K-γ | IPI-549 | IPI-549 vs.IPI-549 + Nivolumab | Nonsmall Cell Lung Cancer | 219 | Ongoing | Active, not recruiting | [164] |

**Table 1.** *Cont.*

| Clinical Trials.gov Identifier | Target | Drug | Study Design | Type | Patients | Outcomes | Status | References |
|---|---|---|---|---|---|---|---|---|
| NCT02953782 | CD47 | Hu5F9-G4 | Hu5F9-G4 + Cetuximab | Colorectal Cancer | 78 | ORR↑ | Completed | [173] |
| NCT04458259 | TAMK | PF-07265807 | PF-07265807 vs. PF-07265807 + Sasanlimab vs. PF-07265807 + Sasanlimab + Axitinib | Neoplasm Metastasis | 67 | Ongoing | Active, not recruiting | [175] |
| NCT02777710 | CSF-1R | Pexidartinib | Pexidartinib + Durvalumab | Colorectal Cancer | 48 | ORR↑ | Completed | [176] |
| NCT02807844 | CSF-1R | MCS110 | MCS110 vs.MCS110 + PDR001 | Pancreatic Carcinoma Melanoma Endometrial Carcinoma | 141 | Safe, Well-tolerated | Completed | [178] |
| NCT01676831 | TLR7/8 | Resiquimod | Resiquimod | Cutaneous T Cell Lymphoma | 13 | Safe | Completed | [179] |
| NCT00537368 | CCL2 | CNTO 888 | CNTO 888 | Cancer | 44 | Safe | Completed | [180] |
| NCT00992186 | CCL2 | Carlumab | Carlumab | Prostate Cancer | 46 | OS↑PFS↑ | Completed | [182] |
| NCT03389802 | CD40 | APX005M | APX005M | Central Nervous System Tumor | 32 | Ongoing | Recruiting | [183] |
| NCT00134043 | Histone Deacetylase Inhibitor | Vorinostat | Vorinostat | Thyroid Cancer | 19 | No Relief | Completed | [185] |
| NCT02371369 | CSF-1R | Pexidartinib | Pexidartinib vs. Placebo | Pigmented Villonodular Synovitis Giant Cell Tumors of the Tendon Sheath Tenosynovial Giant Cell Tumor | 120 | CR↑ PR↑ | Completed | [186] |
| NCT01444404 | CSF-1R | AMG 820 | AMG 820 | Advanced Solid Tumors | 25 | Safe | Completed | [187] |

Abbreviations: tumor control rate (TCR), progression-free survival (PFS), overall survival (OS), objective response rate (ORR), partial response (PR), and complete response (CR).

Clinical studies and scientific research are helping us to gain a deeper understanding of the relationship between TAMs and different types of cancer. These studies are expected to provide an important theoretical basis for the exploitation of new drugs and immunotherapeutic approaches. In the future, more personalized and effective treatment options can be provided to patients.

## 4. Conclusions and Future Directions

TAMs represent a major category of innate immune cells in TME, and they are broadly expressed in a diverse range of tumor tissues [188]. A large infiltration of TAMs or the abundance of TAM-related genes generally predicts tumor advancement or a worse outcome of the disease. There are two main forms of TAM: M1-type macrophages with tumor growth suppression, and the M2-type macrophages with a tumor-promoting effect, which can be transformed through multiple signaling pathways. In addition, extensive findings have indicated that TAMs are closely related to various tumor-related processes, promoting oncogenesis and proliferation, speeding up angiogenesis, facilitating invasion and metastasis, and triggering drug tolerance and immunosuppression. Therefore, multiple tumor-promoting mechanisms in TAMs offer many attractive new targets in cancer therapy. Tumor immunotherapies that target TAMs, involving the suppression of TAMs recruitment, the acceleration of TAMs apoptosis, and the modulation of TAMs anti-tumor polarity, display tremendous potential in both basic and clinical oncology studies.

It is inspiring that drugs against TAMs are undergoing clinical trials and displaying anti-tumor benefits. The CSF-1R inhibitor pexidartinib shrank tumor size and improved symptoms in patients with tenosynovial giant cell tumor (TGCT), with encouraging results in the phase III clinical study (NCT02371369) of CSF1/CSF1R-targeted therapy for benign diffuse TGCT [186]. Results from the ENLIVEN trial prompted the FDA to approve pexidartinib for the treatment of asymptomatic TGCT patients with serious comorbidities or functional limitations TGCT, which originated in the synovium and was marked by CSF-1 overexpression, and this supported a successful response to treatment [189]. However, some poor therapeutic outcomes also exist. In a phase I/II trial of AMG 820-pembrolizumab co-therapy, 37.1% had rash and maculopapular rash, 48.3% had periorbital and facial oedema, and 59.5% of patients had elevated aminotransferase of aspartic acid [190]. Furthermore, in a phase I trial [187] of AMG 820 monotherapy (NCT01444404), periorbital oedema was present in 44% of participants and aspartate aminotransferase was elevated in 28%. It has been argued that the limited success of the current published data may be attributed to acquired disease resistance mediated through the activation of phosphatidylinositol-3-kinase [191]. Taken together, these data indicate that targeting macrophage subpopulations rather than all macrophage populations may have a prospective therapeutic effect. Therapeutic strategies targeting CCL2-CCR2 signaling to kill TAMs have proved promising in existing studies, but there are some problems, e.g., monocytes require CCL2-CCR2 signaling to enter the bloodstream from the skeleton, the inhibition of CCL2 leads to the severe depletion of monocytes, and macrophages in the tissues may undergo compensatory proliferation if TAMs recruitment is blocked. In fact, the discovery of molecules required to inhibit monocyte retention (e.g., CCL3) or to induce monocyte differentiation may be a superior approach [192]. Taken together, these observations suggest that repolarization of macrophages is the most promising therapeutic strategy available. It is well known that TAMs are typically tumor-friendly, however, they can be converted to a tumor cell-killing state under certain conditions, and repolarization can rebalance microenvironmental immunity from a therapeutic pro-tumor immune infiltration to a state of active tumor-rejecting immune infiltration. Furthermore, this approach does not have the drawbacks caused by the inhibition of TAMs recruitment and the long-term toxicity associated with a lack of TAMs. Currently, imiquimod (TLR7 agonist) is permitted by the FDA for topical application in squamous cell carcinoma and basal cell carcinoma. Furthermore, the emerging therapeutic technology CAR-M has created a new paradigm for the exploitation of macrophage-based cancer immunopharmaceuticals. On 27 July 2020, the US

Food and Drug Administration granted new drug approval for anti-human HER2-CARM (CT-0508) for the treatment of recurrent or metastatic HER2 overexpressing solid tumors. It marks a meaningful advance in cell-based cancer immunotherapy.

As far as I am concerned, for different cancers, targeted therapy with TAMs in HCC is promising because TAMs are known to infiltrate to a high degree in HCC, which correlates with the prognosis of the tumor. Secondly, recent studies have found that xanthine oxidoreductase (XOR) deficiency in TAMs increased isocitrate dehydrogenase (IDH)-3$\alpha$ activity, which polarized TAMs towards alternatively activated M2 phenotypes, exacerbated CD8 + T cell depletion, and promoted HCC progression. Among them, XOR was usually considered to be a promoter of M1 macrophages activation, therefore, XOR-IDH3$\alpha$ was a key axis controlling TAMs polarization and HCC progression [193]. The discovery of this potential target provides novel insights into the treatment of HCC. Moreover, recent findings have linked a number of genetic mutations in thyroid cancer that are associated with the polarization of TAMs, for instance, mutations in the *BRAF* gene have been shown to result in the conversion of TAMs to the M2 phenotype [194], and targeted therapies can be much better exploited with the benefit of this gene. Immunotherapies targeting TAMs have different immunotherapeutic effects in different tumors due to the heterogeneity of tumors and differences in the individual immune microenvironment of patients. TAMs immunotherapies also do not show good therapeutic efficacy in all individuals and on all tumors, and the occurrence of adverse events is not the same.

In conclusion, TAMs hold high promise as targets for cancer immunotherapy. Currently, targeted therapeutic drugs for TAMs are still in the research and development stage, and the targeting and selectivity of the drugs need to be further improved, while the diversity and plasticity of TAMs in TME also increase the challenge of drug therapy. TAMs play an immunosuppressive part in tumors, and can inhibit the killing function of immune cells; M2 TAMs are especially key to tumor refractoriness and the development of drug resistance. Therefore, overcoming tumor immune escape is crucial for therapies targeting TAMs. Tumor cells and TAMs can acquire drug resistance through multiple mechanisms, which poses a challenge for therapies targeting TAMs. More effective drugs and combination therapy strategies need to be developed to overcome resistance. Going forward, better strategies would be to specifically target tumor-promoting macrophages, enhance the anti-tumor activity of macrophages, or depolarize existing macrophages. Currently among the strategies targeting TAMs complexes, exosomes and CAR-M therapies show potential for treating solid tumors. Although some therapeutic strategies targeting TAMs have displayed some effectiveness in the data from clinical trials, there is a dearth of adequate clinical data and evidence to support their widespread use. Further large-scale clinical studies are needed to address the safety and tolerability issues associated with the treatment, with the ultimate goal of optimizing treatment options for patients.

**Author Contributions:** M.-Y.L. wrote the original manuscript and drew the table; W.Y. reviewed the literature; K.-W.L. revised the manuscript and created the figures. All authors have read and agreed to the published version of the manuscript.

**Funding:** We acknowledge the support from the National Natural Science Foundation of China [82104457], the Shenzhen Longhua District Science and Technology Innovation Fund [SZLHQJ-CYJ2021001], and the Open Project of Scientific Research Workstation of the Chinese Disease Control Journal [IMMDL20220002].

**Informed Consent Statement:** Not applicable.

**Data Availability Statement:** Not applicable.

**Conflicts of Interest:** The authors declare no conflicts of interest.

## References


1. De Visser, K.E.; Joyce, J.A. The evolving tumor microenvironment: From cancer initiation to metastatic outgrowth. *Cancer Cell* **2023**, *41*, 374–403. [CrossRef] [PubMed]
2. Gordon, S.; Martinez, F.O. Alternative Activation of Macrophages: Mechanism and Functions. *Immunity* **2010**, *32*, 593–604. [CrossRef] [PubMed]
3. Boutilier, A.J.; Elsawa, S.F. Macrophage Polarization States in the Tumor Microenvironment. *Int. J. Mol. Sci.* **2021**, *22*, 6995. [CrossRef] [PubMed]
4. Murray, P.J.; Wynn, T.A. Protective and pathogenic functions of macrophage subsets. *Nat. Rev. Immunol.* **2011**, *11*, 723–737. [CrossRef] [PubMed]
5. Lee, J.-H.; Chen, T.W.-W.; Hsu, C.-H.; Yen, Y.-H.; Yang, J.C.-H.; Cheng, A.-L.; Sasaki, S.I.; Chiu, L.L.; Sugihara, M.; Ishizuka, T.; et al. A phase I study of pexidartinib, a colony-stimulating factor 1 receptor inhibitor, in Asian patients with advanced solid tumors. *Investig. New Drugs* **2020**, *38*, 99–110. [CrossRef] [PubMed]
6. Qian, B.-Z.; Li, J.; Zhang, H.; Kitamura, T.; Zhang, J.; Campion, L.R.; Kaiser, E.A.; Snyder, L.A.; Pollard, J.W. CCL2 recruits inflammatory monocytes to facilitate breast-tumour metastasis. *Nature* **2011**, *475*, 222–225. [CrossRef] [PubMed]
7. Zhang, X.-M.; Chen, D.-G.; Li, S.C.; Zhu, B.; Li, Z.-J. Embryonic Origin and Subclonal Evolution of Tumor-Associated Macrophages Imply Preventive Care for Cancer. *Cells* **2021**, *10*, 903. [CrossRef] [PubMed]
8. Loyher, P.-L.; Hamon, P.; Laviron, M.; Meghraoui-Kheddar, A.; Goncalves, E.; Deng, Z.; Torstensson, S.; Bercovici, N.; Baudesson de Chanville, C.; Combadière, B.; et al. Macrophages of distinct origins contribute to tumor development in the lung. *J. Exp. Med.* **2018**, *215*, 2536–2553. [CrossRef]
9. van de Laar, L.; Saelens, W.; De Prijck, S.; Martens, L.; Scott, C.L.; Van Isterdael, G.; Hoffmann, E.; Beyaert, R.; Saeys, Y.; Lambrecht, B.N.; et al. Yolk Sac Macrophages, Fetal Liver, and Adult Monocytes Can Colonize an Empty Niche and Develop into Functional Tissue-Resident Macrophages. *Immunity* **2016**, *44*, 755–768. [CrossRef]
10. Franklin, R.A.; Liao, W.; Sarkar, A.; Kim, M.V.; Bivona, M.R.; Liu, K.; Pamer, E.G.; Li, M.O. The cellular and molecular origin of tumor-associated macrophages. *Science* **2014**, *344*, 921–925. [CrossRef]
11. Shand, F.H.W.; Ueha, S.; Otsuji, M.; Koid, S.S.; Shichino, S.; Tsukui, T.; Kosugi-Kanaya, M.; Abe, J.; Tomura, M.; Ziogas, J.; et al. Tracking of intertissue migration reveals the origins of tumor-infiltrating monocytes. *Proc. Natl. Acad. Sci. USA* **2014**, *111*, 7771–7776. [CrossRef] [PubMed]
12. Noy, R.; Pollard, J.W. Tumor-Associated Macrophages: From Mechanisms to Therapy. *Immunity* **2014**, *41*, 49–61. [CrossRef] [PubMed]
13. Bonavita, E.; Gentile, S.; Rubino, M.; Maina, V.; Papait, R.; Kunderfranco, P.; Greco, C.; Feruglio, F.; Molgora, M.; Laface, I.; et al. PTX3 Is an Extrinsic Oncosuppressor Regulating Complement-Dependent Inflammation in Cancer. *Cell* **2015**, *160*, 700–714. [CrossRef]
14. Bonavita, E.; Galdiero, M.R.; Jaillon, S.; Mantovani, A. Phagocytes as Corrupted Policemen in Cancer-Related Inflammation. In *Advances in Cancer Research*; Elsevier: Amsterdam, The Netherlands, 2015; pp. 141–171.
15. Bowman, R.L.; Klemm, F.; Akkari, L.; Pyonteck, S.M.; Sevenich, L.; Quail, D.F.; Dhara, S.; Simpson, K.; Gardner, E.E.; Iacobuzio-Donahue, C.A.; et al. Macrophage Ontogeny Underlies Differences in Tumor-Specific Education in Brain Malignancies. *Cell Rep.* **2016**, *17*, 2445–2459. [CrossRef] [PubMed]
16. Ye, Y.-C.; Zhao, J.-L.; Lu, Y.-T.; Gao, C.-C.; Yang, Y.; Liang, S.-Q.; Lu, Y.Y.; Wang, L.; Yue, S.Q.; Dou, K.F.; et al. NOTCH Signaling via WNT Regulates the Proliferation of Alternative, CCR2-Independent Tumor-Associated Macrophages in Hepatocellular Carcinoma. *Cancer Res.* **2019**, *79*, 4160–4172. [CrossRef]
17. DeNardo, D.G.; Ruffell, B. Macrophages as regulators of tumour immunity and immunotherapy. *Nat. Rev. Immunol.* **2019**, *19*, 369–382. [CrossRef] [PubMed]
18. Duan, Z.; Luo, Y. Targeting macrophages in cancer immunotherapy. *Signal Transduct. Target. Ther.* **2021**, *6*, 127. [CrossRef]
19. Song, W.; Mazzieri, R.; Yang, T.; Gobe, G.C. Translational Significance for Tumor Metastasis of Tumor-Associated Macrophages and Epithelial-Mesenchymal Transition. *Front. Immunol.* **2017**, *8*, 1106. [CrossRef] [PubMed]
20. Pan, Y.; Yu, Y.; Wang, X.; Zhang, T. Tumor-Associated Macrophages in Tumor Immunity. *Front. Immunol.* **2020**, *11*, 583084. [CrossRef]
21. Lee, M.; Park, C.-S.; Lee, Y.-R.; Im, S.-A.; Song, S.; Lee, C.-K. Resiquimod, a TLR7/8 agonist, promotes differentiation of myeloid-derived suppressor cells into macrophages and dendritic cells. *Arch. Pharm. Res.* **2014**, *37*, 1234–1240. [CrossRef]
22. Murray, P.J.; Allen, J.E.; Biswas, S.K.; Fisher, E.A.; Gilroy, D.W.; Goerdt, S.; Gordon, S.; Hamilton, J.A.; Ivashkiv, L.B.; Lawrence, T.; et al. Macrophage Activation and Polarization: Nomenclature and Experimental Guidelines. *Immunity* **2014**, *41*, 14–20. [CrossRef] [PubMed]
23. Mosser, D.M.; Edwards, J.P. Exploring the full spectrum of macrophage activation. *Nat. Rev. Immunol.* **2008**, *8*, 958–969. [CrossRef] [PubMed]
24. Liang, Y.-B.; Tang, H.; Chen, Z.-B.; Zeng, L.-J.; Wu, J.-G.; Yang, W.; Li, Z.Y.; Ma, Z.F. Downregulated SOCS1 expression activates the JAK1/STAT1 pathway and promotes polarization of macrophages into M1 type. *Mol. Med. Rep.* **2017**, *16*, 6405–6411. [CrossRef]
25. Wu, L.; Yan, J.; Bai, Y.; Chen, F.; Zou, X.; Xu, J.; Huang, A.; Hou, L.; Zhong, Y.; Jing, Z.; et al. An invasive zone in human liver cancer identified by Stereo-seq promotes hepatocyte-tumor cell crosstalk, local immunosuppression and tumor progression. *Cell Res.* **2023**, *33*, 585–603. [CrossRef]

26. Gong, M.; Zhuo, X.; Ma, A. STAT6 Upregulation Promotes M2 Macrophage Polarization to Suppress Atherosclerosis. *Med. Sci. Monit. Basic Res.* **2017**, *23*, 240–249. [CrossRef]
27. Oh, H.; Park, S.-H.; Kang, M.-K.; Kim, Y.-H.; Lee, E.-J.; Kim, D.Y.; Kim, S.I.; Oh, S.; Lim, S.S.; Kang, Y.H. Asaronic Acid Attenuates Macrophage Activation toward M1 Phenotype through Inhibition of NF-κB Pathway and JAK-STAT Signaling in Glucose-Loaded Murine Macrophages. *J. Agric. Food Chem.* **2019**, *67*, 10069–10078. [CrossRef] [PubMed]
28. Chang, Q.; Bournazou, E.; Sansone, P.; Berishaj, M.; Gao, S.P.; Daly, L.; Wels, J.; Theilen, T.; Granitto, S.; Zhang, X.; et al. The IL-6/JAK/Stat3 Feed-Forward Loop Drives Tumorigenesis and Metastasis. *Neoplasia* **2013**, *15*, 848–862, IN40–IN45. [CrossRef] [PubMed]
29. Szanto, A.; Balint, B.L.; Nagy, Z.S.; Barta, E.; Dezso, B.; Pap, A.; Szeles, L.; Poliska, S.; Oros, M.; Evans, R.M.; et al. STAT6 Transcription Factor Is a Facilitator of the Nuclear Receptor PPARγ-Regulated Gene Expression in Macrophages and Dendritic Cells. *Immunity* **2010**, *33*, 699–712. [CrossRef] [PubMed]
30. Satoh, T.; Takeuchi, O.; Vandenbon, A.; Yasuda, K.; Tanaka, Y.; Kumagai, Y.; Miyake, T.; Matsushita, K.; Okazaki, T.; Saitoh, T.; et al. The Jmjd3-Irf4 axis regulates M2 macrophage polarization and host responses against helminth infection. *Nat. Immunol.* **2010**, *11*, 936–944. [CrossRef]
31. Takaoka, A.; Yanai, H.; Kondo, S.; Duncan, G.; Negishi, H.; Mizutani, T.; Kano, S.I.; Honda, K.; Ohba, Y.; Mak, T.W.; et al. Integral role of IRF-5 in the gene induction programme activated by Toll-like receptors. *Nature* **2005**, *434*, 243–249. [CrossRef]
32. Savitsky, D.; Tamura, T.; Yanai, H.; Taniguchi, T. Regulation of immunity and oncogenesis by the IRF transcription factor family. *Cancer Immunol. Immunother.* **2010**, *59*, 489–510. [CrossRef] [PubMed]
33. Huang, F.; Zhao, J.-L.; Wang, L.; Gao, C.-C.; Liang, S.-Q.; An, D.-J.; Bai, J.; Chen, Y.; Han, H.; Qin, H.Y. miR-148a-3p Mediates Notch Signaling to Promote the Differentiation and M1 Activation of Macrophages. *Front. Immunol.* **2017**, *8*, 1327. [CrossRef] [PubMed]
34. Lin, Y.; Zhao, J.-L.; Zheng, Q.-J.; Jiang, X.; Tian, J.; Liang, S.-Q.; Guo, H.W.; Qin, H.Y.; Liang, Y.M.; Han, H. Notch Signaling Modulates Macrophage Polarization and Phagocytosis Through Direct Suppression of Signal Regulatory Protein α Expression. *Front. Immunol.* **2018**, *9*, 1744. [CrossRef] [PubMed]
35. Covarrubias, A.J.; Aksoylar, H.I.; Yu, J.; Snyder, N.W.; Worth, A.J.; Iyer, S.S.; Wang, J.; Ben-Sahra, I.; Byles, V.; Polynne-Stapornkul, T.; et al. Akt-mTORC1 signaling regulates Acly to integrate metabolic input to control of macrophage activation. *eLife* **2016**, *5*, e11612. [CrossRef] [PubMed]
36. Linton, M.F.; Moslehi, J.J.; Babaev, V.R. Akt Signaling in Macrophage Polarization, Survival, and Atherosclerosis. *Int. J. Mol. Sci.* **2019**, *20*, 2703. [CrossRef] [PubMed]
37. Yang, F.; Tong, J.H.; Li, H.; Chen, J.; Dai, L.M. BTK inhibitor GDC-0853 inhibits M1macmphage polarization and alleviates UUO kidney injury via TLR4/NF-κB pathway. *Immunological* **2021**, *37*, 107–114. (In Chinese)
38. Porta, C.; Riboldi, E.; Ippolito, A.; Sica, A. Molecular and epigenetic basis of macrophage polarized activation. *Semin. Immunol.* **2015**, *27*, 237–248. [CrossRef] [PubMed]
39. Yunna, C.; Mengru, H.; Lei, W.; Weidong, C. Macrophage M1/M2 polarization. *Eur. J. Pharmacol.* **2020**, *877*, 173090. [CrossRef] [PubMed]
40. Lin, E.Y.; Li, J.-F.; Gnatovskiy, L.; Deng, Y.; Zhu, L.; Grzesik, D.A.; Qian, H.; Xue, X.N.; Pollard, J.W. Macrophages Regulate the Angiogenic Switch in a Mouse Model of Breast Cancer. *Cancer Res.* **2006**, *66*, 11238–11246. [CrossRef]
41. Kujawski, M.; Kortylewski, M.; Lee, H.; Herrmann, A.; Kay, H.; Yu, H. Stat3 mediates myeloid cell-dependent tumor angiogenesis in mice. *J. Clin. Investig.* **2008**, *118*, 3367–3377. [CrossRef]
42. Shantsila, E.; Wrigley, B.; Tapp, L.; Apostolakis, S.; Montoro-Garcia, S.; Drayson, M.T.; Lip, G.Y.H. Immunophenotypic characterization of human monocyte subsets: Possible implications for cardiovascular disease pathophysiology. *J. Thromb. Haemost.* **2011**, *9*, 1056–1066. [CrossRef] [PubMed]
43. De Palma, M.; Naldini, L. Angiopoietin-2 TIEs Up Macrophages in Tumor Angiogenesis. *Clin. Cancer Res.* **2011**, *17*, 5226–5232. [CrossRef] [PubMed]
44. Savagner, P. The epithelial-mesenchymal transition (EMT) phenomenon. *Ann. Oncol.* **2010**, *21*, vii89–vii92. [CrossRef] [PubMed]
45. Bonde, A.-K.; Tischler, V.; Kumar, S.; Soltermann, A.; Schwendener, R.A. Intratumoral macrophages contribute to epithelial-mesenchymal transition in solid tumors. *BMC Cancer* **2012**, *12*, 35. [CrossRef] [PubMed]
46. Lee, S.; Lee, E.; Ko, E.; Ham, M.; Lee, H.M.; Kim, E.-S.; Koh, M.; Lim, H.K.; Jung, J.; Park, S.Y.; et al. Tumor-associated macrophages secrete CCL2 and induce the invasive phenotype of human breast epithelial cells through upregulation of ERO1-α and MMP-9. *Cancer Lett.* **2018**, *437*, 25–34. [CrossRef] [PubMed]
47. Jeong, H.; Kim, S.; Hong, B.-J.; Lee, C.-J.; Kim, Y.-E.; Bok, S.; Oh, J.-M.; Gwak, S.-H.; Yoo, M.Y.; Lee, M.S.; et al. Tumor-Associated Macrophages Enhance Tumor Hypoxia and Aerobic Glycolysis. *Cancer Res.* **2019**, *79*, 795–806. [CrossRef] [PubMed]
48. Chen, F.; Chen, J.; Yang, L.; Liu, J.; Zhang, X.; Zhang, Y.; Tu, Q.; Yin, D.; Lin, D.; Wong, P.P.; et al. Extracellular vesicle-packaged HIF-1α-stabilizing lncRNA from tumour-associated macrophages regulates aerobic glycolysis of breast cancer cells. *Nat. Cell Biol.* **2019**, *21*, 498–510. [CrossRef] [PubMed]
49. Bronte, V.; Serafini, P.; Mazzoni, A.; Segal, D.M.; Zanovello, P. L-arginine metabolism in myeloid cells controls T-lymphocyte functions. *Trends Immunol.* **2003**, *24*, 301–305. [CrossRef] [PubMed]

50. Duluc, D.; Corvaisier, M.; Blanchard, S.; Catala, L.; Descamps, P.; Gamelin, E.; Ponsoda, S.; Delneste, Y.; Hebbar, M.; Jeannin, P. Interferon-γ reverses the immunosuppressive and protumoral properties and prevents the generation of human tumor-associated macrophages. *Int. J. Cancer* **2009**, *125*, 367–373. [CrossRef]
51. Porta, C.; Rimoldi, M.; Raes, G.; Brys, L.; Ghezzi, P.; Di Liberto, D.; Dieli, F.; Ghisletti, S.; Natoli, G.; De Baetselier, P.; et al. Tolerance and M2 (alternative) macrophage polarization are related processes orchestrated by p50 nuclear factor κB. *Proc. Natl. Acad. Sci. USA* **2009**, *106*, 14978–14983. [CrossRef]
52. Mantovani, A.; Marchesi, F.; Malesci, A.; Laghi, L.; Allavena, P. Tumour-associated macrophages as treatment targets in oncology. *Nat. Rev. Clin. Oncol.* **2017**, *14*, 399–416. [CrossRef] [PubMed]
53. Komohara, Y.; Fujiwara, Y.; Ohnishi, K.; Takeya, M. Tumor-associated macrophages: Potential therapeutic targets for anti-cancer therapy. *Adv. Drug Deliv. Rev.* **2016**, *99*, 180–185. [CrossRef]
54. Mantovani, A.; Sica, A. Macrophages, innate immunity and cancer: Balance, tolerance, and diversity. *Curr. Opin. Immunol.* **2010**, *22*, 231–237. [CrossRef]
55. Flavell, R.A.; Sanjabi, S.; Wrzesinski, S.H.; Licona-Limón, P. The polarization of immune cells in the tumour environment by TGFβ. *Nat. Rev. Immunol.* **2010**, *10*, 554–567. [CrossRef] [PubMed]
56. Thomas, D.A.; Massagué, J. TGF-β directly targets cytotoxic T cell functions during tumor evasion of immune surveillance. *Cancer Cell* **2005**, *8*, 369–380. [CrossRef] [PubMed]
57. Matsuda, M.; Salazar, F.; Petersson, M.; Masucci, G.; Hansson, J.; Pisa, P.; Zhang, Q.J.; Masucci, M.G.; Kiessling, R. Interleukin 10 pretreatment protects target cells from tumor- and allo-specific cytotoxic T cells and downregulates HLA class I expression. *J. Exp. Med.* **1994**, *180*, 2371–2376. [CrossRef] [PubMed]
58. Sica, A.; Saccani, A.; Bottazzi, B.; Polentarutti, N.; Vecchi, A.; Damme, J.V.; Mantovani, A. Autocrine Production of IL-10 Mediates Defective IL-12 Production and NF-κB Activation in Tumor-Associated Macrophages. *J. Immunol.* **2000**, *164*, 762–767. [CrossRef]
59. Bak, S.P.; Alonso, A.; Turk, M.J.; Berwin, B. Murine ovarian cancer vascular leukocytes require arginase-1 activity for T cell suppression. *Mol. Immunol.* **2008**, *46*, 258–268. [CrossRef]
60. Marigo, I.; Dolcetti, L.; Serafini, P.; Zanovello, P.; Bronte, V. Tumor-induced tolerance and immune suppression by myeloid derived suppressor cells. *Immunol. Rev.* **2008**, *222*, 162–179. [CrossRef]
61. Sarkar, T.; Dhar, S.; Chakraborty, D.; Pati, S.; Bose, S.; Panda, A.K.; Basak, U.; Chakraborty, S.; Mukherjee, S.; Guin, A.; et al. FOXP3/HAT1 Axis Controls Treg Infiltration in the Tumor Microenvironment by Inducing CCR4 Expression in Breast Cancer. *Front. Immunol.* **2022**, *13*, 740588. [CrossRef]
62. Solinas, G.; Germano, G.; Mantovani, A.; Allavena, P. Tumor-associated macrophages (TAM) as major players of the cancer-related inflammation. *J. Leukoc. Biol.* **2009**, *86*, 1065–1073. [CrossRef] [PubMed]
63. Guo, Q.; Jin, Z.; Yuan, Y.; Liu, R.; Xu, T.; Wei, H.; Xu, X.; He, S.; Chen, S.; Shi, Z.; et al. New Mechanisms of Tumor-Associated Macrophages on Promoting Tumor Progression: Recent Research Advances and Potential Targets for Tumor Immunotherapy. *J. Immunol. Res.* **2016**, *2016*, 9720912. [CrossRef]
64. Bhusal, R.P.; Foster, S.R.; Stone, M.J. Structural basis of chemokine and receptor interactions: Key regulators of leukocyte recruitment in inflammatory responses. *Protein Sci.* **2020**, *29*, 420–432. [CrossRef] [PubMed]
65. Van Coillie, E.; Van Damme, J.; Opdenakker, G. The MCP/eotaxin subfamily of CC chemokines. *Cytokine Growth Factor Rev.* **1999**, *10*, 61–86. [CrossRef]
66. Hoesel, B.; Schmid, J.A. The complexity of NF-κB signaling in inflammation and cancer. *Mol. Cancer* **2013**, *12*, 86. [CrossRef]
67. Wang, X.; Wang, J.; Zhao, J.; Wang, H.; Chen, J.; Wu, J. HMGA2 facilitates colorectal cancer progression via STAT3-mediated tumor-associated macrophage recruitment. *Theranostics* **2022**, *12*, 963–975. [CrossRef] [PubMed]
68. Wang, Y.; Yu, L.; Hu, Z.; Fang, Y.; Shen, Y.; Song, M.; Chen, Y. Regulation of CCL2 by EZH2 affects tumor-associated macrophages polarization and infiltration in breast cancer. *Cell Death Dis.* **2022**, *13*, 748. [CrossRef] [PubMed]
69. Nywening, T.M.; Wang-Gillam, A.; Sanford, D.E.; Belt, B.A.; Panni, R.Z.; Cusworth, B.M.; Toriola, A.T.; Nieman, R.K.; Worley, L.A.; Yano, M.; et al. Targeting tumour-associated macrophages with CCR2 inhibition in combination with FOLFIRINOX in patients with borderline resectable and locally advanced pancreatic cancer: A single-centre, open-label, dose-finding, non-randomised, phase 1b trial. *Lancet Oncol.* **2016**, *17*, 651–662. [CrossRef] [PubMed]
70. Linehan, D.; Noel, M.S.; Hezel, A.F.; Wang-Gillam, A.; Eskens, F.; Sleijfer, S.; Desar, I.M.E.; Erdkamp, F.; Wilmink, J.; Diehl, J.; et al. Overall survival in a trial of orally administered CCR2 inhibitor CCX872 in locally advanced/metastatic pancreatic cancer: Correlation with blood monocyte counts. *J. Clin. Oncol.* **2018**, *36*, 92. [CrossRef]
71. Bonapace, L.; Coissieux, M.-M.; Wyckoff, J.; Mertz, K.D.; Varga, Z.; Junt, T.; Bentires-Alj, M. Cessation of CCL2 inhibition accelerates breast cancer metastasis by promoting angiogenesis. *Nature* **2014**, *515*, 130–133. [CrossRef]
72. Walens, A.; DiMarco, A.V.; Lupo, R.; Kroger, B.R.; Damrauer, J.S.; Alvarez, J.V. CCL5 promotes breast cancer recurrence through macrophage recruitment in residual tumors. *eLife* **2019**, *8*, e43653. [CrossRef] [PubMed]
73. Hughes, R.; Qian, B.-Z.; Rowan, C.; Muthana, M.; Keklikoglou, I.; Olson, O.C.; Tazzyman, S.; Danson, S.; Addison, C.; Clemons, M.; et al. Perivascular M2 Macrophages Stimulate Tumor Relapse after Chemotherapy. *Cancer Res.* **2015**, *75*, 3479–3491. [CrossRef] [PubMed]
74. Teicher, B.A.; Fricker, S.P. CXCL12 (SDF-1)/CXCR4 Pathway in Cancer. *Clin. Cancer Res.* **2010**, *16*, 2927–2931. [CrossRef] [PubMed]
75. Scala, S. Molecular Pathways: Targeting the CXCR4-CXCL12 Axis—Untapped Potential in the Tumor Microenvironment. *Clin. Cancer Res.* **2015**, *21*, 4278–4285. [CrossRef] [PubMed]

76. Eli Lilly and Company. A Phase 1a/1b Study of CXCR4 Peptide Antagonist (LY2510924) Administered in Combination with the Anti-PD-L1 Antibody, Durvalumab (MEDI4736), in Advanced Refractory Solid Tumors. NCT02737072. 2016. Available online: https://classic.clinicaltrials.gov/ProvidedDocs/72/NCT02737072/Prot_000.pdf (accessed on 27 April 2024).
77. Huang, Y.; Yuan, J.; Righi, E.; Kamoun, W.S.; Ancukiewicz, M.; Nezivar, J.; Santosuosso, M.; Martin, J.D.; Martin, M.R.; Vianello, F.; et al. Vascular normalizing doses of antiangiogenic treatment reprogram the immunosuppressive tumor microenvironment and enhance immunotherapy. *Proc. Natl. Acad. Sci. USA* **2012**, *109*, 17561–17566. [CrossRef] [PubMed]
78. Dineen, S.P.; Lynn, K.D.; Holloway, S.E.; Miller, A.F.; Sullivan, J.P.; Shames, D.S.; Beck, A.W.; Barnett, C.C.; Fleming, J.B.; Brekken, R.A. Vascular Endothelial Growth Factor Receptor 2 Mediates Macrophage Infiltration into Orthotopic Pancreatic Tumors in Mice. *Cancer Res.* **2008**, *68*, 4340–4346. [CrossRef] [PubMed]
79. Chen, D.S.; Mellman, I. Oncology Meets Immunology: The Cancer-Immunity Cycle. *Immunity* **2013**, *39*, 1–10. [CrossRef] [PubMed]
80. Kubli, S.P.; Berger, T.; Araujo, D.V.; Siu, L.L.; Mak, T.W. Beyond immune checkpoint blockade: Emerging immunological strategies. *Nat. Rev. Drug Discov.* **2021**, *20*, 899–919. [CrossRef] [PubMed]
81. Hamilton, J.A. CSF-1 signal transduction. *J. Leukoc. Biol.* **1997**, *62*, 145–155. [CrossRef]
82. Yeung, Y.-G.; Wang, Y.; Einstein, D.B.; Lee, P.S.W.; Stanley, E.R. Colony-stimulating Factor-1 Stimulates the Formation of Multimeric Cytosolic Complexes of Signaling Proteins and Cytoskeletal Components in Macrophages. *J. Biol. Chem.* **1998**, *273*, 17128–17137. [CrossRef]
83. Li, M.; He, L.; Zhu, J.; Zhang, P.; Liang, S. Targeting tumor-associated macrophages for cancer treatment. *Cell Biosci.* **2022**, *12*, 85. [CrossRef]
84. Liu, Y.-Q.; Wang, Y.-N.; Lu, X.-Y.; Tong, L.-J.; Li, Y.; Zhang, T.; Xun, Q.J.; Feng, F.; Chen, Y.Z.; Su, Y.; et al. Identification of compound D2923 as a novel anti-tumor agent targeting CSF1R. *Acta Pharmacol. Sin.* **2018**, *39*, 1768–1776. [CrossRef] [PubMed]
85. Kuemmel, S.; Campone, M.; Loirat, D.; Lopez, R.L.; Beck, J.T.; De Laurentiis, M.; Im, S.A.; Kim, S.B.; Kwong, A.; Steger, G.G.; et al. A Randomized Phase II Study of Anti-CSF1 Monoclonal Antibody Lacnotuzumab (MCS110) Combined with Gemcitabine and Carboplatin in Advanced Triple-Negative Breast Cancer. *Clin. Cancer Res.* **2022**, *28*, 106–115. [CrossRef] [PubMed]
86. Dowlati, A.; Harvey, R.D.; Carvajal, R.D.; Hamid, O.; Klempner, S.J.; Kauh, J.S.W.; Peterson, D.A.; Yu, D.; Chapman, S.C.; Szpurka, A.M.; et al. LY3022855, an anti-colony stimulating factor-1 receptor (CSF-1R) monoclonal antibody, in patients with advanced solid tumors refractory to standard therapy: Phase 1 dose-escalation trial. *Investig. New Drugs* **2021**, *39*, 1057–1071. [CrossRef] [PubMed]
87. Pfizer. A Phase 1b/2 Study of ARRY-382 in Combination with Pembrolizumab, a Programmed Cell Death Receptor 1 (PD-1) Antibody, for the Treatment of Patients with Advanced Solid Tumors. NCT02880371. 2016. Available online: https://clinicaltrials.gov/study/NCT02880371 (accessed on 27 April 2024).
88. Holen, I.; Coleman, R.E. Anti-tumour activity of bisphosphonates in preclinical models of breast cancer. *Breast Cancer Res.* **2010**, *12*, 214. [CrossRef]
89. Germano, G.; Frapolli, R.; Belgiovine, C.; Anselmo, A.; Pesce, S.; Liguori, M.; Erba, E.; Uboldi, S.; Zucchetti, M.; Pasqualini, F.; et al. Role of Macrophage Targeting in the Antitumor Activity of Trabectedin. *Cancer Cell* **2013**, *23*, 249–262. [CrossRef] [PubMed]
90. Borgoni, S.; Iannello, A.; Cutrupi, S.; Allavena, P.; D'Incalci, M.; Novelli, F.; Cappello, P. Depletion of tumor-associated macrophages switches the epigenetic profile of pancreatic cancer infiltrating T cells and restores their anti-tumor phenotype. *OncoImmunology* **2018**, *7*, e1393596. [CrossRef]
91. Molgora, M.; Colonna, M. Turning enemies into allies—Reprogramming tumor-associated macrophages for cancer therapy. *Med* **2021**, *2*, 666–681. [CrossRef]
92. Zhang, J.Q.; Zeng, S.; Vitiello, G.A.; Seifert, A.M.; Medina, B.D.; Beckman, M.J.; Loo, J.K.; Santamaria-Barria, J.; Maltbaek, J.H.; Param, N.J.; et al. Macrophages and CD8+ T Cells Mediate the Antitumor Efficacy of Combined CD40 Ligation and Imatinib Therapy in Gastrointestinal Stromal Tumors. *Cancer Immunol. Res.* **2018**, *6*, 434–447. [CrossRef]
93. Chand Dakal, T.; Dhabhai, B.; Agarwal, D.; Gupta, R.; Nagda, G.; Meena, A.R.; Dhakar, R.; Menon, A.; Mathur, R.; Mona; et al. Mechanistic basis of co-stimulatory CD40-CD40L ligation mediated regulation of immune responses in cancer and autoimmune disorders. *Immunobiology* **2020**, *225*, 151899. [CrossRef]
94. Liu, P.-S.; Chen, Y.-T.; Li, X.; Hsueh, P.-C.; Tzeng, S.-F.; Chen, H.; Shi, P.Z.; Xie, X.; Parik, S.; Planque, M.; et al. CD40 signal rewires fatty acid and glutamine metabolism for stimulating macrophage anti-tumorigenic functions. *Nat. Immunol.* **2023**, *24*, 452–462. [CrossRef] [PubMed]
95. Byrd, J.C.; Kipps, T.J.; Flinn, I.W.; Cooper, M.; Odenike, O.; Bendiske, J.; Rediske, J.; Bilic, S.; Dey, J.; Baeck, J.; et al. Phase I study of the anti-CD40 humanized monoclonal antibody lucatumumab (HCD122) in relapsed chronic lymphocytic leukemia. *Leuk. Lymphoma* **2012**, *53*, 2136–2142. [CrossRef] [PubMed]
96. Oflazoglu, E.; Stone, I.J.; Brown, L.; Gordon, K.A.; Van Rooijen, N.; Jonas, M.; Law, C.L.; Grewal, I.S.; Gerber, H.P. Macrophages and Fc-receptor interactions contribute to the antitumour activities of the anti-CD40 antibody SGN-40. *Br. J. Cancer* **2009**, *100*, 113–117. [CrossRef] [PubMed]
97. Vonderheide, R.H.; Flaherty, K.T.; Khalil, M.; Stumacher, M.S.; Bajor, D.L.; Hutnick, N.A.; Sullivan, P.; Mahany, J.J.; Gallagher, M.; Kramer, A.; et al. Clinical Activity and Immune Modulation in Cancer Patients Treated With CP-870,893, a Novel CD40 Agonist Monoclonal Antibody. *J. Clin. Oncol.* **2007**, *25*, 876–883. [CrossRef] [PubMed]

98. Vonderheide, R.H.; Burg, J.M.; Mick, R.; Trosko, J.A.; Li, D.; Shaik, M.N.; Tolcher, A.W.; Hamid, O. Phase I study of the CD40 agonist antibody CP-870,893 combined with carboplatin and paclitaxel in patients with advanced solid tumors. *OncoImmunology* **2013**, *2*, e23033. [CrossRef] [PubMed]
99. Wiehagen, K.R.; Girgis, N.M.; Yamada, D.H.; Smith, A.A.; Chan, S.R.; Grewal, I.S.; Quigley, M.; Verona, R.I. Combination of CD40 Agonism and CSF-1R Blockade Reconditions Tumor-Associated Macrophages and Drives Potent Antitumor Immunity. *Cancer Immunol. Res.* **2017**, *5*, 1109–1121. [CrossRef] [PubMed]
100. Kaczanowska, S.; Joseph, A.M.; Davila, E. TLR agonists: Our best *frenemy* in cancer immunotherapy. *J. Leukoc. Biol.* **2013**, *93*, 847–863. [CrossRef] [PubMed]
101. Patra, M.C.; Choi, S. Recent progress in the development of Toll-like receptor (TLR) antagonists. *Expert Opin. Ther. Pat.* **2016**, *26*, 719–730. [CrossRef] [PubMed]
102. Van Dalen, F.; Van Stevendaal, M.; Fennemann, F.; Verdoes, M.; Ilina, O. Molecular Repolarisation of Tumour-Associated Macrophages. *Molecules* **2018**, *24*, 9. [CrossRef]
103. Huang, Z.; Yang, Y.; Jiang, Y.; Shao, J.; Sun, X.; Chen, J.; Dong, L.; Zhang, J. Anti-tumor immune responses of tumor-associated macrophages via toll-like receptor 4 triggered by cationic polymers. *Biomaterials* **2013**, *34*, 746–755. [CrossRef]
104. Liu, Z.; Xie, Y.; Xiong, Y.; Liu, S.; Qiu, C.; Zhu, Z.; Mao, H.; Yu, M.; Wang, X. TLR 7/8 agonist reverses oxaliplatin resistance in colorectal cancer via directing the myeloid-derived suppressor cells to tumoricidal M1-macrophages. *Cancer Lett.* **2020**, *469*, 173–185. [CrossRef]
105. Klinman, D.M. Immunotherapeutic uses of CpG oligodeoxynucleotides. *Nat. Rev. Immunol.* **2004**, *4*, 249–259. [CrossRef]
106. Wang, D.; Jiang, W.; Zhu, F.; Mao, X.; Agrawal, S. Modulation of the tumor microenvironment by intratumoral administration of IMO-2125, a novel TLR9 agonist, for cancer immunotherapy. *Int. J. Oncol.* **2018**, *53*, 1193–1203. [CrossRef] [PubMed]
107. Veillette, A.; Chen, J. SIRPα-CD47 Immune Checkpoint Blockade in Anticancer Therapy. *Trends Immunol.* **2018**, *39*, 173–184. [CrossRef] [PubMed]
108. McCracken, M.N.; Cha, A.C.; Weissman, I.L. Molecular Pathways: Activating T Cells after Cancer Cell Phagocytosis from Blockade of CD47 "Don't Eat Me" Signals. *Clin. Cancer Res.* **2015**, *21*, 3597–3601. [CrossRef] [PubMed]
109. Matlung, H.L.; Szilagyi, K.; Barclay, N.A.; Van Den Berg, T.K. The CD47-SIRPα signaling axis as an innate immune checkpoint in cancer. *Immunol. Rev.* **2017**, *276*, 145–164. [CrossRef]
110. Liu, J.; Wang, L.; Zhao, F.; Tseng, S.; Narayanan, C.; Shura, L.; Willingham, S.; Howard, M.; Prohaska, S.; Volkmer, J.; et al. Pre-Clinical Development of a Humanized Anti-CD47 Antibody with Anti-Cancer Therapeutic Potential. *PLoS ONE* **2015**, *10*, e0137345. [CrossRef] [PubMed]
111. Gilead Sciences. A Phase 1b/2 Trial of Hu5F9-G4 in Combination with Rituximab or Rituximab + Chemotherapy in Patients with Relapsed/Refractory B-cell Non-Hodgkin's Lymphoma. NCT02953509. 2016. Available online: https://clinicaltrials.gov/study/NCT02953509 (accessed on 27 April 2024).
112. Munagala, R.; Aqil, F.; Jeyabalan, J.; Agrawal, A.K.; Mudd, A.M.; Kyakulaga, A.H.; Singh, I.P.; Vadhanam, M.V.; Gupta, R.C. Exosomal formulation of anthocyanidins against multiple cancer types. *Cancer Lett.* **2017**, *393*, 94–102. [CrossRef]
113. Zhang, Y.; Tang, S.; Gao, Y.; Lu, Z.; Yang, Y.; Chen, J.; Li, T. Application of exosomal miRNA mediated macrophage polarization in colorectal cancer: Current progress and challenges. *Oncol. Res.* **2024**, *32*, 61–71. [CrossRef]
114. Li, H.; Jiang, T.; Li, M.-Q.; Zheng, X.-L.; Zhao, G.-J. Transcriptional Regulation of Macrophages Polarization by MicroRNAs. *Front. Immunol.* **2018**, *9*, 1175. [CrossRef]
115. Wu, H.; Ye, C.; Ramirez, D.; Manjunath, N. Alternative Processing of Primary microRNA Transcripts by Drosha Generates 5′ End Variation of Mature microRNA. *PLoS ONE* **2009**, *4*, e7566. [CrossRef]
116. Boeri, M.; Milione, M.; Proto, C.; Signorelli, D.; Lo Russo, G.; Galeone, C.; Verri, C.; Mensah, M.; Centonze, G.; Martinetti, A.; et al. Circulating miRNAs and PD-L1 Tumor Expression Are Associated with Survival in Advanced NSCLC Patients Treated with Immunotherapy: A Prospective Study. *Clin. Cancer Res.* **2019**, *25*, 2166–2173. [CrossRef] [PubMed]
117. Thulin, P.; Wei, T.; Werngren, O.; Cheung, L.; Fisher, R.M.; Grandér, D.; Corcoran, M.; Ehrenborg, E. MicroRNA-9 regulates the expression of peroxisome proliferator-activated receptor δ in human monocytes during the inflammatory response. *Int. J. Mol. Med.* **2013**, *31*, 1003–1010. [CrossRef]
118. Chaudhuri, A.A.; So, A.Y.-L.; Sinha, N.; Gibson, W.S.J.; Taganov, K.D.; O'Connell, R.M.; Baltimore, D. MicroRNA-125b Potentiates Macrophage Activation. *J. Immunol.* **2011**, *187*, 5062–5068. [CrossRef]
119. Qian, M.; Wang, S.; Guo, X.; Wang, J.; Zhang, Z.; Qiu, W.; Gao, X.; Chen, Z.; Xu, J.; Zhao, R.; et al. Hypoxic glioma-derived exosomes deliver microRNA-1246 to induce M2 macrophage polarization by targeting TERF2IP via the STAT3 and NF-κB pathways. *Oncogene* **2020**, *39*, 428–442. [CrossRef] [PubMed]
120. Chen, J.; Zhang, K.; Zhi, Y.; Wu, Y.; Chen, B.; Bai, J.; Wang, X. Tumor-derived exosomal miR-19b-3p facilitates M2 macrophage polarization and exosomal LINC00273 secretion to promote lung adenocarcinoma metastasis via Hippo pathway. *Clin. Transl. Med.* **2021**, *11*, e478. [CrossRef] [PubMed]
121. Su, M.-J.; Aldawsari, H.; Amiji, M. Pancreatic Cancer Cell Exosome-Mediated Macrophage Reprogramming and the Role of MicroRNAs 155 and 125b2 Transfection using Nanoparticle Delivery Systems. *Sci. Rep.* **2016**, *6*, 30110. [CrossRef]
122. Trivedi, M.; Talekar, M.; Shah, P.; Ouyang, Q.; Amiji, M. Modification of tumor cell exosome content by transfection with wt-p53 and microRNA-125b expressing plasmid DNA and its effect on macrophage polarization. *Oncogenesis* **2016**, *5*, e250. [CrossRef]

123. Larson, R.C.; Maus, M.V. Recent advances and discoveries in the mechanisms and functions of CAR T cells. *Nat. Rev. Cancer* **2021**, *21*, 145–161. [CrossRef]
124. Wang, S.; Yang, Y.; Ma, P.; Zha, Y.; Zhang, J.; Lei, A.; Li, N. CAR-macrophage: An extensive immune enhancer to fight cancer. *eBioMedicine* **2022**, *76*, 103873. [CrossRef]
125. Klichinsky, M.; Ruella, M.; Shestova, O.; Lu, X.M.; Best, A.; Zeeman, M.; Schmierer, M.; Gabrusiewicz, K.; Anderson, N.R.; Petty, N.E.; et al. Human chimeric antigen receptor macrophages for cancer immunotherapy. *Nat. Biotechnol.* **2020**, *38*, 947–953. [CrossRef] [PubMed]
126. Kang, M.; Lee, S.H.; Kwon, M.; Byun, J.; Kim, D.; Kim, C.; Koo, S.; Kwon, S.P.; Moon, S.; Jung, M.; et al. Nanocomplex-Mediated In Vivo Programming to Chimeric Antigen Receptor-M1 Macrophages for Cancer Therapy. *Adv. Mater.* **2021**, *33*, 2103258. [CrossRef] [PubMed]
127. MaxCyte, Inc. A Phase 1 Study of Intraperitoneal MCY-M11 Therapy for Women with Platinum Resistant High Grade Serous Adenocarcinoma of the Ovary, Primary Peritoneum, or Fallopian Tube, or Subjects with Peritoneal Mesothelioma with Recurrence after Prior Chemotherapy. NCT03608618. 2018. Available online: https://clinicaltrials.gov/study/NCT03608618 (accessed on 27 April 2024).
128. Zheng, H.; Peng, X.; Yang, S.; Li, X.; Huang, M.; Wei, S.; Zhang, S.; He, G.; Liu, J.; Fan, Q.; et al. Targeting tumor-associated macrophages in hepatocellular carcinoma: Biology, strategy, and immunotherapy. *Cell Death Discov.* **2023**, *9*, 65. [CrossRef] [PubMed]
129. Bao, D.; Zhao, J.; Zhou, X.; Yang, Q.; Chen, Y.; Zhu, J.; Yuan, P.; Yang, J.; Qin, T.; Wan, S.; et al. Mitochondrial fission-induced mtDNA stress promotes tumor-associated macrophage infiltration and HCC progression. *Oncogene* **2019**, *38*, 5007–5020. [CrossRef] [PubMed]
130. Sidney Kimmel Comprehensive Cancer Center at Johns Hopkins. A Phase II Study of Durvalumab (MEDI4736) in Combination with a CSF-1R Inhibitor (SNDX-6532) Following Chemo or Radio-Embolization for Patients with Intrahepatic Cholangiocarcinoma. NCT04301778. 2021. Available online: https://clin.larvol.com/trial-detail/NCT04301778 (accessed on 27 April 2024).
131. Cherney, R.J.; Anjanappa, P.; Selvakumar, K.; Batt, D.G.; Brown, G.D.; Rose, A.V.; Vuppugalla, R.; Chen, J.; Pang, J.; Xu, S.; et al. BMS-813160: A Potent CCR2 and CCR5 Dual Antagonist Selected as a Clinical Candidate. *ACS Med. Chem. Lett.* **2021**, *12*, 1753–1758. [CrossRef] [PubMed]
132. Icahn School of Medicine at Mount Sinai. Tisch Cancer Institute—BMS Study # CA027-005: Neoadjuvant Nivolumab + BMS-813160 (CCR2/5-inhibitor) or BMS-986253 (Anti-IL-8) for NSCLC or HCC. NCT04123379. 2020. Available online: https://www.mountsinai.org/clinical-trials/tisch-cancer-institute-bms-study-ca027-0055 (accessed on 27 April 2024).
133. Wilhelm, S.M.; Adnane, L.; Newell, P.; Villanueva, A.; Llovet, J.M.; Lynch, M. Preclinical overview of sorafenib, a multikinase inhibitor that targets both Raf and VEGF and PDGF receptor tyrosine kinase signaling. *Mol. Cancer Ther.* **2008**, *7*, 3129–3140. [CrossRef]
134. Hage, C.; Hoves, S.; Strauss, L.; Bissinger, S.; Prinz, Y.; Pöschinger, T.; Kiessling, F.; Ries, R.H. Sorafenib Induces Pyroptosis in Macrophages and Triggers Natural Killer Cell-Mediated Cytotoxicity Against Hepatocellular Carcinoma. *Hepatology* **2019**, *70*, 1280–1297. [CrossRef]
135. Zhang, W.; Zhu, X.-D.; Sun, H.-C.; Xiong, Y.-Q.; Zhuang, P.-Y.; Xu, H.-X.; Kong, L.-Q.; Wang, L.; Wu, W.-Z.; Tang, Z.-Y. Depletion of Tumor-Associated Macrophages Enhances the Effect of Sorafenib in Metastatic Liver Cancer Models by Antimetastatic and Antiangiogenic Effects. *Clin. Cancer Res.* **2010**, *16*, 3420–3430. [CrossRef] [PubMed]
136. Ain Shams University. Sorafenib Versus Best Supportive Care in Egyptian Hepatocellular Carcinoma Patients. Prospective Phase III Study. NCT02971696. 2016. Available online: https://clinicaltrials.gov/study/NCT02971696 (accessed on 8 March 2024).
137. Fudan University. Phase II Study of Sorafenib and Zoledronic Acid in Advanced HCC. NCT01259193. 2010. Available online: https://clinicaltrials.gov/study/NCT01259193 (accessed on 27 April 2024).
138. Kato, Y.; Tabata, K.; Kimura, T.; Yachie-Kinoshita, A.; Ozawa, Y.; Yamada, K.; Ito, J.; Tachino, S.; Hori, Y.; Matsuki, M.; et al. Lenvatinib plus anti-PD-1 antibody combination treatment activates CD8 + T cells through reduction of tumor-associated macrophage and activation of the interferon pathway. *PLoS ONE* **2019**, *14*, e0212513. [CrossRef]
139. Tan, H.-Y.; Wang, N.; Man, K.; Tsao, S.-W.; Che, C.-M.; Feng, Y. Autophagy-induced RelB/p52 activation mediates tumour-associated macrophage repolarisation and suppression of hepatocellular carcinoma by natural compound baicalin. *Cell Death Dis.* **2015**, *6*, e1942. [CrossRef]
140. Carisma Therapeutics Inc. A Phase 1, First in Human Study of Adenovirally Transduced Autologous Macrophages Engineered to Contain an Anti-HER2 Chimeric Antigen Receptor in Subjects with HER2 Overexpressing Solid Tumors. NCT04660929. 2021. Available online: https://clinicaltrials.gov/study/NCT04660929 (accessed on 27 April 2024).
141. Sung, H.; Ferlay, J.; Siegel, R.L.; Laversanne, M.; Soerjomataram, I.; Jemal, A.; Bray, F. Global Cancer Statistics 2020: GLOBOCAN Estimates of Incidence and Mortality Worldwide for 36 Cancers in 185 Countries. *CA Cancer J. Clin.* **2021**, *71*, 209–249. [CrossRef] [PubMed]
142. Qiu, S.-Q.; Waaijer, S.J.H.; Zwager, M.C.; De Vries, E.G.E.; Van Der Vegt, B.; Schröder, C.P. Tumor-associated macrophages in breast cancer: Innocent bystander or important player? *Cancer Treat. Rev.* **2018**, *70*, 178–189. [CrossRef] [PubMed]
143. Wen, J.; Wang, S.; Guo, R.; Liu, D. CSF1R inhibitors are emerging immunotherapeutic drugs for cancer treatment. *Eur. J. Med. Chem.* **2023**, *245*, 114884. [CrossRef] [PubMed]

144. Rugo, H. Enhancing Efficacy of Chemotherapy in Triple Negative/Basal-Like Breast Cancer by Targeting Macrophages: A Multicenter Phase Ib/II Study of PLX 3397 and Eribulin in Patients with Metastatic Breast Cancer. NCT01596751. 2012. Available online: https://clinicaltrials.gov/study/NCT01596751 (accessed on 27 April 2024).
145. Daiichi Sankyo. A Phase 1b Study to Assess the Safety of PLX3397 and Paclitaxel in Patients with Advanced Solid Tumors. NCT01525602. 2012. Available online: https://clinicaltrials.gov/study/NCT01525602 (accessed on 27 April 2024).
146. Djureinovic, D.; Wang, M.; Kluger, H.M. Agonistic CD40 Antibodies in Cancer Treatment. *Cancers* **2021**, *13*, 1302. [CrossRef] [PubMed]
147. Hoffmann-La Roche. An Open-Label, Multicenter, Dose-Escalation Phase Ib Study with Expansion Phase to Investigate the Safety, Pharmacokinetics, Pharmacodynamics, and Therapeutic Activity of Emactuzumab and RO7009789 Administered in Combination in Patients with Advanced Solid Tumors. NCT02760797. 2016. Available online: https://clinicaltrials.gov/study/NCT02760797 (accessed on 27 April 2024).
148. Machiels, J.-P.; Gomez-Roca, C.; Michot, J.-M.; Zamarin, D.; Mitchell, T.; Catala, G.; Eberst, L.; Jacob, W.; Jegg, A.M.; Cannarile, M.A.; et al. Phase Ib study of anti-CSF-1R antibody emactuzumab in combination with CD40 agonist selicrelumab in advanced solid tumor patients. *J. ImmunoTherapy Cancer* **2020**, *8*, e001153. [CrossRef] [PubMed]
149. NYU Langone Health. Phase II Evaluation of Imiquimod, a Topical Toll-like Receptor 7 (TLR7) Agonist in Breast Cancer Patients With Chest Wall Recurrence or Skin Metastases. NCT00899574. 2009. Available online: https://classic.clinicaltrials.gov/ct2/history/NCT00899574?V_6=View (accessed on 27 April 2024).
150. Adams, S.; Kozhaya, L.; Martiniuk, F.; Meng, T.-C.; Chiriboga, L.; Liebes, L.; Hochman, T.; Shuman, N.; Axelrod, D.; Speyer, J.; et al. Topical TLR7 Agonist Imiquimod Can Induce Immune-Mediated Rejection of Skin Metastases in Patients with Breast Cancer. *Clin. Cancer Res.* **2012**, *18*, 6748–6757. [CrossRef]
151. Masonic Cancer Center, University of Minnesota. Phase II Study of 852A Administered Subcutaneously in Patients with Metastatic Refractory Breast, Ovarian, Endometrial and Cervical Cancers. NCT00319748. 2006. Available online: https://clinicaltrials.gov/study/NCT00319748 (accessed on 27 April 2024).
152. Geller, M.A.; Cooley, S.; Argenta, P.A.; Downs, L.S.; Carson, L.F.; Judson, P.L.; Ghebre, R.; Weigel, B.; Panoskaltsis-Mortari, A.; Curtsinger, J.; et al. Toll-like receptor-7 agonist administered subcutaneously in a prolonged dosing schedule in heavily pretreated recurrent breast, ovarian, and cervix cancers. *Cancer Immunol. Immunother.* **2010**, *59*, 1877–1884. [CrossRef]
153. Li, L.; Yang, L.; Yang, S.; Wang, R.; Gao, H.; Lin, Z.; Zhao, Y.Y.; Tang, W.W.; Han, R.; Wang, W.J.; et al. Andrographolide suppresses breast cancer progression by modulating tumor-associated macrophage polarization through the Wnt/$\beta$-catenin pathway. *Phytother. Res.* **2022**, *36*, 4587–4603. [CrossRef]
154. Li, J.; Cai, H.; Sun, H.; Qu, J.; Zhao, B.; Hu, X.; Li, W.; Qian, Z.; Yu, X.; Kang, F.; et al. Extracts of Cordyceps sinensis inhibit breast cancer growth through promoting M1 macrophage polarization via NF-κB pathway activation. *J. Ethnopharmacol.* **2020**, *260*, 112969. [CrossRef]
155. Shiri, S.; Alizadeh, A.M.; Baradaran, B.; Farhanghi, B.; Shanehbandi, D.; Khodayari, S.; Khodayari, H.; Tavassoli, A. Dendrosomal Curcumin Suppresses Metastatic Breast Cancer in Mice by Changing M1/M2 Macrophage Balance in the Tumor Microenvironment. *Asian Pac. J. Cancer Prev.* **2015**, *16*, 3917–3922. [CrossRef]
156. Li, C.; Lei, S.; Ding, L.; Xu, Y.; Wu, X.; Wang, H.; Zhang, Z.; Gao, T.; Zhang, Y.; Li, L. Global burden and trends of lung cancer incidence and mortality. *Chin. Med. J.* **2023**, *136*, 1583–1590. [CrossRef] [PubMed]
157. Casanova-Acebes, M.; Dalla, E.; Leader, A.M.; LeBerichel, J.; Nikolic, J.; Morales, B.M.; Brown, M.; Chang, C.; Troncoso, L.; Chen, S.T.; et al. Tissue-resident macrophages provide a pro-tumorigenic niche to early NSCLC cells. *Nature* **2021**, *595*, 578–584. [CrossRef] [PubMed]
158. Gil-Bernabé, A.M.; Ferjančič, Š.; Tlalka, M.; Zhao, L.; Allen, P.D.; Im, J.H.; Watson, K.; Hill, S.A.; Amirkhosravi, A.; Francis, J.L.; et al. Recruitment of monocytes/macrophages by tissue factor-mediated coagulation is essential for metastatic cell survival and premetastatic niche establishment in mice. *Blood* **2012**, *119*, 3164–3175. [CrossRef] [PubMed]
159. Hoffmann-La Roche. Open-Label, Multicenter, Dose Escalation Phase Ib Study with Expansion Phase to Evaluate the Safety, Pharmacokinetics, and Activity of RO5509554 (Emactuzumab) and MPDL3280A (Atezolizumab) Administered in Combination in Patients with Advanced Solid Tumors. NCT02323191. 2015. Available online: https://clinicaltrials.gov/study/NCT02323191 (accessed on 27 April 2024).
160. Xia, L.; Zhu, X.; Zhang, L.; Xu, Y.; Chen, G.; Luo, J. EZH2 enhances expression of CCL5 to promote recruitment of macrophages and invasion in lung cancer. *Biotechnol. Appl. Biochem.* **2020**, *67*, 1011–1019. [CrossRef] [PubMed]
161. VA Office of Research and Development. Phase Ib/II Study of Safety and Efficacy of EZH2 Inhibitor, Tazemetostat, and PD-1 Blockade for Treatment of Advanced Non-small Cell Lung Cancer. NCT05467748. 2024. Available online: https://clinicaltrials.gov/study/NCT05467748 (accessed on 27 April 2024).
162. De Henau, O.; Rausch, M.; Winkler, D.; Campesato, L.F.; Liu, C.; Cymerman, D.H.; Budhu, S.; Ghosh, A.; Pink, M.; Tchaicha, J.; et al. Overcoming resistance to checkpoint blockade therapy by targeting PI3K$\gamma$ in myeloid cells. *Nature* **2016**, *539*, 443–447. [CrossRef] [PubMed]
163. Kaneda, M.M.; Messer, K.S.; Ralainirina, N.; Li, H.; Leem, C.J.; Gorjestani, S.; Woo, G.; Nguyen, A.V.; Figueiredo, C.C.; Foubert, P.; et al. PI3K$\gamma$ is a molecular switch that controls immune suppression. *Nature* **2016**, *539*, 437–442. [CrossRef] [PubMed]

164. Infinity Pharmaceuticals, Inc. A Phase 1/1b First-In-Human, Dose-Escalation Study to Evaluate the Safety, Tolerability, Pharmacokinetics, and Pharmacodynamics of IPI-549 Monotherapy and in Combination with Nivolumab in Subjects with Advanced Solid Tumors. NCT02637531. 2015. Available online: https://clinicaltrials.gov/study/NCT02637531 (accessed on 27 April 2024).
165. Wei, H.; Guo, C.; Zhu, R.; Zhang, C.; Han, N.; Liu, R.; Hua, B.; Li, Y.; Lin, H.; Yu, J. Shuangshen granules attenuate lung metastasis by modulating bone marrow differentiation through mTOR signalling inhibition. *J. Ethnopharmacol.* **2021**, *281*, 113305. [CrossRef] [PubMed]
166. Xu, F.; Cui, W.Q.; Wei, Y.; Cui, J.; Qiu, J.; Hu, L.L.; Gong, W.Y.; Dong, J.C.; Liu, B.J. Astragaloside IV inhibits lung cancer progression and metastasis by modulating macrophage polarization through AMPK signaling. *J. Exp. Clin. Cancer Res.* **2018**, *37*, 207. [CrossRef] [PubMed]
167. Kou, Y.; Li, Z.; Sun, Q.; Yang, S.; Wang, Y.; Hu, C.; Gu, H.; Wang, H.; Xu, H.; Li, Y.; et al. Prognostic value and predictive biomarkers of phenotypes of tumour-associated macrophages in colorectal cancer. *Scand. J. Immunol.* **2022**, *95*, e13137. [CrossRef]
168. Ålgars, A.; Irjala, H.; Vaittinen, S.; Huhtinen, H.; Sundström, J.; Salmi, M.; Ristamäki, R.; Jalkanen, S. Type and location of tumor-infiltrating macrophages and lymphatic vessels predict survival of colorectal cancer patients. *Int. J. Cancer* **2012**, *131*, 864–873. [CrossRef]
169. Jedinak, A.; Dudhgaonkar, S.; Sliva, D. Activated macrophages induce metastatic behavior of colon cancer cells. *Immunobiology* **2010**, *215*, 242–249. [CrossRef] [PubMed]
170. Majeti, R.; Chao, M.P.; Alizadeh, A.A.; Pang, W.W.; Jaiswal, S.; Gibbs, K.D.; van Rooijen, N.; Weissman, I.L. CD47 Is an Adverse Prognostic Factor and Therapeutic Antibody Target on Human Acute Myeloid Leukemia Stem Cells. *Cell* **2009**, *138*, 286–299. [CrossRef] [PubMed]
171. Chao, M.P.; McKenna, K.M.; Cha, A.; Feng Dd Liu, J.; Sikic, B.; Majeti, R.; Weissman, I.; Takimoto, C.; Volkmer, J. The anti-CD47 antibody Hu5F9-G4 is a novel immune checkpoint inhibitor with synergistic efficacy in combination with clinically active cancer targeting antibodies. *Cancer Immunol. Res.* **2016**, *4* (Suppl. 11), PR13. [CrossRef]
172. Willingham, S.B.; Volkmer, J.-P.; Gentles, A.J.; Sahoo, D.; Dalerba, P.; Mitra, S.S.; Wang, J.; Contreras-Trujillo, H.; Martin, R.; Cohen, J.D.; et al. The CD47-signal regulatory protein alpha (SIRPa) interaction is a therapeutic target for human solid tumors. *Proc. Natl. Acad. Sci. USA* **2012**, *109*, 6662–6667. [CrossRef]
173. Gilead Sciences. A Phase 1b/2 Trial of Hu5F9-G4 in Combination with Cetuximab in Patients with Solid Tumors and Advanced Colorectal Cancer. NCT02953782. 2016. Available online: https://clinicaltrials.gov/study/NCT02953782 (accessed on 27 April 2024).
174. Myers, K.V.; Amend, S.R.; Pienta, K.J. Targeting Tyro3, Axl and MerTK (TAM receptors): Implications for macrophages in the tumor microenvironment. *Mol. Cancer* **2019**, *18*, 94. [CrossRef] [PubMed]
175. Pfizer. A Phase 1, Open-Label, Multi-Center, Dose-Finding, Pharmacokinetic, Safety and Tolerability Study of PF 07265807 in Participants with Selected Advanced or Metastatic Solid Tumor Malignancies. NCT04458259. 2020. Available online: https://www.clinicaltrials.gov/study/NCT04458259 (accessed on 27 April 2024).
176. Centre Leon Berard. A Dose Escalation Phase I Study with an Extension Part Evaluating the Safety and Activity of an Anti-PDL1 Antibody (DURVALUMAB) Combined with a Small Molecule CSF-1R Tyrosine Kinase Inhibitor (PEXIDARTINIB) in Patients with Metastatic/Advanced Pancreatic or Colorectal Cancers. NCT02777710. 2016. Available online: https://clinicaltrials.gov/study/NCT02777710 (accessed on 27 April 2024).
177. Lee, N.Y.; Kim, Y.; Kim, Y.S.; Shin, J.-H.; Rubin, L.P.; Kim, Y. β-Carotene exerts anti-colon cancer effects by regulating M2 macrophages and activated fibroblasts. *J. Nutr. Biochem.* **2020**, *82*, 108402. [CrossRef] [PubMed]
178. Novartis Pharmaceuticals. A Phase Ib/II, Open Label, Multicenter Study of MCS110 in Combination with PDR001 in Patients with Advanced Malignancies. NCT02807844. 2016. Available online: https://clinicaltrials.gov/study/NCT02807844 (accessed on 27 April 2024).
179. Abramson Cancer Center at Penn Medicine. A Phase I/IIa, Dose-Ranging Safety and Efficacy Study of Topical Resiquimod for the Treatment of Early Stage Cutaneous T Cell Lymphoma. NCT01676831. 2012. Available online: https://clinicaltrials.gov/study/NCT01676831 (accessed on 27 April 2024).
180. Centocor, Inc. A Phase 1 Study of CNTO 888, a Human Monoclonal Antibody Against CC-Chemokine Ligand 2 in Subjects with Solid Tumors. NCT00537368. 2007. Available online: https://clinicaltrials.gov/study/NCT00537368 (accessed on 27 April 2024).
181. Sandhu, S.K.; Papadopoulos, K.; Fong, P.C.; Patnaik, A.; Messiou, C.; Olmos, D.; Wang, G.; Tromp, B.J.; Puchalski, T.A.; Balkwill, F.; et al. A first-in-human, first-in-class, phase I study of carlumab (CNTO 888), a human monoclonal antibody against CC-chemokine ligand 2 in patients with solid tumors. *Cancer Chemother. Pharmacol.* **2013**, *71*, 1041–1050. [CrossRef] [PubMed]
182. Centocor Research & Development, Inc. An Open-Label, Multicenter, Phase 2 Study of Single-Agent CNTO 888 (an Anti-CCL2 Monoclonal Antibody) for the Treatment of Subjects with Metastatic Castrate-Resistant Prostate Cancer. NCT00992186. 2009. Available online: https://clinicaltrials.gov/study/NCT00992186 (accessed on 27 April 2024).
183. Pediatric Brain Tumor Consortium. Phase I Study to Evaluate the Safety and Tolerability of the CD40 Agonistic Monoclonal Antibody APX005M in Pediatric Subjects with Recurrent/Refractory Brain Tumors and Newly Diagnosed Brain Stem Glioma. NCT03389802. 2018. Available online: https://clinicaltrials.gov/study/NCT03389802 (accessed on 27 April 2024).
184. Kim, Y.-D.; Park, S.-M.; Ha, H.C.; Lee, A.R.; Won, H.; Cha, H.; Cho, S.; Cho, J.M. HDAC Inhibitor, CG-745, Enhances the Anti-Cancer Effect of Anti-PD-1 Immune Checkpoint Inhibitor by Modulation of the Immune Microenvironment. *J. Cancer* **2020**, *11*, 4059–4072. [CrossRef] [PubMed]

185. National Cancer Institute. Phase II Study of Histone Deacetylase Inhibitor SAHA (Vorinostat) in Patients with Metastatic Thyroid Carcinoma. NCT00134043. 2005. Available online: https://clinicaltrials.gov/study/NCT00134043 (accessed on 27 April 2024).
186. Daiichi Sankyo. A Double-Blind, Randomized, Placebo-Controlled Phase 3 Study of Orally Administered PLX3397 in Subjects with Pigmented Villonodular Synovitis or Giant Cell Tumor of the Tendon Sheath. NCT02371369. 2015. Available online: https://clinicaltrials.gov/study/NCT02371369 (accessed on 27 April 2024).
187. AmMax Bio, Inc. A Phase 1, First-In-Human Study Evaluating the Safety, Tolerability, Pharmacokinetics, and Pharmacokinetics of AMG 820 in Adult Subjects with Advanced Solid Tumors. NCT01444404. 2008. Available online: https://clinicaltrials.gov/study/NCT01444404 (accessed on 27 April 2024).
188. Petty, A.J.; Owen, D.H.; Yang, Y.; Huang, X. Targeting Tumor-Associated Macrophages in Cancer Immunotherapy. *Cancers* **2021**, *13*, 5318. [CrossRef]
189. Spierenburg, G.; Van Der Heijden, L.; Van Langevelde, K.; Szuhai, K.; Bovée, J.V.G.M.; Van De Sande, M.A.J.; Gelderblom, H. Tenosynovial giant cell tumors (TGCT): Molecular biology, drug targets and non-surgical pharmacological approaches. *Expert Opin. Ther. Targets* **2022**, *26*, 333–345. [CrossRef]
190. Razak, A.R.; Cleary, J.M.; Moreno, V.; Boyer, M.; Calvo Aller, E.; Edenfield, W.; Tie, J.; Harvey, R.D.; Rutten, A.; Shah, M.A.; et al. Safety and efficacy of AMG 820, an anti-colony-stimulating factor 1 receptor antibody, in combination with pembrolizumab in adults with advanced solid tumors. *J. Immunother. Cancer* **2020**, *8*, e001006. [CrossRef]
191. Quail, D.F.; Bowman, R.L.; Akkari, L.; Quick, M.L.; Schuhmacher, A.J.; Huse, J.T.; Holland, E.C.; Sutton, J.C.; Joyce, J.A. The tumor microenvironment underlies acquired resistance to CSF-1R inhibition in gliomas. *Science* **2016**, *352*, aad3018. [CrossRef]
192. Cassetta, L.; Pollard, J.W. Targeting macrophages: Therapeutic approaches in cancer. *Nat. Rev. Drug Discov.* **2018**, *17*, 887–904. [CrossRef]
193. Lu, Y.; Sun, Q.; Guan, Q.; Zhang, Z.; He, Q.; He, J.; Ji, Z.; Tian, W.; Xu, X.; Liu, Y.; et al. The XOR-IDH3α axis controls macrophage polarization in hepatocellular carcinoma. *J. Hepatol.* **2023**, *79*, 1172–1184. [CrossRef]
194. Zhu, L.; Li, X.J.; Gangadaran, P.; Jing, X.; Ahn, B.-C. Tumor-associated macrophages as a potential therapeutic target in thyroid cancers. *Cancer Immunol. Immunother.* **2023**, *72*, 3895–3917. [CrossRef]

*pharmaceutics*

MDPI

*Review*

# Therapies Targeting Immune Cells in Tumor Microenvironment for Non-Small Cell Lung Cancer

**Wei Ye [1], Meiye Li [1] and Kewang Luo [1,2,*]**

[1] School of Pharmaceutical Sciences, Southern Medical University, Guangzhou 510091, China; yeyewei2023@gmail.com (W.Y.); MeiyeLi2023@gmail.com (M.L.)

[2] People's Hospital of Longhua, Affiliated Longhua People's Hospital, Southern Medical University, Shenzhen 518109, China

* Correspondence: kewangluo@126.com or kewangluo@smu.edu.cn

**Abstract:** The tumor microenvironment (TME) plays critical roles in immune modulation and tumor malignancies in the process of cancer development. Immune cells constitute a significant component of the TME and influence the migration and metastasis of tumor cells. Recently, a number of therapeutic approaches targeting immune cells have proven promising and have already been used to treat different types of cancer. In particular, PD-1 and PD-L1 inhibitors have been used in the first-line setting in non-small cell lung cancer (NSCLC) with PD-L1 expression $\geq$1%, as approved by the FDA. In this review, we provide an introduction to the immune cells in the TME and their efficacies, and then we discuss current immunotherapies in NSCLC and scientific research progress in this field.

**Keywords:** NSCLC; TME; immune cells; immunotherapies

## 1. Introduction

Cancer is one of the leading causes of mortality worldwide [1], contributing to a reduction in life expectancy in many nations [2]. The Global Burden of Cancer 2020 (GLOBOCAN 2020) database from the World Health Organization estimates the most recent incidence and mortality rates for 36 varieties of cancer as well as cancer trends in 185 nations. This latest cancer report demonstrated that there were almost 19.3 million new cases of cancer and close to 10 million cancer-related deaths in 2020, and that by 2040 there would be 28.4 million new cancer cases worldwide [3,4]. The most recent edition of the International Agency for Research on Cancer (IARC) World Cancer Report shows that cancer is the primary cause of death among people aged 30 to 69 [5]. Lung cancer is the leading cause of cancer-related deaths and ranks second in terms of cancer incidence worldwide, with an estimated 1.8 million deaths (18%) in 2020 [4]. Non-small cell lung cancer (NSCLC) accounts for 85% of all lung cancer cases and is one of the most fatal tumors worldwide [6]. According to the Chinese National Cancer Center's statistics for 2016, the number of lung cancer cases was about 787,000 and the number of deaths was about 630,000, making it the primary cause of mortality (21.7%) in China [7]. In recent years, the survival rate of NSCLC patients has increased due to the development of surgery, radiotherapy, and other treatments. However, the 5-year survival rate remains low, with a rate of 15% [8].

The tumor microenvironment (TME) is widely considered to be vital in dynamically modulating tumor growth and affecting therapeutic effectiveness, and numerous therapeutic approaches targeting components of the TME have been designed recently. The TME is defined as the cellular environment. It is composed of various cell types, such as cancer cells, immune cells, stromal cells, and cytokines as well as chemokines [9,10]. Much scientific research indicates that regulating a particular TME component can increase cancer survival rates. Garon et al., revealed that the combination of docetaxel and ramucirumab, which targeted vascular endothelial growth factor receptor-2 (VEGFR-2), could effectively prolong the lifetime of NSCLC patients [11]. Gocheva et al., illustrated that Tenascin-C, one of the components of the extracellular matrix, was much more prevalent in primary and metastatic lung cancers than in normal tissue, which was closely related to lung cancer patient survival [12]. Moreover, a study by Lambrechts analyzed the TME cell profile of lung cancer and discovered that a subpopulation of Tregs from NSCLC was related to a poor prognosis for lung adenocarcinoma [13].

Immune cells have been shown to be crucial in the TME. Tumor cells can develop a variety of immunosuppressive mechanisms, causing cancer cells to evade immune surveillance and undergo immune escape, resulting in tumor proliferation after treatment [14]. Different types of immune cells within the TME are able to activate an immune response through a number of interactions, and lead to a substantial impact on tumor progression and metastasis [15]. In the past few decades, a number of immunotherapies have already been used to treat different types of cancer. Immunotherapy is an essential part of cancer therapy, with better efficacy and fewer side effects than conventional chemotherapies. Rodriguez-Garcia demonstrated that CAR-T cell therapy, which was approved by the FDA for use in clinical treatment for B cell acute lymphoblastic leukemia, is an extremely successful therapy for hematological malignancies [16,17]. There is also increased promise for treatment of tumors with immunotherapies targeting Dendritic Cells (DCs), such as DC vaccines. DCs can induce tumor-directed immune responses in cancer patients by activating cytotoxic T cells [18]. The treatment of advanced NSCLC has undergone a fundamental change due to the advent of immunotherapy in recent years. The use of immune checkpoint inhibitors (ICIs) alone or in combination with chemotherapy has become the primary immunotherapy strategy for advanced or metastatic NSCLC without driver mutations [19]. The FDA has approved the use of ICI therapies such as nivolumab, pembrolizumab and atezolizumab as first-line therapy for NSCLC patients with high PD-L1 expression [20]. Nevertheless, a large proportion of patients still suffer from disease progression.

In this review, we focus on the immune cells in the TME and tumor development. We also discuss the mainstream immunotherapies currently used to treat NSCLC and some novel therapeutic approaches used in the clinic, highlighting therapies that are under clinical trials or that have been approved.

## 2. Immune Cells in Tumor Microenvironment

Immune cells are a fundamental part of the TME and are essential for both pro- and antitumor immune responses [21]. The cells of the immune system include both innate immune cells, such as macrophages, neutrophils, mast cells, DCs, and MDSC and NK cells, and adaptive T and B lymphatic immune cells [22]. Early studies using immunohistochemistry to identify immune cells in NSCLC found that NSCLC tumors contain multiple types of immune cells, including T cells, B cells, macrophages, NK cells, and DCs, and many studies have demonstrated a crucial link between immune cells and the survival of NSCLC patients [23,24]. It is clear that immune cells are a non-negligible presence in the TME. Most importantly, the immune system is normally capable of monitoring, recognizing, and destroying cancerous cells [25]. However, due to their close proximity to tumor cells, or as a result of chemokine and cytokine communication, the immune cells within the TME are able to evade identification and annihilation by the host immune system [26]. The occurrence of lung cancer and the entire process from early lung cancer to metastatic lung cancer are considered to depend on the immune escape mechanism [27,28]. Therefore, the role that immune cells play in the TME and the mechanisms by which they influence tumor growth deserve to be discussed. In the following part, we introduce the main immune cells in the TME, including T cells, tumor-associated macrophages, dendritic cells, and natural killer cells (Figure 1).

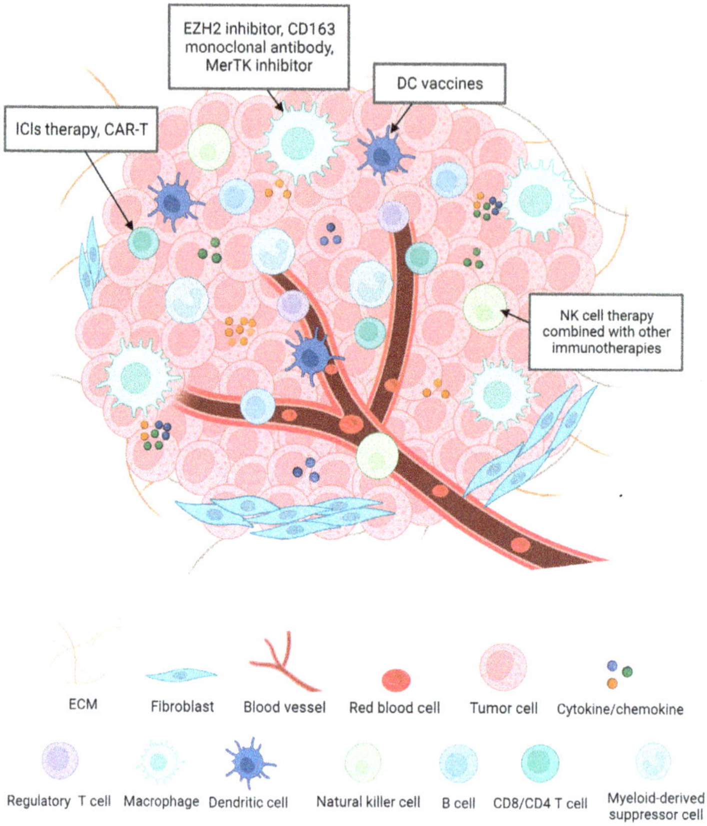


**Figure 1.** Tumor microenvironment and immunotherapies. The TME is composed of various cell types, such as cancer cells, immune cells, and stromal cells, and cytokines as well as chemokines. These growth factors and cytokines are essential for communication between the TME and other cell types. Due to the importance of immune cells in the TME and in tumor progression, a number of immunotherapies have been developed against tumors in recent years. Immunotherapies that have been approved for use or that are undergoing clinical trials focus on TAMs, DCs, T cells, and NK cells as their main targets.

### 2.1. T Cells

T cells are an essential part of the immune system, which is responsible for defending cells against cancer and viruses [29]. T cells can be further divided into three subpopulations: cytotoxic T lymphocytes (CTLs), T helper cells (Ths), and Tregs [30]. CTLs are the cells in the TME with direct tumor-killing power, Ths cells help to postpone tumor growth, and Treg cells are typically associated with poor outcomes in tumor patients.

CTLs (which include cytotoxic CD8$^+$ T cells and CD4$^+$ T cells) in the TME can directly destroy malignant tumors. As major killers of pathogens and cancers, CD8$^+$ T cells are the preferred immune cells in the fight against cancer [31,32]. The presence of cytotoxic CD8$^+$ T lymphocytes is also linked to better outcomes in NSCLC patients [33]. When CD8$^+$ T cells develop into cytotoxic T cells, naive CD8$^+$ T cells are connected to the peptide major histocompatibility complex (MHC) on antigen-presenting cells (APCs) via their T-cell receptors (TCRs), and are activated by co-stimulatory signals and extracellular cytokines. These CD8$^+$ T cells subsequently become effectors, and their activation enables them to attack cancer cells directly [34]. In addition to actively destroying tumor cells, CD8$^+$ T cells have the capacity to prevent tumor angiogenesis by secreting interferon-$\gamma$

(IFN-$\gamma$) [35]. However, prolonged antigenic stimulation transforms $CD8^+$ T cells in the TME into a T cell-depleted hypoactive state (including progressive loss of effector function and persistent expression of inhibitory receptors), which prevents the tumor cell-killing function of $CD8^+$ T cells from proceeding normally [36,37]. Apart from $CD8^+$ T cells, $CD4^+$ T cells are essential for tumor elimination. $CD4^+$ T cells can directly contribute to $CD8^+$ T cell activation, support $CD8^+$ T cells in the formation of memory CTL, and enhance $CD8^+$ T cell proliferation by generating interleukin(IL)-2 [38,39]. Furthermore, $CD4^+$ T cells can help activate $CD8^+$ T cells by delivering tumor antigens to $CD8^+$ T cells or by triggering the production of cytokines and suppressor molecules [40].

Ths cells are generated by cytokine-specific polarization or TCR-signaling activation in the TME, and they can assist $CD4^+$ T lymphocytes in producing cytotoxicity and destroying tumor cells [41]. Th1 and Th9 cells in the TME boost $CD8^+$ T cells' ability to fight tumors, mainly by secreting IL-4 and IFN-$\gamma$, which are linked to a favorable prognosis in various cancer types [9,42].

Tregs normally inhibit autoimmunity by restricting the immune system's reaction to autoantigens [43]. However, Tregs in the TME can promote cancer growth by reducing the function of lymphatic and bone marrow immune cells [44]. Many studies have reported that Treg cells in the TME suppress effector T cells directly by generating higher levels of cytokines than those associated with T-cell activation, resulting in immunosuppressive TME and the progression of tumors [45–48]. On the other hand, Treg cells are capable of promoting tumor growth and metastasis by secreting growth factors, interacting with stromal cells, and undergoing immune escape [43]. A higher Treg-to-effector T-cell ratio in NSCLC tumor tissue has been linked to a worse prognosis [49].

### *2.2. Tumor-Associated Macrophages (TAMs)*

The majority of immune cells that infiltrate the TME are tumor-associated macrophages, which influence tumor angiogenesis and metastasis and are related to a poor prognosis for various cancers [50,51]. In the TME, TAMs may be differentiated into classical activated macrophages (M1) or, alternatively, activated macrophages (M2) [52,53]. Phenotype M1 is able to directly kill tumor cells by producing nitric oxide and reactive oxygen species, or by secreting pro-inflammatory cytokines such as tumor necrosis factor-$\alpha$ (TNF-$\alpha$), IL-6, and IFN-$\gamma$ [50,54,55]. Additionally, through the process of antibody-dependent cell-mediated cytotoxicity (ADCC), M1 has the capacity to eradicate malignant cells [56]. In contrast, M2 stimulates angiogenesis, tissue healing, and cancer-cell proliferation by secreting anti-inflammatory cytokines such as IL-4, IL-1, and VEGF [57–59]. As macrophages are highly plastic in the TME, they convert between M1 and M2 in response to microenvironmental factors (cytokines, growth factors, chemokines, inflammation, hypoxia, and infection), thereby inhibiting the antitumor response and producing immunosuppressive TME. This is a process known as macrophage polarization [52,59,60]. It has been found that tumor cells express significant amounts of colony-stimulating factor 1, C-C pattern ligand 2 (CCL2), and monocyte chemotactic protein-1, something which contributes to TAMs' function in tumor development [61]. At the same time, TAMs activate tumor cells by activating transcription factors (STAT3 and NF-κB) to produce VEGF and matrix metalloproteinases (MMPs) to promote tumor angiogenesis [51,62]. As the relationship between TAMs and cancer becomes clearer, TAMs have become a desirable target for the development of novel immunotherapies. It has been demonstrated that activation of TAM receptors reduces resistance to ICI treatment in NSCLC patients, indicating that the combination of the two strategies may be beneficial for these patients [63].

### *2.3. Dendritic Cells (DCs)*

As the most powerful APCs, DCs serve as central regulators of the adaptive immune response and connect innate and adaptive immunity [64–66]. DCs are inherently plastic and can be stratified into a variety of subtypes [15]. According to their phenotypes and their functions in the TME, DCs are typically divided into two major subgroups: plasmacytoid DCs (pDCs) and myeloid DCs (mDCs) [67,68].

A primary function of pDCs is to produce IFN-I, which is needed to counteract the antiviral immune response [65,69]. It has also been suggested that pDCs may have potential as APCs due to the MHC-II and co-stimulatory molecules they express at steady state [70]. In the TME, the function of pDCs is controversial. Tumor-infiltrating pDCs are reported to produce immunosuppressive and carcinogenic effects; however, due to their ability to secrete INF-I and TNF-α, pDCs are potential therapeutic targets for combating cancer [71,72].

In the TME, conventional DCs (cDCs), as the typical representatives of mDCs, can be further subdivided into cDC1 and cDC2 spectrums [73]. cDC1 is regulated by transcription factors IRF8, ID2, and BATF3, while cDC2 is regulated by transcription factors IRF4, ID2, ZEB2, and Notch2 [74]. cDC1 is able to cross-present antigens and present exogenous antigens to $CD8^+$ T cells on MHC-I, activating $CD8^+$ T cells and making them the primary mediators of antitumor immunity [75]. Hence, cDC1 has the unique ability to induce intracellular infections and encourage the immune system to reject malignant cells [15,65,76]. The cDC2 exhibits enhanced presentation of the MHC II antigen. In contrast to cDC1, cDC2 presents only exogenous antigens without cross-presentation and activates $CD4^+$ T cells selectively, making it the most effective activation and expansion agent for $CD4^+$ T cells [77,78].

It has been shown that immunogenic DCs secrete substantial quantities of inflammatory cytokines, including TNF-α, IL-12, IL-6, and IL-8, which may improve the clinical outcomes of tumor patients [79,80]. Despite this, the uptake of antigen by DCs in the TME is often insufficient. The phenomenon is caused by aberrant expression of some tumor-derived chemokines on DCs within the TME, resulting in the suppression of DC invasion [67]. The maturation state of DCs and specific markers expressed by different subgroups of DCs have been considered significant indicators of prognosis and prediction in human cancer. DC-based vaccines have been developed to induce and maintain immune responses [78]. Consequently, the use of DC therapy in conjunction with other immunotherapies to reduce immunosuppressive TME can serve as a future treatment strategy for cancer. Zhong et al., found that chemotherapy combined with a DC vaccine significantly inhibited tumor growth in a mouse model of NSCLC [81].

### 2.4. Natural Killer Cells (NK Cells)

As innate lymphocytes, NK cells can stimulate the immune system to destroy cancer cells [82]. It has been demonstrated that NK cells can kill tumors by direct cytotoxic killing of target cells [83]. Besides, NK cells can inhibit tumor growth by inducing pro-inflammatory cytokines, which include IFN-α, TNF-α, and granulocyte macrophage colony-stimulating factor [84].

NK cells have been divided into two distinct subpopulations based on CD56 expression levels, $CD56^{bright}CD16^-$ and $CD56^{dim}CD16$ [85]. When $CD56^{bright}$ NK cells are exposed to pro-inflammatory cytokines including IL-12, IL-15, and IL-18, they produce additional cytokines to regulate adaptive immunity and cause cytotoxicity [86,87]. $CD56^{dim}$ NK cells can directly mediate the death of infected and cancer cells via cytotoxicity and cytokine production [86,88]. NK cells may also eliminate MHC class I tumors and carry out antigen presentation on their own, creating a connection between innate and adaptive immunity [89].

NK cells are associated with both the killing of tumor cells and the prevention of cancer progression. However, NK cell toxicity is decreased in the TME [9,90]. A change in angiogenesis may be responsible for this, as well as insufficient access to nutrients and oxygen. Many studies have reported that hypoxia and the secretion of transforming growth factor-β (TGF-β) and other cytokines in the TME limit the activity of NK cells [91–93]. TGF-β can reduce the antitumor effect of NK cells by transforming peripheral $CD4^+$ T cells activated into Treg cells [92,94]. One study found that delivering TGF-β inhibitors and selenocysteine to breast cancer cells can reduce TGF-β in the TME, improve NK cell activity, and increase antitumor capability, suggesting that NK-targeted immunotherapies may be promising [95].

### *2.5. Other Types of Immune Cells That Affect Tumor Development*

Apart from the immune cells discussed above, neutrophils, MDSCs, and B cells also play crucial roles in the TME.

Neutrophils, the most abundant innate immune cells in the bone marrow and peripheral blood, serve a complex and important function in cancer development [96]. In many cancer patients, neutrophil peripheral blood counts are elevated, and neutrophil-to-lymphocyte ratios are independent prognostic factors [97,98]. In the TME, neutrophils produce MMP-9 to stimulate angiogenesis, boosting cancer growth and offering extra immune-escape pathways for cancer cells [97]. The neutrophil extracellular trap (NET) can promote tumor progression, metastasis, invasion, and angiogenesis [99,100]. Several studies have shown that mice with lung cancer, breast cancer, and chronic myeloid leukemia are more likely to release NET than healthy mice [100–102].

MDSCs are a heterogeneous cell population composed of progenitor cells derived from bone marrow, immature macrophages, immature granulocytes, and immature DCs [103]. As part of the TME, they promote tumor angiogenesis and metastasis [104]. In Hinshaw's study, it was found that MDSC could be stimulated in the TME and released chemokines including NO, CCL3, and CCL4, which inhibited innate and adaptive immune responses [15]. In addition, MDSCs promote epithelial mesenchymal transition by secreting IL-6, which increases angiogenesis and speeds up tumor progression [105,106].

Tumor-infiltrating B cells are responsible for antibody production, antigen presentation, and cytokine secretion in tumors, as well as for complementing T-cell-mediated antitumor immunity [9,107]. Recent studies demonstrated that B cells in the TME have prognostic value in various tumors [108,109].

## 3. Target Immune Cells against NSCLC

Given the crucial roles of immune cells in immunomodulation and tumor progression in the TME, strategies to target immune cells in the TME hold significant promise. In the past few decades, a number of immunotherapies have already been used to treat different types of cancer. Current research indicates that immunotherapies targeting ICIs when utilized in NSCLC patients have exhibited promising results in terms of five-year survival and progression-free survival (PFS) when compared with previous treatments [110,111].

In the following part of our review, the immunotherapies (Figure 1) used in NSCLC in clinical trials and in scientific research are discussed.

### *3.1. Target T Cells against NSCLC*

T cells are usually recognized as the most essential immune cells in attacking malignancies [112]. Among T-cell-targeted immunotherapies, treatments using ICIs have undergone the most extensive research and been approved by the FDA. This strategy keeps the antitumor immune response in the TME, bringing a new era of cancer immunotherapy [113,114]. An ICI is an immune checkpoint protein that maintains the ability of T cells to destroy tumors by binding to their partner proteins. Immune checkpoint molecules include CTLA-4, PD-1, etc. (Figure 2), and their role is to maintain an immune balance and prevent an immune response from attacking normal tissues and cells in the body. Immunotherapy drugs are mainly monoclonal antibodies, which can block immunosuppressive effect, allowing T cells to recognize and attack cancer cells, thereby enhancing immune responses, by binding with their partner proteins. These drugs (antibodies) are preferentially designed as ICIs [115]. The main agents undergoing clinical trial and research are nivolumab and pembrolizumab (PD-1 antibody), atezolizumab (PD-L1 antibody), and ipilimumab (CTLA-4 antibody) [116].

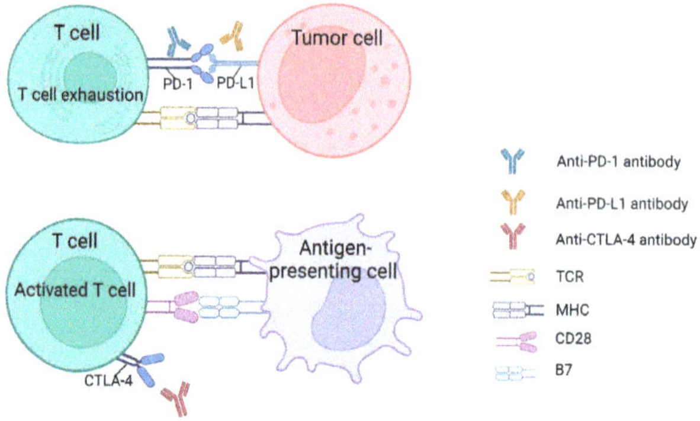


**Figure 2.** Two of the most common targeting pathways for ICIs (anti-CTLA-4 and anti-PD-1/PD-L1). PD-1 receptor on T cells leads to T cell exhaustion by binding to its ligand PD-L1 on tumor cells. Targeted antibodies that block PD-1 or PD-L1 prevent T cell exhaustion and maintain the ability of T cells to destroy tumors. T cells can be activated through two primary mechanisms. T cell receptors (TCRs) on antigen-presenting cells (APCs) present antigens with the major histocompatibility complex (MHC) and activate T lymphocytes. Additionally, the binding of CD28 on T cells and B7 on APCs can result in T-cell activation and antitumor activity. CTLA-4 antigen limits T cell-activation by competing for CD28 binding to B7 on the T cell surface, resulting in a decrease in T cell antitumor capacity. Therefore, the use of anti-CTLA-4 drugs can prevent the competitive behavior of CTLA-4 antibodies and support normal T cell-activation.

According to scientific studies, ICIs have a significant impact on patients' prognoses, and have become the first-line therapy for most individuals with advanced lung cancer [117–119]. PD-1 receptor is mainly expressed on activated T cells, and by adhering to ligands PD-L1 and PD-L2, it suppresses the antitumor activity of T cells [120,121]. Expression of PD-L1 is widespread in cancer cells and elevated in the TME, leading to suppression of the antitumor immune response by limiting the signals that activate T cells [112,121]. Nivolumab is an antibody against PD-1. As demonstrated in a clinical trial (NCT01642004), among patients with metastatic NSCLC (mNSCLC) (stage III patients) for whom platinum-based chemotherapy had failed, improved overall survival (OS) and substantially improved PFS were seen in individuals treated with nivolumab [122]. An additional study comparing the efficacy of nivolumab and docetaxel (a chemotherapy drug) in patients with mNSCLC (NCT01673867) also discovered positive results for nivolumab [123]. As a result, nivolumab is the first ICI targeting PD-1 to receive FDA approval for use in the treatment of patients with mNSCLC. Pembrolizumab is also an anti-PD-1 antibody. Patients with mNSCLC who participated in a randomized, phase III trial (NCT02142738) demonstrated significant improvements in 6-month PFS, OS, and objective response rate (ORR) when compared with platinum-based chemotherapy [124]. Furthermore, a phase III trial (NCT03850444) comparing pembrolizumab to platinum-based chemotherapy in patients with advanced or mNSCLC found that pembrolizumab had a meaningful effect in individuals whose PD-L1 expression was higher than 50% [125]. The FDA has approved pembrolizumab as a first-line treatment for patients with PD-L1 levels $\geq$ 1%, and these results have led to the authorization of pembrolizumab by the European Medicines Agency (EMA) as a first-line treatment for patients with PD-L1 levels $\geq$ 50% [20]. Atezolizumab, a PD-L1 antibody, has also been approved by the FDA and the EMA as a single-agent treatment for patients with mNSCLC with high PD-L1 expression [20,126], having shown significant benefits in treating patients with NSCLC in clinical trial NCT02409342 (Table 1).

Moreover, ICIs includes antibodies against CTLA-4, which inhibits T-cell proliferation by competing binding with CD28 on the cell surface [127]. Since the antitumor effect of CTLA-4 antibodies is mainly related to T-cell initiation in lymph nodes and the TME, this may offset some ICI resistance [120,128,129]. Ipilimumab is a therapeutic antibody targeting

CTLA-4 [130]. A trial (NCT02477826) has been carried out on patients with stage IV NSCLC to compare the efficacies of three different strategies: nivolumab alone, the combination of nivolumab and ipilimumab, and the combination of chemotherapy with nivolumab plus platinum [131]. Recent findings from this trial indicated that the combination of nivolumab and ipilimumab enhanced OS for those patients with PD-L1 expression levels of more than 1%, suggesting that the ICI two-drug combination could be considered as a first-line therapy for NSCLC. Meanwhile, the results of this trial also implied a positive outcome from the combination of chemotherapy and anti-PD-1 drugs [132]. In addition, in a clinical trial of patients with metastatic squamous NSCLC treated with carboplatin-paclitaxel/nab-paclitaxel with or without pembrolizumab (NCT03875092), it was found that PFS and OS improved significantly when anti-PD-1 medications were taken in conjunction with chemotherapy [133] (Table 1). Combination therapy with ICIs has been shown to have great potential in terms of antitumor response. Apart from chemotherapy and ICIs, many studies indicate that inhibitors targeting IDO, VEGF, lymphocyte activation3 and T-cell immunoglobulin mucin 3 may also be considered as future combination options [134–137].

In addition to the immunotherapy of ICIs against NSCLC, chimeric antigen receptor-modified T cells (CAR-T cells, a type of genetically engineered T cells) treatment is another very rapidly developing form of cellular immunotherapy [138]. Synthetic CAR vectors are genetically engineered to recognize and bind specifically to tumor cell surface antigens (such as CD19) to achieve antitumor effects in this therapy [139,140]. However, the presence of tumor-associated antigens (TAAs) in NSCLC has been heterogeneous in terms of both intensity and distribution, severely limiting the clinical efficacy of CAR-T therapy [141].

Recently, understanding of the molecular typing of NSCLC has been significantly enhanced, because of research into the causative genes of NSCLC patients [142,143]. It is clear that the molecular typing of NSCLC can be classified into three groups. The first category refers to genes with clinical relevance, such as KRAS, HER2, ROS1, TP53, BRAF, and NTRK, and relevant medications targeting these genes are currently being researched [142,144]. Several studies have demonstrated that patients with mutant NSCLC, such as KRAS, BRAF, and TP53, can benefit from ICIs [145–147]. The second category consists of treatable mutation-driver genes. The current focus of therapies based on mutation-driver genes in NSCLC are epidermal growth factor receptor (EGFR) and anaplastic lymphoma kinase (ALK) [142]. Because of the mutations in EGRF or ALK, the efficacy of ICI treatment in these NSCLC patients is not obvious [19,148]. Many targeted medicines that target the driver genes of EGFR and ALK have had some success [143]. The third category includes biomarkers that have some association efficacy, such as PD-L1 and TMB [149,150]. In NSCLC patients with mutations in EGFR, the PD-L1 expression is predominantly reduced. Consequently, anti-PD-1 ICIs are ineffective in this group of patients [151]. However, EGFR-tyrosine kinase inhibitors (EGFR-TKIs) have been developed to treat NSCLC patients. First-generation EGFR-TKIs, such as gefitinib, erlotinib, and ecotinib, have been shown to be effective in treating patients with EGFR-sensitive mutant NSCLC. Afatinib is a second-generation EGFR-TKI that was approved by the FDA and the EMA in 2013 used to treat adults with advanced, EGFR mutation-positive NSCLC [152]. However, long-term use of EGFR-TKI would result in drug resistance and the loss of the original therapeutic effect [142]. Osimertinib, a third-generation EGFR-TKI, was developed to treat NSCLC patients who acquired the EGFR T790M resistance mutation [153]. Due to the drug resistance of EGFR-TKIs, future strategies must be developed to cope with resistance to next generation EGFR-TKIs, including conventional combinations of EGFR-TKIs and other agents and treatments combined with ICIs.

Although ICIs targeting PD-1 and CTLA4 have been shown to be beneficial in mNSCLC, the efficiency in NSCLC is, however, only 8–30% [154]. Emerging evidence indicates that driver oncogenes have different effects on the TME that influence the potential benefit from treatment with ICIs. For instance, patients harboring BRAF, KRAS or TP53 co-mutations benefit from ICIs [155,156]. However, certain patient populations do not respond to these drugs targeting ICIs [112]. Further strategies to enlarge the efficacy of ICIs are to synergistically combine them with CAR-T, EGFR-TKIs and other agents.

**Table 1.** Relevant immunotherapies for the treatment of NSCLC.

| ClinicalTrials.gov Identifier | Target | Drug | Study Design | Cancer Types | Phase | Status | Enroll-ment | Outcomes | Refe-rences |
|---|---|---|---|---|---|---|---|---|---|
| NCT01642004 | T cells, PD-1 | Nivolumab | Nivolumab vs. Docetaxel | Advanced or metastatic squamous cell NSCLC | III | Completed | 352 | OS↑ | [122] |
| NCT01673867 | T cells, PD-1 | Nivolumab | Nivolumab vs. Docetaxel | Metastatic non-squamous NSCLC | III | Completed | 792 | OS↑ | [123] |
| NCT02142738 | T cells, PD-1 | Pembrolizumab | Pembrolizumab vs. Paclitaxel + Carboplatin vs. Pemetrexed + Carboplatin vs. Pemetrexed + Cisplatin vs. Gemcitabine + Carboplatin vs. Gemcitabine + Cisplatin | Metastatic NSCLC | III | Completed | 305 | PFS↑ | [124] |
| NCT03850444 | T cells, PD-1 | Pembrolizumab | Pembrolizumab vs. Carboplatin + Paclitaxel + Pemetrexed | PD-L1 positive advanced or metastatic NSCLC | III | Active, not recruiting | 262 | Undergoing | [125] |
| NCT02409342 | Tumor cells, PD-L1 | Atezolizumab | (Carboplatin/Cisplatin) + (Pemetrexed/Gemcitabine) vs. Atezolizumab | Stage IV non-squamous or squamous NSCLC | III | Completed | 572 | OS↑, PFS↑ | [126] |
| NCT02477826 | T cells, CTLA-4 | Ipilimumab | Nivolumab vs. Nivolumab + Ipilimumab | Stage IV or recurrent NSCLC | III | Active, not recruiting | 2748 | Undergoing | [131] |
| NCT03875092 | T cells, PD-1 | Pembrolizumab | Pembrolizumab + Chemotherapy vs. Chemotherapy | Metastatic squamous NSCLC | III | Active, not recruiting | 125 | Undergoing | [133] |
| NCT05467748 | TAMs, EZH2 | Tazemetostat | Tazemetostat + Pembrolizumab | Advanced NSCLC | Ib/II | Not yet recruiting | 66 | Undergoing | [157] |
| NCT05094804 | TAMs, CD163 | OR2805 | OR2805 vs. OR2805 + PD-1 inhibitor | Advanced malignancies | I/II | Recruiting | 130 | Undergoing | [158] |
| NCT04762199 | TAMs, MerTK | MRX-2843 | Osimertinib + MRX-2843 | Advanced EGFR mutant NSCLC | III | Recruiting | 69 | Undergoing | [159] |

**Table 1.** *Cont.*

| ClinicalTrials.gov Identifier | Target | Drug | Study Design | Cancer Types | Phase | Status | Enrollment | Outcomes | References |
|---|---|---|---|---|---|---|---|---|---|
| NCT00103116 | DC | Autologous dendritic cell cancer vaccine | Autologous dendritic cell cancer vaccine | Stage I, Stage II, or Stage III NSCLC | II | Completed | 32 | Safety, no related adverse events | [160] |
| NCT02808416 | DC | Personalized cellular vaccine | Personalized cellular vaccine | Patients with brain metastases from solid tumors | I | Completed | 10 | Induced specific $CD4^+$ and $CD8^+$ T cell responses | [161] |
| NCT02843204 | NK cells | Pembrolizumab and NK immunotherapy | Pembrolizumab + NK immunotherapy vs. Pembrolizumab | Malignant solid tumor | I/II | Completed | 110 | OS↑, PFS↑ | [162] |
| NCT02843815 | NK cells | NK immunotherapy and cryosurgery | Cryosurgery + NK immunotherapy vs. Cryosurgery | Advanced NSCLC | I/II | Completed | 30 | Relief degree↑ | [163] |
| NCT02118415 | NK cells | Hsp70-peptide TKD/IL-2 activated, autologous NK cells | (Hsp70-peptide TKD/IL-2 activated, autologous NK cells) vs. Control group | NSCLC Stage IIIA/B | II | Suspended | 90 | Undergoing | [164] |

↑ means an improvement in the outcomes.

### 3.2. Target TAMs against NSCLC

Crosstalk between TAMs and other cells in the TME results in an immunosuppression that promotes tumor cell proliferation, angiogenesis, tumor metastasis, and the development of cancer-therapy resistance [165]. It is widely known that macrophage polarization may cause a direct switch between M1 and M2 in the TME, while subtype M1 could kill tumor cells and M2 can promote tumor progression [52]. Small molecule inhibitors or monoclonal antibodies against TAM signaling can consequently inhibit the progression and metastasis of cancer [129]. Recently, the main immunotherapies targeting TAMs and undergoing clinical or scientific trials are tazemetostat, OR2805, and MRX-2843.

Tazemetostat, an enhancer of zeste homolog 2 (EZH2) inhibitor, has been used individually or in combination with ICIs against advanced NSCLC in clinical trials. It has been demonstrated that EZH2 could stimulate the expression of CCL5 and result in the recruitment of macrophages and the invasion of lung cancer [166]. When EZH2 is inhibited, the quantity of M2 decreases, thereby preventing the progression of lung cancer [166]. An open-label, single-arm, phase Ib/II clinical trial (NCT05467748) is underway, in which pembrolizumab in combination with tazemetostat is used to treat patients with advanced NSCLC who have relapsed following initial or second-line therapy (Table 1) [157].

OR2805 is a monoclonal antibody against CD163. CD163 is one of the biomarkers of M2 macrophage polarization, which can inhibit PD-1 and PD-L1 signaling and stimulate macrophage polarization to the M1 phenotype, resulting in enhanced antitumor activity [167,168]. Therefore, OR2805 can be used as a monotherapy or in combination with PD-1 inhibitors to treat patients with advanced solid tumors, and is a valuable targeted TAMs therapy. An open-label, multicenter, first-in-human dose escalation and extension phase I, II trial (NCT05094804) to verify the safety, tolerability, pharmacokinetics, pharmacodynamics, and preliminary anticancer activity of OR2805 is at the recruitment stage, with individuals with NSCLC being expected to enroll (Table 1) [158].

MRX-2843 is a mer tyrosine kinase (MerTK) inhibitor. MerTK is a macrophage-specific tyrosine kinase receptor (RTK) that can induce tumor immunological tolerance by inducing macrophage death, polarizing macrophages towards the M2 phenotype, and inhibiting the secretion of inflammatory factors [169,170]. In contrast, blocking MerTK signaling repolarizes macrophages to M1 phenotypes and enhances antitumor immunity [171]. MerTK antibodies stimulate T-cell activation and are synergistic with anti-PD-1 and anti-PD-L1 treatments [172]. Blocking the macrophage MerTK protein may increase antitumor immunity and induce tumor immunogenicity, a promising method for treating cancer. An ongoing phase Ib safety and pharmacodynamic study is being conducted with MRX-2843 in conjunction with osimertinib in patients with advanced EGFR-mutated NSCLC (NCT04762199) (Table 1) [159]. Melittin (MEL-dKLA) is a promising option for NSCLC patients because it selectively induces cell death in M2 macrophages in vitro without interacting with the normal function of other cell types [173,174]. In addition, a preclinical study showed that the construction of targeted nano-micelles (called 'nano-dandelion') for simultaneous delivery of curcumin (Cur) and baicalin (Bai) was effective in overcoming tumor resistance, which resulted in the transforming of TAMs to tumor-killing M1-type macrophages, indicating an adjuvant therapy for tumors [175].

Due to the high level of macrophage infiltration, the prognosis for NSCLC patients is poor. Macrophage polarization promotes the cancer development in the TME, thus targeting TAMs has emerged as a promising therapeutic strategy and has led to the development of numerous relevant drugs undergoing clinical trials.

### 3.3. Target DCs against NSCLC

As the primary APCs, DCs trigger antigen-specific $CD8^+$ T lymphocyte activation, which initiates innate and adaptive immune responses that are capable of killing tumors [176,177]. Usually, DC-targeted treatments include autologous DC vaccination and individualized cellular vaccination. In the majority of studies, patients are vaccinated with DCs via numerous subcutaneous injections of primed DCs [177]. Moreover, combination therapy with DC and cytokine-induced killer cells (DC-CIK) has been confirmed to be an effective treatment for NSCLC patients.

In a clinical trial (NCT00103116), an autologous DC vaccine was involved in the treatment of individuals with stage I, II, and III NSCLC. Specific T-cell activity in the blood was compared before and six months after vaccination. As a result of the trial, there are 22 out of 32 patients who demonstrated an immune response to the vaccine six months after vaccination, and 20 patients out of 32 who were still alive five years after dual vaccination. These pieces of evidence suggest that the DC vaccine has a favorable safety profile [160]. Moreover, one study was conducted in ten patients with tumor brain metastases (BM) (NCT02808416), five of whom were NSCLC patients. The trial was to examine the security and effectiveness of an individualized cellular tumor vaccination (DC vaccine) in patients with BM [161]. These patients had a good OS rate and an excellent objective response; however, due to the limited number of samples, additional clinical trials are required in the future [178]. Details of the above two tests are shown in Table 1. Based on the outcomes of the aforementioned trials, DC vaccines have demonstrated significant potential for treating NSCLC patients.

In mouse models, DC vaccination was found to be effective when used in combination with chemotherapy and radiotherapy for the treatment of NSCLC [81,179]. Studies have compared the combined effects of chemotherapy or radiotherapy, DC vaccination, and cytokine-induced killer cells (CIK) in humans [180–183]. Consequently, a combination therapy consisting of DC-CIK may have a stronger antitumor effect. Clinical trials have shown that DC-CIK immunotherapy is effective in controlling the disease, improving immune function, and delaying the progression of advanced NSCLC without increasing adverse effects, indicating a promising future in the treatment of NSCLC patients [184].

DC-related immunotherapy for NSCLC patients focuses on DC vaccines and DC-CIK therapy. The safety of these treatments has been recognized, but their exact efficacy still needs to be further determined.

### 3.4. Target NK Cells against NSCLC

NK cells can destroy tumor cells directly or indirectly through the release of pro-inflammatory factors [83,185]. Many researchers have discovered that $CD56^{bright}$ $CD16^{-}$ NK cells that release high levels of cytokines (such as VEGF, placental growth factor, and IL-8/CXCL8) which promote tumor neoangiogenesis exhibit low cytotoxicity in the lung TME [89,185,186]. In addition, recent research has demonstrated that NK cells can identify and eliminate cancer progenitor cells in solid tumors, and have a beneficial effect on lung cancer [187,188].

Immunotherapies targeting NK cells are mostly utilized as an additional therapy with other treatments and are seldom used alone in clinical studies. It has been revealed that the mixture of NK and T lymphocytes cells (NKTm) improves OS and 2-year survival among patients with NSCLC [189]. In addition, NK immunotherapy in combination with cryosurgery or the PD-1 representative drug Pembrolizumab is currently under research. Hsp70-peptide TKD/IL-2 activated autologous NK cells are being considered as a new treatment for NSCLC patients after demonstrating their potential to treat cancer in preclinical models.

In a clinical trial (NCT02843204), NK immunotherapy combined with ICI pembrolizumab was used to treat patients with advanced relapsed NSCLC. Results from the study indicated that pembrolizumab combined with NK cell therapy improved OS and PFS in patients with previously treated advanced PD-L1 NSCLC without causing any serious adverse effects compared to pembrolizumab alone, showing significant potential for NK cell immunotherapy (Table 1) [162,190]. In a separate trial (NCT02843815), the safety and efficacy of cryosurgery combined with allogeneic NK cell immunotherapy for advanced NSCLC were initially determined (Table 1) [163,191]. Preclinical models demonstrated that the combination of NK cells and anti-PD-1 therapy provides long-term tumor control with a substantial infiltration of $CD8^{+}$ T cells and NK cells [192]. A combination-therapy study using anti-PD-1 antibodies and autologous NK cells has made significant progress in view of the enormous potential NK cells have demonstrated in tumor therapy.

Currently, a trial (NCT02118415) is taking place to test the efficacy of sequential immunotherapy using autologous NK cells and Hsp70-peptide TKD/IL-2 in patients with NSCLC (stage IIIa, b) after radiotherapy and chemotherapy (Table 1) [164]. It has been shown in a preclinical model of lung cancer that autologous NK cells-based therapies are highly effective against tumors selectively expressing membrane-type Hsp70 [193]. When combined with other ICIs or modulators, autologous NK cell therapy or other therapies that target tumors expressing mHsp70 may be effective in inhibiting tumor growth and progression [194]. In current NSCLC research, relay transfer of NK cells is being evaluated as a potential treatment method.

Furthermore, CAR-NK therapy has emerged as one of the most promising new research topics targeting NK cells for the treatment of NSCLC patients over the past few years [195]. CAR-NK cells have a number of benefits over CAR-T cells due to the fact that they can be produced from pre-existing cell lines or allogeneic NK cells with mismatched MHC. Moreover, they can kill cancer cells through CAR-dependent and CAR-independent pathways with less toxicity [196]. However, CAR-NK cells still have some limitations, such as the short half-life of NK cells and the extra-tumor toxicity [196,197]. Optimizing the CAR-NK structure and prolonging the survival of CAR-NK cells in vivo are the main research goals for the future.

The efficacy of NK cells immunotherapies in combination with other therapies has demonstrated promising results for NSCLC patients. The benefits of recently developed CAR-NK immunotherapies have also been recognized. However, immunotherapies associated with NK cells are still immature, and further research is needed to increase the treatment options for NSCLC patients.

## 4. Conclusions and Future Directions

The TME is engaged in the whole process of tumor growth and serves a crucial role. Different immune cells in the TME are required to mediate pro- and antitumor immune responses, which affect tumor destiny and the capacity for tumors to become aggressive and grow [21,198]. Due to the significance of immune cells in tumor progression, several immunotherapies have been designed for use in different types of cancer. Over the decades, there have been breakthroughs in immunotherapy, especially ICI immunotherapy applied to NSCLC patients, suggesting immunotherapy's enormous potential for cancer treatment.

Anti-PD-1/PD-L1 immunotherapies are some of the most common ICIs. The FDA has authorized the representative PD-1- or PD-L1-blocking antibodies nivolumab, pembrolizumab, and atezolizumab for the treatment of NSCLC patients, and pembrolizumab has been used as a first-line treatment for patients with PD-L1 levels $\geq 1\%$. Recent clinical trial studies targeting PD-L1 include avelumab and durvalumab, and the most recent follow-up results for avelumab and the positive results shown with durvalumab in NSCLC patients after radiotherapy provide a potential treatment option [116]. In addition, it has been demonstrated that the anti-PD-1 drug cemiplimab substantially improved clinical outcomes in advanced NSCLC patients with more than 50% PD-L1 expression, indicating that this drug may be beneficial for NSCLC patients [116]. ICIs also contain antibodies against CTLA-4, such as ipilimumab. In the treatment of NSCLC, two-drug combinations of ICIs (e.g., nivolumab and ipilimumab) have the potential to be first-line therapies. Combination regimens of multiple ICIs offer additional options for future NSCLC patients. In addition, CAR-T genetically engineered T cell-related immunotherapy is being studied to improve the adverse effects seen in patients during the current trials as well as to make the treatment more effective for NSCLC patients in the future. For patients with EGRF-mutant NSCLC for whom ICIs therapy is ineffective, some EGRF-TKI drugs have been developed which have improved the survival rate among these patients. However, the long-term use of these drugs may result in a resistance; future research may focus on developing new drugs to reduce such resistance. TAMs-related immunotherapies are often used in combination with other immunotherapies to treat patients with NSCLC. ICIs with tazemetostat (an EZH2 inhibitor which targets TAMs) is an option for patients with NSCLC whose disease has progressed following first- or second-line therapy. Other TAMs-targeting cancer immunotherapies, such as MRX-2843, OR2805, and related nanotherapies, are currently undergoing clinical testing as promising NSCLC treatments.

NSCLC patients with DC-related immunotherapies are mainly vaccinated with autologous DCs, and studies have shown that they are both safe and effective, though their exact efficacy remains unclear.

Targeted NK cells therapies are mostly used in combination with other therapies for patients with NSCLC. The efficacy of NKTm cell transplantation, as well as cryosurgery combined with allogeneic NK immunotherapy, has been demonstrated. Autologous NK cells treatment or other medicines targeting mHsp70-expressing tumors, in conjunction with ICIs, may be beneficial in preventing the progression of NSCLC. Genetically engineered CAR-NK immunotherapies are being developed to improve NSCLC treatment in the future.

However, immunotherapy still has some drawbacks. ICIs boost T-cell activation in NSCLC patients by blocking negative regulators of T-cell function, which leads to an uncontrolled immune response and results in immune-related adverse events, including colitis, hypophysis, and pneumonitis [199]. Furthermore, checkpoint inhibitor pneumonia seems to be an uncommon but harmful side effect of anti-PD-1 and PD-L1 ICIs [193,200]. Thus, more scientific research and clinical studies are needed to improve treatment plans, reduce side effects, and control the immune response.

Moreover, sitravatinib (a TAM-targeting MerTK inhibitor) has exhibited an antitumor effect and modification of the TME in preclinical trials [201]. A retrospective analysis of NSCLC patients with tumor progression after ICI treatment showed that sitravatinib does not have significant antitumor activity when used singly. On the basis of its immunomodulatory effect on the TME, studies of sitravatinib in combination with ICI will be one of the primary areas of future research.

In summary, immune cells within the TME not only affect tumor growth and metastasis but are also used for therapy against tumors. For patients with advanced NSCLC, a number of immunotherapeutic strategies have been suggested as first-line therapies, and preclinical and clinical studies have proven their effectiveness. The combination of multiple medicines and the development of new therapeutic targets for NSCLC should be investigated in greater depth in the future, along with existing immunotherapy strategies, in order to increase the survival rate of cancer patients.

**Author Contributions:** W.Y. provided the idea and wrote the manuscript. M.L. searched the literature. K.L. illustrated the figures and revised the manuscript. All authors contributed to the article and approved the submitted version. All authors have read and agreed to the published version of the manuscript.

**Funding:** This work was supported by the National Natural Science Foundation of China [82104457] and the Shenzhen Longhua District Science and Technology Innovation Fund [SZLHQJCYJ2021001].

**Institutional Review Board Statement:** Exclude this statement.

**Informed Consent Statement:** Not applicable.

**Data Availability Statement:** Not applicable.

**Conflicts of Interest:** All authors declare that there is no conflict of interest.

## References

1. Bray, F.; Laversanne, M.; Weiderpass, E.; Soerjomataram, I. The ever-increasing importance of cancer as a leading cause of premature death worldwide. *Cancer* **2021**, *127*, 3029–3030. [CrossRef] [PubMed]
2. Brustugun, O.T.; Møller, B.; Helland, Å. Years of life lost as a measure of cancer burden on a national level. *Br. J. Cancer* **2014**, *111*, 1014–1020. [CrossRef] [PubMed]
3. Deo, S.V.S.; Sharma, J.; Kumar, S. GLOBOCAN 2020 Report on Global Cancer Burden: Challenges and Opportunities for Surgical Oncologists. *Ann. Surg. Oncol.* **2022**, *29*, 6497–6500. [CrossRef] [PubMed]

4. Sung, H.; Ferlay, J.; Siegel, R.L.; Laversanne, M.; Soerjomataram, I.; Jemal, A.; Bray, F. Global Cancer Statistics 2020: GLOBOCAN Estimates of Incidence and Mortality Worldwide for 36 Cancers in 185 Countries. *CA Cancer J. Clin.* **2021**, *71*, 209–249. [CrossRef]
5. Wild, C.P.; Weiderpass, E.; Stewart, B.W. *World Cancer Report: Cancer Research for Cancer Prevention*; IARC: Lyon, France, 2020.
6. Siegel, R.L.; Miller, K.D.; Jemal, A. Cancer statistics, 2020. *CA Cancer J. Clin.* **2020**, *70*, 7–30. [CrossRef] [PubMed]
7. Chen, W.; Zheng, R.; Baade, P.D.; Zhang, S.; Zeng, H.; Bray, F.; Jemal, A.; Yu, X.Q.; He, J. Cancer statistics in China, 2015. *CA Cancer J. Clin.* **2016**, *66*, 115–132. [CrossRef]
8. Bray, F.; Ferlay, J.; Soerjomataram, I.; Siegel, R.L.; Torre, L.A.; Jemal, A. Global cancer statistics 2018: GLOBOCAN estimates of incidence and mortality worldwide for 36 cancers in 185 countries. *CA Cancer J. Clin.* **2018**, *68*, 394–424. [CrossRef]
9. Anderson, N.M.; Simon, M.C. Tumor Microenvironment. *Curr. Biol.* **2020**, *30*, R921–R925. [CrossRef]
10. Arneth, B. Tumor Microenvironment. *Medicina* **2019**, *56*, 15. [CrossRef]
11. Garon, E.B.; Ciuleanu, T.-E.; Arrieta, O.; Prabhash, K.; Syrigos, K.N.; Goksel, T.; Park, K.; Gorbunova, V.; Kowalyszyn, R.D.; Pikiel, J.; et al. Ramucirumab plus docetaxel versus placebo plus docetaxel for second-line treatment of stage IV non-small-cell lung cancer after disease progression on platinum-based therapy (REVEL): A multicentre, double-blind, randomised phase 3 trial. *Lancet* **2014**, *384*, 665–673. [CrossRef]
12. Gocheva, V.; Naba, A.; Bhutkar, A.; Guardia, T.; Miller, K.M.; Li, C.M.-C.; Dayton, T.L.; Sanchez-Rivera, F.J.; Kim-Kiselak, C.; Jailkhani, N.; et al. Quantitative proteomics identify Tenascin-C as a promoter of lung cancer progression and contributor to a signature prognostic of patient survival. *Proc. Natl. Acad. Sci. USA* **2017**, *114*, E5625–E5634. [CrossRef]
13. Lambrechts, D.; Wauters, E.; Boeckx, B.; Aibar, S.; Nittner, D.; Burton, O.; Bassez, A.; Decaluwé, H.; Pircher, A.; Van den Eynde, K.; et al. Phenotype molding of stromal cells in the lung tumor microenvironment. *Nat. Med.* **2018**, *24*, 1277–1289. [CrossRef]
14. Jiang, X.; Wang, J.; Deng, X.; Xiong, F.; Ge, J.; Xiang, B.; Wu, X.; Ma, J.; Zhou, M.; Li, X.; et al. Role of the tumor microenvironment in PD-L1/PD-1-mediated tumor immune escape. *Mol. Cancer* **2019**, *18*, 10. [CrossRef]
15. Hinshaw, D.C.; Shevde, L.A. The Tumor Microenvironment Innately Modulates Cancer Progression. *Cancer Res.* **2019**, *79*, 4557–4566. [CrossRef] [PubMed]
16. Rodriguez-Garcia, A.; Palazon, A.; Noguera-Ortega, E.; Powell, D.J.; Guedan, S. CAR-T Cells Hit the Tumor Microenvironment: Strategies to Overcome Tumor Escape. *Front. Immunol.* **2020**, *11*, 1109. [CrossRef] [PubMed]
17. Ma, S.; Li, X.; Wang, X.; Cheng, L.; Li, Z.; Zhang, C.; Ye, Z.; Qian, Q. Current Progress in CAR-T Cell Therapy for Solid Tumors. *Int. J. Biol. Sci.* **2019**, *15*, 2548–2560. [CrossRef] [PubMed]
18. Wculek, S.K.; Cueto, F.J.; Mujal, A.M.; Melero, I.; Krummel, M.F.; Sancho, D. Dendritic cells in cancer immunology and immunotherapy. *Nat. Rev. Immunol.* **2020**, *20*, 7–24. [CrossRef]
19. Doroshow, D.B.; Sanmamed, M.F.; Hastings, K.; Politi, K.; Rimm, D.L.; Chen, L.; Melero, I.; Schalper, K.A.; Herbst, R.S. Immunotherapy in Non-Small Cell Lung Cancer: Facts and Hopes. *Clin. Cancer Res.* **2019**, *25*, 4592–4602. [CrossRef]
20. Reck, M.; Remon, J.; Hellmann, M.D. First-Line Immunotherapy for Non-Small-Cell Lung Cancer. *J. Clin. Oncol.* **2022**, *40*, 586–597. [CrossRef]
21. Pansy, K.; Uhl, B.; Krstic, J.; Szmyra, M.; Fechter, K.; Santiso, A.; Thüminger, L.; Greinix, H.; Kargl, J.; Prochazka, K.; et al. Immune Regulatory Processes of the Tumor Microenvironment under Malignant Conditions. *Int. J. Mol. Sci.* **2021**, *22*, 13311. [CrossRef]
22. Wu, T.; Dai, Y. Tumor microenvironment and therapeutic response. *Cancer Lett.* **2017**, *387*, 61–68. [CrossRef] [PubMed]
23. Donnem, T.; Kilvaer, T.K.; Andersen, S.; Richardsen, E.; Paulsen, E.E.; Hald, S.M.; Al-Saad, S.; Brustugun, O.T.; Helland, A.; Lund-Iversen, M.; et al. Strategies for clinical implementation of TNM-Immunoscore in resected nonsmall-cell lung cancer. *Ann. Oncol.* **2016**, *27*, 225–232. [CrossRef] [PubMed]
24. Banat, G.-A.; Tretyn, A.; Pullamsetti, S.S.; Wilhelm, J.; Weigert, A.; Olesch, C.; Ebel, K.; Stiewe, T.; Grimminger, F.; Seeger, W.; et al. Immune and Inflammatory Cell Composition of Human Lung Cancer Stroma. *PLoS ONE* **2015**, *10*, e0139073. [CrossRef] [PubMed]
25. Saab, S.; Zalzale, H.; Rahal, Z.; Khalifeh, Y.; Sinjab, A.; Kadara, H. Insights Into Lung Cancer Immune-Based Biology, Prevention, and Treatment. *Front. Immunol.* **2020**, *11*, 159. [CrossRef]
26. Hanahan, D.; Weinberg, R.A. Hallmarks of cancer: The next generation. *Cell* **2011**, *144*, 646–674. [CrossRef]
27. Tian, Y.; Zhai, X.; Yan, W.; Zhu, H.; Yu, J. Clinical outcomes of immune checkpoint blockades and the underlying immune escape mechanisms in squamous and adenocarcinoma NSCLC. *Cancer Med.* **2020**, *10*, 3–14. [CrossRef]
28. Qu, J.; Jiang, M.; Wang, L.; Zhao, D.; Qin, K.; Wang, Y.; Tao, J.; Zhang, X. Mechanism and potential predictive biomarkers of immune checkpoint inhibitors in NSCLC. *Biomed. Pharmacother.* **2020**, *127*, 109996. [CrossRef]
29. Khedri, M.; Samei, A.; Fasihi-Ramandi, M.; Taheri, R.A. The immunopathobiology of T cells in stress condition: A review. *Cell Stress Chaperones* **2020**, *25*, 743–752. [CrossRef]
30. Kumar, B.V.; Connors, T.J.; Farber, D.L. Human T Cell Development, Localization, and Function throughout Life. *Immunity* **2018**, *48*, 202–213. [CrossRef]
31. Farhood, B.; Najafi, M.; Mortezaee, K. CD8+ cytotoxic T lymphocytes in cancer immunotherapy: A review. *J. Cell. Physiol.* **2019**, *234*, 8509–8521. [CrossRef]
32. Raskov, H.; Orhan, A.; Christensen, J.P.; Gögenur, I. Cytotoxic CD8+ T cells in cancer and cancer immunotherapy. *Br. J. Cancer* **2021**, *124*, 359–367. [CrossRef] [PubMed]
33. Gueguen, P.; Metoikidou, C.; Dupic, T.; Lawand, M.; Goudot, C.; Baulande, S.; Lameiras, S.; Lantz, O.; Girard, N.; Seguin-Givelet, A.; et al. Contribution of resident and circulating precursors to tumor-infiltrating CD8+ T cell populations in lung cancer. *Sci. Immunol.* **2021**, *6*, eabd5778. [CrossRef] [PubMed]

34. Iwahori, K. Cytotoxic CD8+ Lymphocytes in the Tumor Microenvironment. In *Tumor Microenvironment: Hematopoietic Cells—Part A*; Birbrair, A., Ed.; Advances in Experimental Medicine and Biology; Springer International Publishing: Cham, Switzerland, 2020; pp. 53–62. ISBN 978-3-030-35723-8.
35. Paul, M.S.; Ohashi, P.S. The Roles of CD8+ T Cell Subsets in Antitumor Immunity. *Trends Cell Biol.* **2020**, *30*, 695–704. [CrossRef] [PubMed]
36. Wherry, E.J. T cell exhaustion. *Nat. Immunol.* **2011**, *12*, 492–499. [CrossRef]
37. Jiang, W.; He, Y.; He, W.; Wu, G.; Zhou, X.; Sheng, Q.; Zhong, W.; Lu, Y.; Ding, Y.; Lu, Q.; et al. Exhausted CD8+ T Cells in the Tumor Immune Microenvironment: New Pathways to Therapy. *Front. Immunol.* **2021**, *11*, 622509. [CrossRef]
38. Lei, X.; Lei, Y.; Li, J.-K.; Du, W.-X.; Li, R.-G.; Yang, J.; Li, J.; Li, F.; Tan, H.-B. Immune cells within the tumor microenvironment: Biological functions and roles in cancer immunotherapy. *Cancer Lett.* **2020**, *470*, 126–133. [CrossRef]
39. Borst, J.; Ahrends, T.; Bąbała, N.; Melief, C.J.M.; Kastenmüller, W. CD4+ T cell help in cancer immunology and immunotherapy. *Nat. Rev. Immunol.* **2018**, *18*, 635–647. [CrossRef]
40. Ahrends, T.; Borst, J. The opposing roles of CD4+ T cells in anti-tumour immunity. *Immunology* **2018**, *154*, 582–592. [CrossRef]
41. Basu, A.; Ramamoorthi, G.; Albert, G.; Gallen, C.; Beyer, A.; Snyder, C.; Koski, G.; Disis, M.L.; Czerniecki, B.J.; Kodumudi, K. Differentiation and Regulation of TH Cells: A Balancing Act for Cancer Immunotherapy. *Front. Immunol.* **2021**, *12*, 669474. [CrossRef]
42. Maier, E.; Duschl, A.; Horejs-Hoeck, J. STAT6-dependent and -independent mechanisms in Th2 polarization. *Eur. J. Immunol.* **2012**, *42*, 2827–2833. [CrossRef]
43. Halvorsen, E.C.; Mahmoud, S.M.; Bennewith, K.L. Emerging roles of regulatory T cells in tumour progression and metastasis. *Cancer Metastasis Rev.* **2014**, *33*, 1025–1041. [CrossRef] [PubMed]
44. Beyer, M.; Schultze, J.L. Regulatory T cells in cancer. *Blood* **2006**, *108*, 804–811. [CrossRef]
45. Vignali, D.A.A.; Collison, L.W.; Workman, C.J. How regulatory T cells work. *Nat. Rev. Immunol.* **2008**, *8*, 523–532. [CrossRef] [PubMed]
46. Lim, W.C.; Olding, M.; Healy, E.; Millar, T.M. Human Endothelial Cells Modulate CD4+ T Cell Populations and Enhance Regulatory T Cell Suppressive Capacity. *Front. Immunol.* **2018**, *9*, 565. [CrossRef]
47. Comito, G.; Iscaro, A.; Bacci, M.; Morandi, A.; Ippolito, L.; Parri, M.; Montagnani, I.; Raspollini, M.R.; Serni, S.; Simeoni, L.; et al. Lactate modulates CD4+ T-cell polarization and induces an immunosuppressive environment, which sustains prostate carcinoma progression via TLR8/miR21 axis. *Oncogene* **2019**, *38*, 3681–3695. [CrossRef] [PubMed]
48. Huppert, L.A.; Green, M.D.; Kim, L.; Chow, C.; Leyfman, Y.; Daud, A.I.; Lee, J.C. Tissue-specific Tregs in cancer metastasis: Opportunities for precision immunotherapy. *Cell Mol. Immunol.* **2022**, *19*, 33–45. [CrossRef]
49. Tao, H.; Mimura, Y.; Aoe, K.; Kobayashi, S.; Yamamoto, H.; Matsuda, E.; Okabe, K.; Matsumoto, T.; Sugi, K.; Ueoka, H. Prognostic potential of FOXP3 expression in non-small cell lung cancer cells combined with tumor-infiltrating regulatory T cells. *Lung. Cancer* **2012**, *75*, 95–101. [CrossRef]
50. Cheng, N.; Bai, X.; Shu, Y.; Ahmad, O.; Shen, P. Targeting tumor-associated macrophages as an antitumor strategy. *Biochem. Pharmacol.* **2021**, *183*, 114354. [CrossRef]
51. Lin, Y.; Xu, J.; Lan, H. Tumor-associated macrophages in tumor metastasis: Biological roles and clinical therapeutic applications. *J. Hematol. Oncol.* **2019**, *12*, 76. [CrossRef]
52. Pan, Y.; Yu, Y.; Wang, X.; Zhang, T. Tumor-Associated Macrophages in Tumor Immunity. *Front. Immunol.* **2020**, *11*, 583084. [CrossRef]
53. Biswas, S.K.; Mantovani, A. Macrophage plasticity and interaction with lymphocyte subsets: Cancer as a paradigm. *Nat. Immunol.* **2010**, *11*, 889–896. [CrossRef] [PubMed]
54. Li, M.; He, L.; Zhu, J.; Zhang, P.; Liang, S. Targeting tumor-associated macrophages for cancer treatment. *Cell Biosci.* **2022**, *12*, 85. [CrossRef] [PubMed]
55. Bernsmeier, C.; van der Merwe, S.; Périanin, A. Innate immune cells in cirrhosis. *J. Hepatol.* **2020**, *73*, 186–201. [CrossRef] [PubMed]
56. Bruns, H.; Büttner, M.; Fabri, M.; Mougiakakos, D.; Bittenbring, J.T.; Hoffmann, M.H.; Beier, F.; Pasemann, S.; Jitschin, R.; Hofmann, A.D.; et al. Vitamin D-dependent induction of cathelicidin in human macrophages results in cytotoxicity against high-grade B cell lymphoma. *Sci. Transl. Med.* **2015**, *7*, 282ra47. [CrossRef] [PubMed]
57. Movahedi, K.; Laoui, D.; Gysemans, C.; Baeten, M.; Stangé, G.; Van den Bossche, J.; Mack, M.; Pipeleers, D.; In't Veld, P.; De Baetselier, P.; et al. Different tumor microenvironments contain functionally distinct subsets of macrophages derived from Ly6C(high) monocytes. *Cancer Res.* **2010**, *70*, 5728–5739. [CrossRef] [PubMed]
58. Ngambenjawong, C.; Gustafson, H.H.; Pun, S.H. Progress in tumor-associated macrophage (TAM)-targeted therapeutics. *Adv. Drug Deliv. Rev.* **2017**, *114*, 206–221. [CrossRef]
59. Dallavalasa, S.; Beeraka, N.M.; Basavaraju, C.G.; Tulimilli, S.V.; Sadhu, S.P.; Rajesh, K.; Aliev, G.; Madhunapantula, S.V. The Role of Tumor Associated Macrophages (TAMs) in Cancer Progression, Chemoresistance, Angiogenesis and Metastasis—Current Status. *Curr. Med. Chem.* **2021**, *28*, 8203–8236. [CrossRef]
60. Fu, L.-Q.; Du, W.-L.; Cai, M.-H.; Yao, J.-Y.; Zhao, Y.-Y.; Mou, X.-Z. The roles of tumor-associated macrophages in tumor angiogenesis and metastasis. *Cell Immunol.* **2020**, *353*, 104119. [CrossRef]

61. Gazzaniga, S.; Bravo, A.I.; Guglielmotti, A.; van Rooijen, N.; Maschi, F.; Vecchi, A.; Mantovani, A.; Mordoh, J.; Wainstok, R. Targeting tumor-associated macrophages and inhibition of MCP-1 reduce angiogenesis and tumor growth in a human melanoma xenograft. *J. Investig. Dermatol.* **2007**, *127*, 2031–2041. [CrossRef]
62. Cortese, N.; Soldani, C.; Franceschini, B.; Barbagallo, M.; Marchesi, F.; Torzilli, G.; Donadon, M. Macrophages in Colorectal Cancer Liver Metastases. *Cancers* **2019**, *11*, 633. [CrossRef]
63. Msaouel, P.; Genovese, G.; Gao, J.; Sen, S.; Tannir, N.M. TAM kinase inhibition and immune checkpoint blockade- a winning combination in cancer treatment? *Expert Opin. Ther. Targets* **2021**, *25*, 141–151. [CrossRef] [PubMed]
64. Constantino, J.; Gomes, C.; Falcão, A.; Neves, B.M.; Cruz, M.T. Dendritic cell-based immunotherapy: A basic review and recent advances. *Immunol. Res* **2017**, *65*, 798–810. [CrossRef] [PubMed]
65. Gardner, A.; Ruffell, B. Dendritic Cells and Cancer Immunity. *Trends Immunol.* **2016**, *37*, 855–865. [CrossRef] [PubMed]
66. Salmon, H.; Idoyaga, J.; Rahman, A.; Leboeuf, M.; Remark, R.; Jordan, S.; Casanova-Acebes, M.; Khudoynazarova, M.; Agudo, J.; Tung, N.; et al. Expansion and activation of CD103+ dendritic cell progenitors at the tumor site enhances tumor responses to therapeutic PD-L1 and BRAF inhibition. *Immunity* **2016**, *44*, 924–938. [CrossRef] [PubMed]
67. Zhu, S.; Yang, N.; Wu, J.; Wang, X.; Wang, W.; Liu, Y.-J.; Chen, J. Tumor microenvironment-related dendritic cell deficiency: A target to enhance tumor immunotherapy. *Pharmacol. Res.* **2020**, *159*, 104980. [CrossRef]
68. Escors, D. Tumour immunogenicity, antigen presentation and immunological barriers in cancer immunotherapy. *N. J. Sci.* **2014**, *2014*, 734515. [CrossRef]
69. Mathan, T.S.M.; Figdor, C.G.; Buschow, S.I. Human Plasmacytoid Dendritic Cells: From Molecules to Intercellular Communication Network. *Front. Immunol.* **2013**, *4*, 372. [CrossRef]
70. Bi, E.; Li, R.; Bover, L.C.; Li, H.; Su, P.; Ma, X.; Huang, C.; Wang, Q.; Liu, L.; Yang, M.; et al. E-cadherin expression on multiple myeloma cells activates tumor-promoting properties in plasmacytoid DCs. *J. Clin. Investig.* **2018**, *128*, 4821–4831. [CrossRef]
71. Yang, L.-L.; Mao, L.; Wu, H.; Chen, L.; Deng, W.-W.; Xiao, Y.; Li, H.; Zhang, L.; Sun, Z.-J. pDC depletion induced by CD317 blockade drives the antitumor immune response in head and neck squamous cell carcinoma. *Oral. Oncol.* **2019**, *96*, 131–139. [CrossRef]
72. Kranz, L.M.; Diken, M.; Haas, H.; Kreiter, S.; Loquai, C.; Reuter, K.C.; Meng, M.; Fritz, D.; Vascotto, F.; Hefesha, H.; et al. Systemic RNA delivery to dendritic cells exploits antiviral defence for cancer immunotherapy. *Nature* **2016**, *534*, 396–401. [CrossRef]
73. Mildner, A.; Jung, S. Development and function of dendritic cell subsets. *Immunity* **2014**, *40*, 642–656. [CrossRef]
74. Collin, M.; Bigley, V. Human dendritic cell subsets: An update. *Immunology* **2018**, *154*, 3–20. [CrossRef]
75. Joffre, O.P.; Segura, E.; Savina, A.; Amigorena, S. Cross-presentation by dendritic cells. *Nat. Rev. Immunol.* **2012**, *12*, 557–569. [CrossRef]
76. Fucikova, J.; Palova-Jelinkova, L.; Bartunkova, J.; Spisek, R. Induction of Tolerance and Immunity by Dendritic Cells: Mechanisms and Clinical Applications. *Front. Immunol.* **2019**, *10*, 2393. [CrossRef] [PubMed]
77. Motta, J.M.; Rumjanek, V.M. Sensitivity of Dendritic Cells to Microenvironment Signals. *J. Immunol. Res.* **2016**, *2016*, 4753607. [CrossRef] [PubMed]
78. Verneau, J.; Sautés-Fridman, C.; Sun, C.-M. Dendritic cells in the tumor microenvironment: Prognostic and theranostic impact. *Semin. Immunol.* **2020**, *48*, 101410. [CrossRef] [PubMed]
79. Gkirtzimanaki, K.; Kabrani, E.; Nikoleri, D.; Polyzos, A.; Blanas, A.; Sidiropoulos, P.; Makrigiannakis, A.; Bertsias, G.; Boumpas, D.T.; Verginis, P. IFNα Impairs Autophagic Degradation of mtDNA Promoting Autoreactivity of SLE Monocytes in a STING-Dependent Fashion. *Cell Rep.* **2018**, *25*, 921–933.e5. [CrossRef] [PubMed]
80. Subbiah, V.; Murthy, R.; Hong, D.S.; Prins, R.M.; Hosing, C.; Hendricks, K.; Kolli, D.; Noffsinger, L.; Brown, R.; McGuire, M.; et al. Cytokines Produced by Dendritic Cells Administered Intratumorally Correlate with Clinical Outcome in Patients with Diverse Cancers. *Clin. Cancer Res.* **2018**, *24*, 3845–3856. [CrossRef] [PubMed]
81. Zhong, H.; Han, B.; Tourkova, I.L.; Lokshin, A.; Rosenbloom, A.; Shurin, M.R.; Shurin, G.V. Low-Dose Paclitaxel Prior to Intratumoral Dendritic Cell Vaccine Modulates Intratumoral Cytokine Network and Lung Cancer Growth. *Clin. Cancer Res.* **2007**, *13*, 5455–5462. [CrossRef]
82. Mattiola, I. Immune Circuits to Shape Natural Killer Cells in Cancer. *Cancers* **2021**, *13*, 3225. [CrossRef]
83. Marofi, F.; Al-Awad, A.S.; Sulaiman Rahman, H.; Markov, A.; Abdelbasset, W.K.; Ivanovna Enina, Y.; Mahmoodi, M.; Hassanzadeh, A.; Yazdanifar, M.; Stanley Chartrand, M.; et al. CAR-NK Cell: A New Paradigm in Tumor Immunotherapy. *Front. Oncol.* **2021**, *11*, 673276. [CrossRef] [PubMed]
84. Carnevalli, L.S.; Ghadially, H.; Barry, S.T. Therapeutic Approaches Targeting the Natural Killer-Myeloid Cell Axis in the Tumor Microenvironment. *Front. Immunol.* **2021**, *12*, 633685. [CrossRef] [PubMed]
85. Jewett, A.; Kos, J.; Kaur, K.; Safaei, T.; Sutanto, C.; Chen, W.; Wong, P.; Namagerdi, A.K.; Fang, C.; Fong, Y.; et al. Natural Killer Cells: Diverse Functions in Tumor Immunity and Defects in Pre-Neoplastic and Neoplastic Stages of Tumorigenesis. *Mol. Ther. Oncolytics* **2019**, *16*, 41–52. [CrossRef] [PubMed]
86. Melaiu, O.; Lucarini, V.; Cifaldi, L.; Fruci, D. Influence of the Tumor Microenvironment on NK Cell Function in Solid Tumors. *Front. Immunol.* **2020**, *10*, 3038. [CrossRef] [PubMed]
87. Wagner, J.A.; Rosario, M.; Romee, R.; Berrien-Elliott, M.M.; Schneider, S.E.; Leong, J.W.; Sullivan, R.P.; Jewell, B.A.; Becker-Hapak, M.; Schappe, T.; et al. CD56bright NK cells exhibit potent antitumor responses following IL-15 priming. *J. Clin. Investig.* **2017**, *127*, 4042–4058. [CrossRef]

88. Prager, I.; Liesche, C.; van Ooijen, H.; Urlaub, D.; Verron, Q.; Sandström, N.; Fasbender, F.; Claus, M.; Eils, R.; Beaudouin, J.; et al. NK cells switch from granzyme B to death receptor–mediated cytotoxicity during serial killing. *J. Exp. Med.* **2019**, *216*, 2113–2127. [CrossRef]
89. Gemelli, M.; Noonan, D.M.; Carlini, V.; Pelosi, G.; Barberis, M.; Ricotta, R.; Albini, A. Overcoming Resistance to Checkpoint Inhibitors: Natural Killer Cells in Non-Small Cell Lung Cancer. *Front. Oncol.* **2022**, *12*, 886440. [CrossRef]
90. Gaggero, S.; Witt, K.; Carlsten, M.; Mitra, S. Cytokines Orchestrating the Natural Killer-Myeloid Cell Crosstalk in the Tumor Microenvironment: Implications for Natural Killer Cell-Based Cancer Immunotherapy. *Front. Immunol.* **2021**, *11*, 621225. [CrossRef]
91. Terrén, I.; Orrantia, A.; Vitallé, J.; Zenarruzabeitia, O.; Borrego, F. NK Cell Metabolism and Tumor Microenvironment. *Front. Immunol.* **2019**, *10*, 2278. [CrossRef]
92. Myers, J.A.; Miller, J.S. Exploring the NK cell platform for cancer immunotherapy. *Nat. Rev. Clin. Oncol.* **2021**, *18*, 85–100. [CrossRef]
93. Vitale, M.; Cantoni, C.; Pietra, G.; Mingari, M.C.; Moretta, L. Effect of tumor cells and tumor microenvironment on NK-cell function. *Eur. J. Immunol.* **2014**, *44*, 1582–1592. [CrossRef] [PubMed]
94. Wahl, S.M.; Wen, J.; Moutsopoulos, N.M. The kiss of death: Interrupted by NK-cell close encounters of another kind. *Trends Immunol.* **2006**, *27*, 161–164. [CrossRef] [PubMed]
95. Liu, C.; Lai, H.; Chen, T. Boosting Natural Killer Cell-Based Cancer Immunotherapy with Selenocystine/Transforming Growth Factor-Beta Inhibitor-Encapsulated Nanoemulsion. *ACS Nano* **2020**, *14*, 11067–11082. [CrossRef]
96. Mollinedo, F. Neutrophil Degranulation, Plasticity, and Cancer Metastasis. *Trends Immunol.* **2019**, *40*, 228–242. [CrossRef]
97. Xiong, S.; Dong, L.; Cheng, L. Neutrophils in cancer carcinogenesis and metastasis. *J. Hematol. Oncol.* **2021**, *14*, 173. [CrossRef]
98. Templeton, A.J.; McNamara, M.G.; Šeruga, B.; Vera-Badillo, F.E.; Aneja, P.; Ocaña, A.; Leibowitz-Amit, R.; Sonpavde, G.; Knox, J.J.; Tran, B.; et al. Prognostic role of neutrophil-to-lymphocyte ratio in solid tumors: A systematic review and meta-analysis. *J. Natl. Cancer Inst.* **2014**, *106*, dju124. [CrossRef] [PubMed]
99. Masucci, M.T.; Minopoli, M.; Del Vecchio, S.; Carriero, M.V. The Emerging Role of Neutrophil Extracellular Traps (NETs) in Tumor Progression and Metastasis. *Front. Immunol.* **2020**, *11*, 1749. [CrossRef] [PubMed]
100. Mouchemore, K.A.; Anderson, R.L.; Hamilton, J.A. Neutrophils, G-CSF and their contribution to breast cancer metastasis. *FEBS J.* **2018**, *285*, 665–679. [CrossRef]
101. Jung, H.S.; Gu, J.; Kim, J.-E.; Nam, Y.; Song, J.W.; Kim, H.K. Cancer cell-induced neutrophil extracellular traps promote both hypercoagulability and cancer progression. *PLoS ONE* **2019**, *14*, e0216055. [CrossRef]
102. Demers, M.; Wagner, D.D. Neutrophil extracellular traps: A new link to cancer-associated thrombosis and potential implications for tumor progression. *Oncoimmunology* **2013**, *2*, e22946. [CrossRef]
103. Gabrilovich, D.I. Myeloid-Derived Suppressor Cells. *Cancer Immunol. Res.* **2017**, *5*, 3–8. [CrossRef] [PubMed]
104. Li, Y.; He, H.; Jihu, R.; Zhou, J.; Zeng, R.; Yan, H. Novel Characterization of Myeloid-Derived Suppressor Cells in Tumor Microenvironment. *Front. Cell Dev. Biol.* **2021**, *9*, 698532. [CrossRef] [PubMed]
105. Condamine, T.; Dominguez, G.A.; Youn, J.-I.; Kossenkov, A.V.; Mony, S.; Alicea-Torres, K.; Tcyganov, E.; Hashimoto, A.; Nefedova, Y.; Lin, C.; et al. Lectin-type oxidized LDL receptor-1 distinguishes population of human polymorphonuclear myeloid-derived suppressor cells in cancer patients. *Sci. Immunol.* **2016**, *1*, aaf8943. [CrossRef] [PubMed]
106. Condamine, T.; Ramachandran, I.; Youn, J.-I.; Gabrilovich, D.I. Regulation of tumor metastasis by myeloid-derived suppressor cells. *Annu. Rev. Med.* **2015**, *66*, 97–110. [CrossRef] [PubMed]
107. Engelhard, V.; Conejo-Garcia, J.R.; Ahmed, R.; Nelson, B.H.; Willard-Gallo, K.; Bruno, T.C.; Fridman, W.H. B cells and cancer. *Cancer Cell* **2021**, *39*, 1293–1296. [CrossRef]
108. Kroeger, D.R.; Milne, K.; Nelson, B.H. Tumor-Infiltrating Plasma Cells Are Associated with Tertiary Lymphoid Structures, Cytolytic T-Cell Responses, and Superior Prognosis in Ovarian Cancer. *Clin. Cancer Res. J. Am. Assoc. Cancer Res.* **2016**, *22*, 3005–3015. [CrossRef]
109. Sautès-Fridman, C.; Petitprez, F.; Calderaro, J.; Fridman, W.H. Tertiary lymphoid structures in the era of cancer immunotherapy. *Nat. Rev. Cancer* **2019**, *19*, 307–325. [CrossRef]
110. West, H.; McCleod, M.; Hussein, M.; Morabito, A.; Rittmeyer, A.; Conter, H.J.; Kopp, H.-G.; Daniel, D.; McCune, S.; Mekhail, T.; et al. Atezolizumab in combination with carboplatin plus nab-paclitaxel chemotherapy compared with chemotherapy alone as first-line treatment for metastatic non-squamous non-small-cell lung cancer (IMpower130): A multicentre, randomised, open-label, phase 3 trial. *Lancet Oncol.* **2019**, *20*, 924–937. [CrossRef]
111. Neoadjuvant Chemo-ICI Boosts NSCLC Survival. *Cancer Discov.* **2022**, *12*, 2228. [CrossRef]
112. Xia, L.; Liu, Y.; Wang, Y. PD-1/PD-L1 Blockade Therapy in Advanced Non-Small-Cell Lung Cancer: Current Status and Future Directions. *Oncologist* **2019**, *24*, S31–S41. [CrossRef]
113. Kono, K.; Nakajima, S.; Mimura, K. Current status of immune checkpoint inhibitors for gastric cancer. *Gastric Cancer* **2020**, *23*, 565–578. [CrossRef] [PubMed]
114. Yi, M.; Jiao, D.; Qin, S.; Chu, Q.; Wu, K.; Li, A. Synergistic effect of immune checkpoint blockade and anti-angiogenesis in cancer treatment. *Mol. Cancer* **2019**, *18*, 60. [CrossRef] [PubMed]
115. Carlino, M.S.; Larkin, J.; Long, G.V. Immune checkpoint inhibitors in melanoma. *Lancet* **2021**, *398*, 1002–1014. [CrossRef]

116. Tang, S.; Qin, C.; Hu, H.; Liu, T.; He, Y.; Guo, H.; Yan, H.; Zhang, J.; Tang, S.; Zhou, H. Immune Checkpoint Inhibitors in Non-Small Cell Lung Cancer: Progress, Challenges, and Prospects. *Cells* **2022**, *11*, 320. [CrossRef] [PubMed]
117. Sharma, P.; Allison, J.P. Immune checkpoint targeting in cancer therapy: Toward combination strategies with curative potential. *Cell* **2015**, *161*, 205–214. [CrossRef] [PubMed]
118. Bravo Montenegro, G.; Farid, S.; Liu, S.V. Immunotherapy in lung cancer. *J. Surg. Oncol.* **2021**, *123*, 718–729. [CrossRef]
119. Grant, M.J.; Herbst, R.S.; Goldberg, S.B. Selecting the optimal immunotherapy regimen in driver-negative metastatic NSCLC. *Nat. Rev. Clin. Oncol.* **2021**, *18*, 625–644. [CrossRef]
120. Keir, M.E.; Butte, M.J.; Freeman, G.J.; Sharpe, A.H. PD-1 and its ligands in tolerance and immunity. *Annu. Rev. Immunol.* **2008**, *26*, 677–704. [CrossRef]
121. Sun, C.; Mezzadra, R.; Schumacher, T.N. Regulation and Function of the PD-L1 Checkpoint. *Immunity* **2018**, *48*, 434–452. [CrossRef]
122. Bristol-Myers Squibb An Open-Label Randomized Phase III Trial of BMS-936558 (Nivolumab) Versus Docetaxel in Previously Treated Advanced or Metastatic Squamous Cell Non-Small Cell Lung Cancer (NSCLC). 2012. Available online: https://ClinicalTrials.gov/show/NCT01642004 (accessed on 13 April 2023).
123. Bristol-Myers Squibb Study of BMS-936558 (Nivolumab) Compared to Docetaxel in Previously Treated Metastatic Non-squamous NSCLC (CheckMate057). 2012. Available online: https://ClinicalTrials.gov/show/NCT01673867 (accessed on 13 April 2023).
124. Merck Sharp & Dohme LLC A Randomized Open-Label Phase III Trial of Pembrolizumab Versus Platinum Based Chemotherapy in 1L Subjects with PD-L1 Strong Metastatic Non-Small Cell Lung Cancer. 2014. Available online: https://ClinicalTrials.gov/show/NCT02142738 (accessed on 13 April 2023).
125. Merck Sharp & Dohme LLC A Randomized, Open Label, Phase III Study of Overall Survival Comparing Pembrolizumab (MK-3475) Versus Platinum Based Chemotherapy in Treatment Naïve Subjects With PD-L1 Positive Advanced or Metastatic Non-Small Cell Lung Cancer (Keynote 042). 2019. Available online: https://ClinicalTrials.gov/show/NCT03850444 (accessed on 13 April 2023).
126. Hoffmann-La Roche A Phase III, Open Label, Randomized Study of Atezolizumab (Anti-PD-L1 Antibody) Compared with a Platinum Agent (Cisplatin or Carboplatin) in Combination with Either Pemetrexed or Gemcitabine for PD-L1-Selected, Chemotherapy-Naive Patients with Stage IV Non-Squamous or Squamous Non-Small Cell Lung Cancer. 2015. Available online: https://ClinicalTrials.gov/show/NCT02409342 (accessed on 13 April 2023).
127. Krummel, M.F.; Allison, J.P. CD28 and CTLA-4 have opposing effects on the response of T cells to stimulation. *J. Exp. Med.* **1995**, *182*, 459–465. [CrossRef]
128. Wei, S.C.; Sharma, R.; Anang, N.-A.A.S.; Levine, J.H.; Zhao, Y.; Mancuso, J.J.; Setty, M.; Sharma, P.; Wang, J.; Pe'er, D.; et al. Negative Co-Stimulation Constrains T Cell Differentiation by Imposing Boundaries on Possible Cell States. *Immunity* **2019**, *50*, 1084–1098. [CrossRef] [PubMed]
129. Buchbinder, E.I.; Desai, A. CTLA-4 and PD-1 Pathways. *Am. J. Clin. Oncol.* **2016**, *39*, 98–106. [CrossRef]
130. Patel, S.A.; Weiss, J. Advances in the Treatment of Non-Small Cell Lung Cancer: Immunotherapy. *Clin. Chest. Med.* **2020**, *41*, 237–247. [CrossRef] [PubMed]
131. Bristol-Myers Squibb An Open-Label, Randomized Phase 3 Trial of Nivolumab, or Nivolumab Plus Ipilimumab, or Nivolumab Plus Platinum Doublet Chemotherapy Versus Platinum Doublet Chemotherapy in Subjects with Chemotherapy-Naïve Stage IV or Recurrent Non-Small Cell Lung Cancer (NSCLC). 2015. Available online: https://ClinicalTrials.gov/show/NCT02477826 (accessed on 13 April 2023).
132. Hellmann, M.D.; Paz-Ares, L.; Bernabe Caro, R.; Zurawski, B.; Kim, S.-W.; Carcereny Costa, E.; Park, K.; Alexandru, A.; Lupinacci, L.; de la Mora Jimenez, E.; et al. Nivolumab plus Ipilimumab in Advanced Non-Small-Cell Lung Cancer. *N. Engl. J. Med.* **2019**, *381*, 2020–2031. [CrossRef] [PubMed]
133. Merck Sharp & Dohme LLC A Randomized, Double-Blind, Phase III Study of Carboplatin-Paclitaxel/Nab-Paclitaxel Chemotherapy with or without Pembrolizumab (MK-3475) in First Line Metastatic Squamous Non-small Cell Lung Cancer Subjects (KEYNOTE-407). 2019. Available online: https://ClinicalTrials.gov/show/NCT03875092 (accessed on 13 April 2023).
134. Epacadostat Shows Value in Two SCCHN Trials. *Cancer Discov.* **2017**, *7*, OF2. [CrossRef]
135. Einstein, D.J.; McDermott, D.F. Combined blockade of vascular endothelial growth factor and programmed death 1 pathways in advanced kidney cancer. *Clin. Adv. Hematol. Oncol.* **2017**, *15*, 478–488.
136. He, Y.; Yu, H.; Rozeboom, L.; Rivard, C.J.; Ellison, K.; Dziadziuszko, R.; Suda, K.; Ren, S.; Wu, C.; Hou, L.; et al. LAG-3 Protein Expression in Non-Small Cell Lung Cancer and Its Relationship with PD-1/PD-L1 and Tumor-Infiltrating Lymphocytes. *J. Thorac. Oncol.* **2017**, *12*, 814–823. [CrossRef]
137. Liu, J.; Ma, S.; Mao, L.; Bu, L.; Yu, G.; Li, Y.; Huang, C.; Deng, W.; Kulkarni, A.B.; Zhang, W.; et al. T-cell immunoglobulin mucin 3 blockade drives an antitumor immune response in head and neck cancer. *Mol. Oncol.* **2017**, *11*, 235–247. [CrossRef] [PubMed]
138. Zhang, L.; Li, H.; Zhang, F.; Wang, S.; Li, G. CAR-T Immunotherapy and Non-small Cell Lung Cancer: Bottleneck and Dawn. *Zhongguo Fei Ai Za Zhi* **2020**, *23*, 916–920. [CrossRef]
139. Srivastava, S.; Riddell, S.R. Engineering CAR-T Cells: Design Concepts. *Trends Immunol.* **2015**, *36*, 494–502. [CrossRef]
140. Ying, Z.; Huang, X.F.; Xiang, X.; Liu, Y.; Kang, X.; Song, Y.; Guo, X.; Liu, H.; Ding, N.; Zhang, T.; et al. A safe and potent anti-CD19 CAR T cell therapy. *Nat. Med.* **2019**, *25*, 947–953. [CrossRef] [PubMed]

141. Qu, J.; Mei, Q.; Chen, L.; Zhou, J. Chimeric antigen receptor (CAR)-T-cell therapy in non-small-cell lung cancer (NSCLC): Current status and future perspectives. *Cancer Immunol. Immunother.* **2021**, *70*, 619–631. [CrossRef] [PubMed]
142. Dong, J.; Li, B.; Lin, D.; Zhou, Q.; Huang, D. Advances in Targeted Therapy and Immunotherapy for Non-small Cell Lung Cancer Based on Accurate Molecular Typing. *Front. Pharmacol.* **2019**, *10*, 230. [CrossRef] [PubMed]
143. Zhao, J.; Xiong, J. Advances on driver oncogenes of non-small cell lung cancer. *Zhongguo Fei Ai Za Zhi* **2015**, *18*, 42–47. [CrossRef] [PubMed]
144. Mogi, A.; Kuwano, H. TP53 mutations in nonsmall cell lung cancer. *J. Biomed. Biotechnol.* **2011**, *2011*, 583929. [CrossRef]
145. Borghaei, H.; Paz-Ares, L.; Horn, L.; Spigel, D.R.; Steins, M.; Ready, N.E.; Chow, L.Q.; Vokes, E.E.; Felip, E.; Holgado, E.; et al. Nivolumab versus Docetaxel in Advanced Non-squamous Non-small Cell Lung Cancer. *N. Engl. J. Med.* **2015**, *373*, 1627. [CrossRef]
146. Mazieres, J.; Drilon, A.; Lusque, A.; Mhanna, L.; Cortot, A.B.; Mezquita, L.; Thai, A.A.; Mascaux, C.; Couraud, S.; Veillon, R.; et al. Immune checkpoint inhibitors for patients with advanced lung cancer and oncogenic driver alterations: Results from the IMMUNOTARGET registry. *Ann. Oncol.* **2019**, *30*, 1321–1328. [CrossRef]
147. Schoenfeld, A.J.; Rizvi, H.; Bandlamudi, C.; Sauter, J.L.; Travis, W.D.; Rekhtman, N.; Plodkowski, A.J.; Perez-Johnston, R.; Sawan, P.; Beras, A.; et al. Clinical and molecular correlates of PD-L1 expression in patients with lung adenocarcinomas. *Ann. Oncol. J. Eur. Soc. Med. Oncol.* **2020**, *31*, 599–608. [CrossRef]
148. Qiao, M.; Jiang, T.; Liu, X.; Mao, S.; Zhou, F.; Li, X.; Zhao, C.; Chen, X.; Su, C.; Ren, S.; et al. Immune Checkpoint Inhibitors in EGFR-Mutated NSCLC: Dusk or Dawn? *J. Thorac. Oncol.* **2021**, *16*, 1267–1288. [CrossRef]
149. Imyanitov, E.N.; Iyevleva, A.G.; Levchenko, E.V. Molecular testing and targeted therapy for non-small cell lung cancer: Current status and perspectives. *Crit. Rev. Oncol. Hematol.* **2021**, *157*, 103194. [CrossRef]
150. Bravaccini, S.; Bronte, G.; Ulivi, P. TMB in NSCLC: A Broken Dream? *Int. J. Mol. Sci.* **2021**, *22*, 6536. [CrossRef] [PubMed]
151. Masuda, K.; Horinouchi, H.; Tanaka, M.; Higashiyama, R.; Shinno, Y.; Sato, J.; Matsumoto, Y.; Okuma, Y.; Yoshida, T.; Goto, Y.; et al. Efficacy of anti-PD-1 antibodies in NSCLC patients with an EGFR mutation and high PD-L1 expression. *J. Cancer Res. Clin. Oncol.* **2021**, *147*, 245–251. [CrossRef] [PubMed]
152. Yang, J.C.-H.; Sequist, L.V.; Geater, S.L.; Tsai, C.-M.; Mok, T.S.K.; Schuler, M.; Yamamoto, N.; Yu, C.-J.; Ou, S.-H.I.; Zhou, C.; et al. Clinical activity of afatinib in patients with advanced non-small-cell lung cancer harbouring uncommon EGFR mutations: A combined post-hoc analysis of LUX-Lung 2, LUX-Lung 3, and LUX-Lung 6. *Lancet Oncol.* **2015**, *16*, 830–838. [CrossRef]
153. Remon, J.; Steuer, C.E.; Ramalingam, S.S.; Felip, E. Osimertinib and other third-generation EGFR TKI in EGFR-mutant NSCLC patients. *Ann. Oncol.* **2018**, *29*, i20–i27. [CrossRef] [PubMed]
154. Park, S.; Choi, Y.; Kim, J.; Kho, B.; Park, C.; Oh, I.; Kim, Y. Efficacy of immune checkpoint inhibitors according to PD-L1 tumor proportion scores in non-small cell lung cancer. *Thorac. Cancer* **2020**, *11*, 408–414. [CrossRef]
155. Uehara, Y.; Watanabe, K.; Hakozaki, T.; Yomota, M.; Hosomi, Y. Efficacy of first-line immune checkpoint inhibitors in patients with advanced NSCLC with KRAS, MET, FGFR, RET, BRAF, and HER2 alterations. *Thorac. Cancer* **2022**, *13*, 1703–1711. [CrossRef]
156. Zhang, L.; Zhang, T.; Shang, B.; Li, Y.; Cao, Z.; Wang, H. Prognostic effect of coexisting TP53 and ZFHX3 mutations in non-small cell lung cancer patients treated with immune checkpoint inhibitors. *Scand. J. Immunol.* **2021**, *94*, e13087. [CrossRef]
157. VA Office of Research and Development Phase Ib/II Study of Safety and Efficacy of EZH2 Inhibitor, Tazemetostat, and PD-1 Blockade for Treatment of Advanced Non-Small Cell Lung Cancer. 2022. Available online: https://ClinicalTrials.gov/show/NCT05467748 (accessed on 13 April 2023).
158. OncoResponse, Inc. A Phase 1-2 Study of OR2805, a Monoclonal Antibody Targeting CD163, Alone and in Combination With a PD-1 Inhibitor in Subjects with Advanced Malignancies. 2021. Available online: https://ClinicalTrials.gov/show/NCT05094804 (accessed on 13 April 2023).
159. Steuer, C. A Phase 1b Safety and Pharmacodynamic Study of MER Tyrosine Kinase Inhibitor, MRX-2843, in Combination with Osimertinib in Advanced EGFR Mutant Non-Small Cell Lung Cancer. 2021. Available online: https://ClinicalTrials.gov/show/NCT04762199 (accessed on 13 April 2023).
160. Hirschowitz, E. Autologous Dendritic Cell Vaccines in Non-Small Cell Lung Cancer (NSCLC). 2005. Available online: https://ClinicalTrials.gov/show/NCT00103116 (accessed on 13 April 2023).
161. Personalized Cellular Vaccine for Brain Metastases (PERCELLVAC3)—Tabular View—ClinicalTrials.gov. Available online: https://clinicaltrials.gov/ct2/show/record/NCT02808416 (accessed on 13 April 2023).
162. Fuda Cancer Hospital, Guangzhou Combination of Anti-PD-1 and NK Immunotherapy for Recurrent Solid Tumors. 2016. Available online: https://ClinicalTrials.gov/show/NCT02843204 (accessed on 13 April 2023).
163. Combination of Cryosurgery and NK Immunotherapy for Advanced Non-Small Cell Lung Cancer—Full Text View—ClinicalTrials.gov. Available online: https://clinicaltrials.gov/ct2/show/NCT02843815 (accessed on 13 April 2023).
164. Targeted Natural Killer (NK) Cell Based Adoptive Immunotherapy for the Treatment of Patients with Non-Small Cell Lung Cancer (NSCLC) after Radiochemotherapy (RCT)—Full Text View—ClinicalTrials.gov. Available online: https://clinicaltrials.gov/ct2/show/NCT02118415 (accessed on 13 April 2023).
165. Wang, N.; Wang, S.; Wang, X.; Zheng, Y.; Yang, B.; Zhang, J. Research trends in pharmacological modulation of tumor-associated macrophages. *Clin. Transl. Med.* **2021**, *11*, e288. [CrossRef]
166. Xia, L.; Zhu, X.; Zhang, L.; Xu, Y.; Chen, G.; Luo, J. EZH2 enhances expression of CCL5 to promote recruitment of macrophages and invasion in lung cancer. *Biotechnol. Appl. Biochem.* **2020**, *67*, 1011–1019. [CrossRef]

167. Sica, A.; Allavena, P.; Mantovani, A. Cancer related inflammation: The macrophage connection. *Cancer Lett.* **2008**, *267*, 204–215. [CrossRef]
168. Van Gorp, H.; Delputte, P.L.; Nauwynck, H.J. Scavenger receptor CD163, a Jack-of-all-trades and potential target for cell-directed therapy. *Mol. Immunol.* **2010**, *47*, 1650–1660. [CrossRef] [PubMed]
169. Davra, V.; Kumar, S.; Geng, K.; Calianese, D.; Mehta, D.; Gadiyar, V.; Kasikara, C.; Lahey, K.C.; Chang, Y.-J.; Wichroski, M.; et al. Axl and Mertk Receptors Cooperate to Promote Breast Cancer Progression by Combined Oncogenic Signaling and Evasion of Host Antitumor Immunity. *Cancer Res.* **2021**, *81*, 698–712. [CrossRef] [PubMed]
170. Zizzo, G.; Hilliard, B.A.; Monestier, M.; Cohen, P.L. Efficient clearance of early apoptotic cells by human macrophages requires "M2c" polarization and MerTK induction. *J. Immunol.* **2012**, *189*, 3508–3520. [CrossRef] [PubMed]
171. Caetano, M.S.; Younes, A.I.; Barsoumian, H.B.; Quigley, M.; Menon, H.; Gao, C.; Spires, T.; Reilly, T.P.; Cadena, A.P.; Cushman, T.R.; et al. Triple Therapy with MerTK and PD1 Inhibition plus Radiotherapy Promotes Abscopal Antitumor Immune Responses. *Clin. Cancer Res.* **2019**, *25*, 7576–7584. [CrossRef]
172. Zhou, Y.; Fei, M.; Zhang, G.; Liang, W.-C.; Lin, W.; Wu, Y.; Piskol, R.; Ridgway, J.; McNamara, E.; Huang, H.; et al. Blockade of the Phagocytic Receptor MerTK on Tumor-Associated Macrophages Enhances P2X7R-Dependent STING Activation by Tumor-Derived cGAMP. *Immunity* **2020**, *52*, 357–373. [CrossRef]
173. Lee, C.; Bae, S.-J.S.; Joo, H.; Bae, H. Melittin suppresses tumor progression by regulating tumor-associated macrophages in a Lewis lung carcinoma mouse model. *Oncotarget* **2017**, *8*, 54951–54965. [CrossRef]
174. Lee, C.; Jeong, H.; Bae, Y.; Shin, K.; Kang, S.; Kim, H.; Oh, J.; Bae, H. Targeting of M2-like tumor-associated macrophages with a melittin-based pro-apoptotic peptide. *J. Immunother. Cancer* **2019**, *7*, 147. [CrossRef]
175. Wang, B.; Zhang, W.; Zhou, X.; Liu, M.; Hou, X.; Cheng, Z.; Chen, D. Development of dual-targeted nano-dandelion based on an oligomeric hyaluronic acid polymer targeting tumor-associated macrophages for combination therapy of non-small cell lung cancer. *Drug Deliv.* **2019**, *26*, 1265–1279. [CrossRef]
176. Wang, J.-B.; Huang, X.; Li, F.-R. Impaired dendritic cell functions in lung cancer: A review of recent advances and future perspectives. *Cancer Commun.* **2019**, *39*, 43. [CrossRef]
177. Van der Hoorn, I.A.E.; Flórez-Grau, G.; van den Heuvel, M.M.; de Vries, I.J.M.; Piet, B. Recent Advances and Future Perspective of DC-Based Therapy in NSCLC. *Front. Immunol.* **2021**, *12*, 704776. [CrossRef]
178. Wang, Q.-T.; Nie, Y.; Sun, S.-N.; Lin, T.; Han, R.-J.; Jiang, J.; Li, Z.; Li, J.-Q.; Xiao, Y.-P.; Fan, Y.-Y.; et al. Tumor-associated antigen-based personalized dendritic cell vaccine in solid tumor patients. *Cancer Immunol. Immunother.* **2020**, *69*, 1375–1387. [CrossRef] [PubMed]
179. Flieswasser, T.; Van Loenhout, J.; Freire Boullosa, L.; Van den Eynde, A.; De Waele, J.; Van Audenaerde, J.; Lardon, F.; Smits, E.; Pauwels, P.; Jacobs, J. Clinically Relevant Chemotherapeutics Have the Ability to Induce Immunogenic Cell Death in Non-Small Cell Lung Cancer. *Cells* **2020**, *9*, 1474. [CrossRef] [PubMed]
180. Hu, R.-H.; Shi, S.-B.; Qi, J.-L.; Tian, J.; Tang, X.-Y.; Liu, G.-F.; Chang, C.-X. Pemetrexed plus dendritic cells as second-line treatment for patients with stage IIIB/IV non-small cell lung cancer who had treatment with TKI. *Med. Oncol* **2014**, *31*, 63. [CrossRef] [PubMed]
181. Zhao, M.; Li, H.; Li, L.; Zhang, Y. Effects of a gemcitabine plus platinum regimen combined with a dendritic cell-cytokine induced killer immunotherapy on recurrence and survival rate of non-small cell lung cancer patients. *Exp. Ther. Med.* **2014**, *7*, 1403–1407. [CrossRef] [PubMed]
182. Zhang, L.; Yang, X.; Sun, Z.; Li, J.; Zhu, H.; Li, J.; Pang, Y. Dendritic cell vaccine and cytokine-induced killer cell therapy for the treatment of advanced non-small cell lung cancer. *Oncol. Lett.* **2016**, *11*, 2605–2610. [CrossRef]
183. Zhao, Y.; Qiao, G.; Wang, X.; Song, Y.; Zhou, X.; Jiang, N.; Zhou, L.; Huang, H.; Zhao, J.; Morse, M.A.; et al. Combination of DC/CIK adoptive T cell immunotherapy with chemotherapy in advanced non-small-cell lung cancer (NSCLC) patients: A prospective patients' preference-based study (PPPS). *Clin. Transl. Oncol.* **2019**, *21*, 721–728. [CrossRef]
184. Zhong, R.; Teng, J.; Han, B.; Zhong, H. Dendritic cells combining with cytokine-induced killer cells synergize chemotherapy in patients with late-stage non-small cell lung cancer. *Cancer Immunol. Immunother.* **2011**, *60*, 1497–1502. [CrossRef]
185. Hamilton, G.; Plangger, A. The Impact of NK Cell-Based Therapeutics for the Treatment of Lung Cancer for Biologics: Targets and Therapy. *Biologics* **2021**, *15*, 265–277. [CrossRef]
186. Bruno, A.; Focaccetti, C.; Pagani, A.; Imperatori, A.S.; Spagnoletti, M.; Rotolo, N.; Cantelmo, A.R.; Franzi, F.; Capella, C.; Ferlazzo, G.; et al. The Proangiogenic Phenotype of Natural Killer Cells in Patients with Non-Small Cell Lung Cancer. *Neoplasia* **2013**, *15*, 133–142. [CrossRef]
187. Luna, J.I.; Grossenbacher, S.K.; Murphy, W.J.; Canter, R.J. Natural Killer Cell Immunotherapy Targeting Cancer Stem Cells. *Expert. Opin. Biol. Ther.* **2017**, *17*, 313–324. [CrossRef]
188. Kim, S.; Iizuka, K.; Aguila, H.L.; Weissman, I.L.; Yokoyama, W.M. In vivo natural killer cell activities revealed by natural killer cell-deficient mice. *Proc. Natl. Acad. Sci. USA* **2000**, *97*, 2731–2736. [CrossRef] [PubMed]
189. Zhang, G.; Zhao, H.; Wu, J.; Li, J.; Xiang, Y.; Wang, G.; Wu, L.; Jiao, S. Adoptive immunotherapy for non-small cell lung cancer by NK and cytotoxic T lymphocytes mixed effector cells: Retrospective clinical observation. *Int. Immunopharmacol.* **2014**, *21*, 396–405. [CrossRef] [PubMed]
190. Lin, M.; Luo, H.; Liang, S.; Chen, J.; Liu, A.; Niu, L.; Jiang, Y. Pembrolizumab plus allogeneic NK cells in advanced non–small cell lung cancer patients. *J. Clin. Investig.* **2020**, *130*, 2560–2569. [CrossRef] [PubMed]

191. Lin, M.; Liang, S.-Z.; Wang, X.-H.; Liang, Y.-Q.; Zhang, M.-J.; Niu, L.-Z.; Chen, J.-B.; Li, H.-B.; Xu, K.-C. Clinical efficacy of percutaneous cryoablation combined with allogenic NK cell immunotherapy for advanced non-small cell lung cancer. *Immunol. Res.* **2017**, *65*, 880–887. [CrossRef]
192. Iliopoulou, E.G.; Kountourakis, P.; Karamouzis, M.V.; Doufexis, D.; Ardavanis, A.; Baxevanis, C.N.; Rigatos, G.; Papamichail, M.; Perez, S.A. A phase I trial of adoptive transfer of allogeneic natural killer cells in patients with advanced non-small cell lung cancer. *Cancer Immunol. Immunother.* **2010**, *59*, 1781–1789. [CrossRef]
193. Shevtsov, M.; Pitkin, E.; Ischenko, A.; Stangl, S.; Khachatryan, W.; Galibin, O.; Edmond, S.; Lobinger, D.; Multhoff, G. Ex vivo Hsp70-Activated NK Cells in Combination With PD-1 Inhibition Significantly Increase Overall Survival in Preclinical Models of Glioblastoma and Lung Cancer. *Front. Immunol.* **2019**, *10*, 454. [CrossRef]
194. Pockley, A.G.; Vaupel, P.; Multhoff, G. NK cell-based therapeutics for lung cancer. *Expert Opin. Biol. Ther.* **2020**, *20*, 23–33. [CrossRef]
195. Daher, M.; Rezvani, K. Outlook for new CAR-based therapies with a focus on CAR-NK cells: What lies beyond CAR-engineered T cells in the race against cancer. *Cancer Discov.* **2021**, *11*, 45–58. [CrossRef]
196. Pan, K.; Farrukh, H.; Chittepu, V.C.S.R.; Xu, H.; Pan, C.; Zhu, Z. CAR race to cancer immunotherapy: From CAR T, CAR NK to CAR macrophage therapy. *J. Exp. Clin. Cancer Res.* **2022**, *41*, 119. [CrossRef]
197. Zhang, Y.; Wallace, D.L.; de Lara, C.M.; Ghattas, H.; Asquith, B.; Worth, A.; Griffin, G.E.; Taylor, G.P.; Tough, D.F.; Beverley, P.C.L.; et al. In vivo kinetics of human natural killer cells: The effects of ageing and acute and chronic viral infection. *Immunology* **2007**, *121*, 258–265. [CrossRef]
198. Roma-Rodrigues, C.; Mendes, R.; Baptista, P.V.; Fernandes, A.R. Targeting Tumor Microenvironment for Cancer Therapy. *Int. J. Mol. Sci.* **2019**, *20*, 840. [CrossRef] [PubMed]
199. Freeman-Keller, M.; Kim, Y.; Cronin, H.; Richards, A.; Gibney, G.; Weber, J.S. Nivolumab in Resected and Unresectable Metastatic Melanoma: Characteristics of Immune-Related Adverse Events and Association with Outcomes. *Clin. Cancer Res.* **2016**, *22*, 886–894. [CrossRef] [PubMed]
200. Suresh, K.; Naidoo, J.; Lin, C.T.; Danoff, S. Immune Checkpoint Immunotherapy for Non-Small Cell Lung Cancer. *Chest* **2018**, *154*, 1416–1423. [CrossRef] [PubMed]
201. Bauer, T.; Cho, B.C.; Heist, R.; Bazhenova, L.; Werner, T.; Goel, S.; Kim, D.-W.; Adkins, D.; Carvajal, R.D.; Alva, A.; et al. First-in-human phase 1/1b study to evaluate sitravatinib in patients with advanced solid tumors. *Investig. New Drugs* **2022**, *40*, 990–1000. [CrossRef]

pharmaceutics

MDPI

Article

# Synergistic Effect of Conditioned Medium from Amniotic Membrane Mesenchymal Stromal Cells Combined with Paclitaxel on Ovarian Cancer Cell Viability and Migration in 2D and 3D In Vitro Models

**Paola Chiodelli [1,*], Patrizia Bonassi Signoroni [2], Elisa Scalvini [2], Serafina Farigu [2], Elisabetta Giuzzi [2], Alice Paini [2], Andrea Papait [1,3], Francesca Romana Stefani [2], Antonietta Rosa Silini [2] and Ornella Parolini [1,4]**

1 Department of Life Science and Public Health, Università Cattolica del Sacro Cuore, 00168 Rome, Italy; andrea.papait@unicatt.it (A.P.); ornella.parolini@unicatt.it (O.P.)
2 Centro di Ricerca E. Menni, Fondazione Poliambulanza Istituto Ospedaliero, 25124 Brescia, Italy; patrizia.bonassi@poliambulanza.it (P.B.S.); elisa.scalvini@poliambulanza.it (E.S.); serafina.farigu@poliambulanza.it (S.F.); elisabetta.giuzzi@poliambulanza.it (E.G.); alice.paini@poliambulanza.it (A.P.); francesca.stefani@poliambulanza.it (F.R.S.); antonietta.silini@poliambulanza.it (A.R.S.)
3 Fondazione Policlinico Universitario "Agostino Gemelli" IRCCS, 00168 Rome, Italy
4 Fondazione IRCCS Casa Sollievo della Sofferenza, Viale Cappuccini 1, San Giovanni Rotondo, 71013 Foggia, Italy
* Correspondence: paola.chiodelli@unicatt.it

**Abstract: Background:** Ovarian cancer accounts for more deaths than any other cancer of the female reproductive system. Despite standard care, recurrence due to tumor spread and chemoresistance is common, highlighting the need for novel therapies. Mesenchymal stromal cells from the human amniotic membrane (hAMSC) and the intact amniotic membrane (hAM) are promising due to their secretion of tumor-modulating bioactive factors, accessibility from biological waste, and ethical favorability. Furthermore, unlike isolated cells, hAM provides an easier, clinically translatable product. We previously demonstrated that hAMSC can inhibit tumor cell proliferation, both in contact and transwell settings, suggesting that hAMSC secrete bioactive factors able to target tumor cells. This study evaluates the anti-tumor effects of bioactive factors from hAMSC and hAM conditioned medium (CM) on ovarian cancer cells in 2D and 3D models, alone or with paclitaxel. **Methods:** The impact of CM, alone or with paclitaxel, was tested on ovarian cancer cell proliferation, migration, invasion, and on angiogenesis. **Results:** hAMSC-CM and hAM-CM inhibited the proliferation and migration in 2D cultures and reduced spheroid growth and invasion in 3D models. Combining CM with paclitaxel enhanced anti-tumor effects in both settings. **Conclusions:** hAMSC-CM and hAM-CM show therapeutic potential against ovarian cancer, with synergistic benefits when combined with paclitaxel.

**Keywords:** human amniotic mesenchymal stromal cell; amniotic membrane; ovarian cancer; 3D model; paclitaxel

## 1. Introduction

Ovarian cancer is among the most lethal gynecological malignancies, characterized by late diagnosis, high recurrence rates, and resistance to conventional therapies [1]. Despite advancements in chemotherapy, including the widespread use of paclitaxel and platinum-based agents, the five-year survival rate remains dismally low (about 31%) for advanced-stage disease [2–4], underscoring the urgent need for novel therapeutic strategies.

 https://doi.org/10.3390/pharmaceutics17040420

Recent studies have highlighted the dual nature of mesenchymal stromal cells (MSC) in cancer biology; while they can promote tumor growth and metastasis under certain conditions, their conditioned media (CM) demonstrate notable anti-tumor effects [5–8]. MSC from different sources are known for their unique ability to secrete a diverse array of bioactive molecules, including cytokines, growth factors, and extracellular vesicles, which collectively form a complex secretome. This secretome plays a pivotal role in mediating the paracrine effects. The therapeutic potential of the MSC secretome, or CM lies in its ability to modulate key biological processes such as proliferation, apoptosis, and migration affecting different cellular pathways including IL-6/JAK2/STAT3, cyclins, FAK/PI3K/Akt/mTOR [9–11].

The human amniotic membrane is a highly favorable source of mesenchymal stromal cells (hAMSC) due to its origin from placental tissue after childbirth, making it an ethically acceptable and non-controversial option. Furthermore, it is obtained from biological waste—the placenta—following routine childbirth, ensuring no harm or risk to the mother or baby. hAMSC meet the established criteria for MSC from all tissues [12], as well as the specific standards for fetal membrane MSC defined during the First International Workshop on Placenta-Derived Stem Cells in 2008 [13]. On the other hand, the intact amniotic membrane (hAM) comprises two cell populations, hAMSC and amniotic epithelial cells (hAEC), both of which exhibit anti-tumor properties [14–16]; hAM is easier to use, as it bypasses the additional step of MSC isolation.

In our previous research, we showed that hAMSC can effectively inhibit tumor cell proliferation in a paracrine manner [17], and that hAM-CM reduces the migration of bladder urothelial cancer cell lines [18]. Notably, both hAMSC-CM and hAM-CM are rich in cytokines, growth factors, and extracellular vesicles (EVs) [19,20].

The aim of this study is to evaluate the anticancer potential of hAMSC-CM and hAM-CM on ovarian cancer cell lines (HEY, OV-90, and SKOV3) using the classical 2D monolayer and the more advanced 3D spheroid culture system, a physiologically relevant environment closely mimicking in vivo tumor architecture and behavior. Given that 3D cell cultures more accurately mimic in vivo tumor conditions, including increased resistance to chemotherapeutic agents such as paclitaxel, we hypothesize that combining paclitaxel with CM might overcome this resistance in 3D ovarian cancer models.

## 2. Materials and Methods

### 2.1. Cell Cultures

HEY and OV-90 human ovarian cancer cell lines were kindly provided by Daniela Gallo (Fondazione Policlinico Universitario "Agostino Gemelli" IRCCS, Rome, Italy). SKOV3 cell line was purchased by ATCC. HEY cells derive from a human ovarian cancer xenograft originally grown from a peritoneal deposit of a patient with moderately differentiated papillary cystadenocarcinoma [21]. OV-90 cells were originally isolated from malignant ascites from patients with ovarian adenocarcinoma and harbor p53 mutations that exhibit genomic features similar to high-grade serous ovarian carcinoma. SKOV3 cells derive from the ascites of a patient with ovarian adenocarcinoma and lack the expression of p53 protein. HEY cells were cultured in RPMI 1640 (Euroclone, Pero, Itlay; ECB9006) supplemented with 10% fetal bovine serum (FBS) (Euroclone; ECS50000LH) and 1% non-essential amino acids (Thermo Fisher, Waltham, MA, USA; 11140-035). OV-90 cells were cultured in a complex medium composed by MCDB (Sigma Aldrich, St. Louis, MO, USA; M-6770) plus M199 (Merk; Whitehouse Station, NJ, USA; M4530) at a 1:1 ratio, and 0.5% MEM (Sigma Aldrich; 56416C-1L), supplemented with 15% FBS. SKOV3 cells were cultured in Mcoy's medium (Euroclone, ECM0210L) supplemented with 10% FBS. All culture media were supplemented with 2 mM L-glutamine (Euroclone; ECB3000D) and 1% penicillin/streptomycin (herein referred to P/S, all from Euroclone; ECB30010D).

Umbilical cords were obtained following the guidelines outlined by the Brescia Provincial Ethics Committee (number NP 2243, 19/01/2016). Human umbilical vein endothelial cells (HUVEC) were isolated from the umbilical cord vein following cannulation, followed by PBS washes to remove blood cells. The vein was then incubated for 1 h at 37 °C in DMEM supplemented with P/S, 0.2% collagenase I (Thermo Fisher; 17018029), and 0.01 mg/mL DNase (Merck, Darmstadt, Germany; 11284932001). After incubation, the detached cells were collected using PBS (Euroclone; ECB4004) with P/S, centrifuged at 300× $g$ for 10 min without braking, resuspended in medium, and seeded into a flask pre-coated with 1.5% porcine gelatin (Merck; G2500). HUVEC at passages I–V were grown in EBM-2 Basal Medium (Lonza, Basilea, Swizerland; CC-3156) supplemented with EGM-2 SingleQuots Supplements (Lonza; CC-4176).

### 2.2. Human Amniotic Membrane (hAM) Fragment Preparation

The study adhered to the principles of the Declaration of Helsinki, and informed consent was obtained following the guidelines outlined by the Brescia Provincial Ethics Committee (number NP 2243, 19 January 2016).

For each placenta, the amniotic membrane was manually separated from the chorion and cut into a 50 cm$^2$ fragments for CM preparation from hAM, or into 9 cm$^2$ for the isolation of hAMSCs. The fragments were decontaminated by placing them in a physiological solution + 0.25% povidone-iodine for 1–2 s, then removed and incubated in PBS + P/S + amphotericin B (Euroclone; ECM0009D) + cefamezin (Teva Italia, Milan, Italy) for 3 min. The fragments were then washed in PBS containing 1% P/S.

### 2.3. Isolation and Culture of Human Amniotic Mesenchymal Stromal Cells (hAMSC)

Cells were isolated and phenotypically characterized as previously described [22]. hAM fragments were digested at 37 °C for 9 min with 2.5 U/mL dispase (VWR, Radnor, PA, USA; 734-1312) and then transferred to RPMI 1640 medium supplemented with 10% heat-inactivated FBS, 1% P/S, and 1% L-glutamine. Afterward, the fragments were treated with 0.9 mg/mL collagenase (Merck; 10103586001) and 0.01 mg/mL DNase I (Merck; 11284932001) for approximately 2.5–3 h at 37 °C. The resulting cell suspensions were centrifuged at 150 g, and the supernatant was filtered through a 100-μm cell strainer (BD Falcon, Bedford, MA, USA), and the cells were collected by centrifugation. Freshly isolated cells were expanded until passage 2 (p2) by plating at a density of 10,000 cells/cm$^2$ in Chang medium D (Irvine Scientific, Santa Ana, CA, USA; 12401340) supplemented with 2 mM L-glutamine and 1% P/S at 37 °C in the incubator at 5% $CO_2$ and phenotypically characterized.

### 2.4. Preparation of Conditioned Medium (CM)

From hAM: two fragments of hAM were placed in 50 mL conical tubes with filter caps (Greiner Bio-One, Kremsmünster, Austria; 227245) containing 20 mL of DMEM/F12 (Thermo Fisher Scientific; 31330038). The fragments were left for 5 days under gentle rotation at 37 °C and 5% $CO_2$. After incubation, the medium was centrifuged at 300× $g$, filtered through a 0.2-μm sterile filter (Sartorius Stedim, Florence, Italy: 16532), and stored at −80 °C until use.

From hAMSC P2: hAMSC were cultured for 5 days in 24-well plates (Euroclone; ET3024) at a density of 5 × 10$^5$ cells/well in 0.5 mL of DMEM/F12 supplemented with 2 mM L-glutamine and 1% P/S as previously described [23]. At the end of incubation, the CM was collected, centrifuged at 300× $g$, filtered through a 0.2-μm sterile filter (Sartorius Stedim), and stored at −80 °C until use.

Pooling of CM for experiments: Each experiment was performed using CM pooled from at least three different hAMSC/hAM donors. The CM were used at varying percentages in DMEM/F12 as required by the experimental protocol. For each experiment, DMEM/F12 served as the negative control. FBS was added to both CM, and the negative control at the concentration specified for each assay. In all assays, CM and the negative control were added simultaneously, using the same volume and experimental procedures.

### *2.5. Determination of Cellular Viability (MTT-Assay and CyQUANT-Assay)*

Cells were plated in 96-well plates at a density of 15,000 cells/cm$^2$ for HEY and SKOV3 or 30,000 cells/cm$^2$ for OV-90. They were then treated with increasing concentrations of different CM (12.5%, 25%, 50%, 75%, 100%) in DMEM/F12 containing 1% FBS for 24, 48, 72, and 96 h.

For the matrix assay, cells were treated for 48 h with increasing concentrations of CM (12.5%, 25%, 50%, 75%, 100%) in combination with increasing concentrations of paclitaxel (Vinci-Biochem, Vinci, Italy; Cod. AG-CN2-0045-M001) (0.6, 1.8, 5.5, 16.6, 50 nM). At the end of incubation, cell viability was assessed using either the MTT or CyQUANT assay.

MTT Assay: MTT (Merck; M2128) was added to each well at a final concentration of 0.5 mg/mL, and the cells were incubated at 37 °C for 3 h. After incubation, 100 µL of lysis buffer [20% SDS (Merck; 1.13760.0100) in a 50% $H_2O$/50% DMF (Thermo Fisher Scientific, 423640010) solution, pH 4.7] was added overnight at 37 °C. The absorbance was measured at 550 nm using a Victor™ X4 plate reader (PerkinElmer, Waltham, MA, USA). Since MTT occurs only in metabolically active cells, the level of activity was considered as an indirect measure of the viability of the cells, without a count of live and death cells.

CyQuant Assay: The CyQUANT™ NF Cell Proliferation Assay (Thermo Fisher Scientific; C35006) was performed according to the manufacturer's instructions. Briefly, the medium was removed from each well, and 100 µL of CyQuant reagent was added. The cells were incubated at 37 °C for 1 h. Fluorescence was then measured using a Victor™ X4 plate reader at 485 nm.

### *2.6. Colony Formation*

Cells were seeded into 12-well plates (Euroclone; ET3012) at the following densities: HEY (250 cells/well), SKOV3 (500 cells/well), and OV-90 (800 cells/well). Cells were allowed to attach overnight. The next day, cells were treated with 50%, 75%, or 100% of the different CM in 1% FBS and cultured for 10–14 days to allow colony formation. After the incubation period, debris was washed twice with PBS, and cells were fixed with cold methanol for 10 min. They were then stained with crystal violet (Merck; V5265). After staining, the cells were solubilized with 400 µL of 30% acetic acid (Carlo Erba, Cornaredo, MI, Italy; 524521). A 100 µL aliquot was transferred to a 96-well plate, and absorbance was measured at 550 nm using a Victor™ X4 plate reader.

### *2.7. Apoptosis Assay*

Cell apoptosis was evaluated using flow cytometry with the Annexin V-fluorescein isothiocyanate (FITC)/Propidium iodide (PI) kit (BD Pharmingen™ FITC Annexin V kit, Cat. No. 556420). Cells were treated with different concentrations of CM (50%, 75%, or 100%) in DMEM/F12 containing 1% FBS. After treatment, the cells were resuspended in buffer and incubated with Annexin V at room temperature for 20 min. Subsequently, PI was added and the cells were further incubated for an additional 10 min at room temperature. Samples were acquired on a BD FACS Symphony A3 flow cytometer (BD Biosciences, Franklin Lakes, NJ, USA), and the data were analyzed using FlowJo 10.8 software (BD Biosciences).

### 2.8. Wound Healing Assay

Cells were seeded in silicone inserts (ibidi GmbH, Gräfelfing, Germany; 81176) in 24-well plates. The following cell densities were used: HEY at 100,000 cells/cm$^2$, SKOV3 at 85,000 cells/cm$^2$, and OV-90 at 150,000 cells/cm$^2$. The day after seeding, the inserts were removed, and the cells were treated with 50%, 75%, or 100% of the different CM in 1% FBS. Microphotographs were taken at Day 0, Day 1, and Day 2 using an Olympus IX50 microscope equipped with an OPTIKA camera (OPTIKA, Ponteranica, Italy; Model 4083.13), using a 4× magnification. The extent of wound repair was evaluated by measuring the wound area at Day 1 and Day 2 relative to Day 0 (T0) using computerized image analysis with ImageJ software (http://rsb.info.nih.gov/ij/).

### 2.9. Single-Cell Migration

Cell motility was assessed by time-lapse videomicroscopy. HEY cells were seeded at a density of 3000 cells/cm$^2$, and SKOV3 and OV-90 cells were seeded at 5000 cells/cm$^2$ in 12-well plates. After 18 h, the cells were treated with 75% of the different CM in 1% FBS. A constant temperature of 37 °C and $pCO_2$ of 5% were maintained throughout the experimental period. Cells were observed under Mica Widefield Live Cell (Leica Microsystems, Wetzlar, Germany), and images (1 frame every 30 min) were digitally recorded for 1380 min. Single-cell migration was analyzed using AIVIA software version 12.1 (Leica Microsystems) through cell tracking recipe. Path lengths (in µm) of cells were recovered for at least 10 frames and were used for analysis. Path Length is the distance traveled by the object along its trajectory over the entire duration of the track and is calculated as the sum of the Euclidean distances between the object's positions at sequential time points.

### 2.10. Transwell Migration Assay

Cells were seeded in 6-well plates at a density of 50,000 cells/cm$^2$ and treated with 50%, 75%, or 100% of the different CM plus 1% FBS for 24 h. After treatment, the cells were detached and seeded in transwell inserts (Corning, Glendale, AZ, USA; CL-β422-48EA) at the following densities: 100,000 cells/insert for HEY and OV-90, 40,000 cells/insert for SKOV3, in a volume of 150 µL of serum-free DMEM/F12. The inserts were then placed into 24-well plates containing 500 µL of DMEM with 10% FBS for HEY and SKOV3, or 20% FBS for OV-90. After 24 h, the inserts were removed, and the upper side of the inserts was gently cleaned with swabs to remove non-migrated cells. Cells on the lower side of the inserts were then fixed with ice-cold methanol for 15 min and left to air dry. Crystal violet (Sigma-Aldrich; V5265) staining was performed by soaking the inserts in the dye for 10 min. The upper side of the inserts was again cleaned with swabs. Once the inserts were dry, three images per insert were acquired using an Olympus IX50 microscope equipped with an OPTIKA camera at 4× magnification. To quantify the migrated cells, crystal violet was solubilized by adding 200 µL of 33% acetic acid (Carlo Erba; 2789) to each insert. Then, 100 µL of the solubilized solution was transferred into a 96-well plate, and absorbance was measured at 595 nm using a Victor™ X4 plate reader (PerkinElmer).

### 2.11. Western Blot

Cells were seeded in 6-well plates at a density of 20,000 cells/cm$^2$ and treated with 75% of the different CM in 1% FBS. After 24 h of treatment, the cells were collected and homogenized in RIPA buffer (supplemented with protease inhibitor, Sigma-Aldrich, P8340, and phosphatase inhibitor, Merck, P0044). Protein extraction was performed by applying 5 cycles of sonication, with cooling on ice between cycles. Protein concentration was determined using the BCA assay (Thermo Fisher Scientific; 23235). Next, 20 µg of protein per sample was loaded onto an SDS-PAGE gel and analyzed by Western blot using specific primary antibodies against phospho-p70 S6 Kinase (Cell Signaling Thecnologies, Danvers, MA, USA; 9205), and GAPDH (Bio-Rad; Hercules, CA, USA; MCA4740). After primary antibody incubation, membranes were probed with the appropriate secondary antibodies: anti-rabbit-HRP (Bio-Rad; 170-6515) or anti-mouse-HRP (Bio-Rad; 170-6516).

### 2.12. Spheroid Generation

Spheroids were generated by seeding 3000 cells for HEY or 6000 cells for SKOV3 and OV-90. To promote spheroid formation, 2% methylcellulose (Sigma Aldrich; M7027) was added to the respective culture medium, comprising 20% of the total volume. The cells were then seeded in U-bottom 96-well plates (Corning; 3788) in a final volume of 100 μL per well. After 24 h, some of the medium was replaced with different conditioned media (CM) to achieve final concentrations of 50% or 75% in 1% FBS. For the matrix assay, spheroids were treated for 6 days with increasing concentrations of CM (12.5%, 25%, 50%, 75%) in combination with increasing concentrations of paclitaxel (1.1, 3.3, 10, 30 nM). Alternatively, 75% CM was added immediately during spheroid formation under the same spheroid-forming conditions.

Spheroid Growth Assessment: To assess spheroid growth, 6–8 images per condition were captured using an Olympus IX50 microscope equipped with an OPTIKA camera at 4× magnification on day 1, day 3, and day 6. The areas of the spheroids were measured using ImageJ software (http://rsb.info.nih.gov/ij/) and reported in $\mu m^2$.

ImageJ Calculations: Spheroid area was calculated using the "Macros" plugin in ImageJ. Images were first converted to grayscale. Images with an area less than 1000 $pixels^2$ were excluded, and any holes within the spheroids were automatically filled. The area of the resulting spheroids was then calculated automatically in ImageJ software [24].

### 2.13. Three-Dimensional Cell Viability Assay (ATPlite)

Three spheroids per condition were harvested with 50 μL of medium after 6 days of treatment and collected into a 96-well plate. The assay was performed according to the manufacturer's instructions (3D ATPlite 1 Step, PerkinElmer; 38221900). After adding 50 μL of lysis buffer to each well, the spheroids were mechanically disaggregated by pipetting 10–15 times. The plate was covered and incubated for 30 min on an orbital shaker in the dark. After incubation, 50 μL from each well was transferred into a 96-well white plate. Luminescence was measured using a Victor™ X4 luminometer (PerkinElmer).

### 2.14. Three-Dimensional Co-Culture Angiogenesis Model

The protocol was adapted from Xiao Wan et al. [25]. HUVEC were labeled with Celltracker green CMFDA 5 μM at 37 °C for 30 min. Then, 40 μL Geltrex was added into a 96-well plate which had been pre-chilled on ice. The plates were incubated at 37 °C for 30 min, allowing the Geltrex to polymerise. Then, 12,800 HUVECs resuspended in 40 μL EBM-2 2% FBS were seeded onto the polymerised gel layer.

After four hours of HUVEC seeding, 5000 ovarian cancer cells in 100 μL hAMSC-CM or hAM-CM with 2% FBS and 10% Geltrex (*v*/*v*), in the presence or absence of 16.6 nM Paclitaxel, were added onto the polymerized Geltrex. The final concentration of CM was 50%. The plate was then incubated at 37 °C to allow the top layer of Matrigel to polymerize. After 24 h, z-stack microphotographs with a step size of 4.75 μm were taken at Mica Widefield Live Cell (Leica Microsystems) using a 10× objective. Image reconstructions were performed using MAX projection of 15–20 images. Images were analyzed with the ImageJ Angiogenesis Analyzer Plugin (https://imagej.net/ij/macros/toolsets/Angiogenesis%20Analyzer.txt, accessed on 15 February 2025) [26]. Total segment length and the number of isolated segments were measured and calculated.

### 2.15. Statistical Analysis

Data report the mean and standard deviation. The parameters were compared using one-way or two-way analysis of variance (ANOVA), with Dunnet multiple comparison test post-analysis. N is reported in each figure legend. Statistical analysis was performed using Prism 9.5 (GraphPad Software, La Jolla, CA, USA). A $p$-value lower than 0.05 was considered statistically significant.

## 3. Results

### 3.1. hAMSC-CM and hAM-CM Inhibit Ovarian Cancer Cell Proliferation

We first characterized the antiproliferative effects of CM derived from hAMSC-CM and hAM-CM on three ovarian cancer cell lines: HEY, SKOV3, and OV-90. CM were collected after five days from pooled samples and assessed for their ability to reduce cell viability using the CyQUANT assay. HEY, SKOV3, and OV-90 cell lines were treated with different concentrations of CM (12.5%, 25%, 50%, 75%, and 100%) for 24, 48, 72, and 96 h. There was a dose-dependent inhibition of proliferation in all three cell lines, with effects becoming apparent after 48 h (Figure 1A,B). HEY cells were most sensitive to both hAMSC-CM and hAM-CM, while OV-90 cells exhibited the least sensitivity. Notably, CM from normal dermal fibroblasts had no effect on cell viability, underscoring the specificity of hAMSC-CM and hAM-CM (Figure S1). Mechanistically, hAM-CM markedly inhibited the phosphorylation of p70 S6 kinase (p-p70 S6), a key regulator of cell growth and cell cycle progression, after 24 h of treatment (Figure 1C).

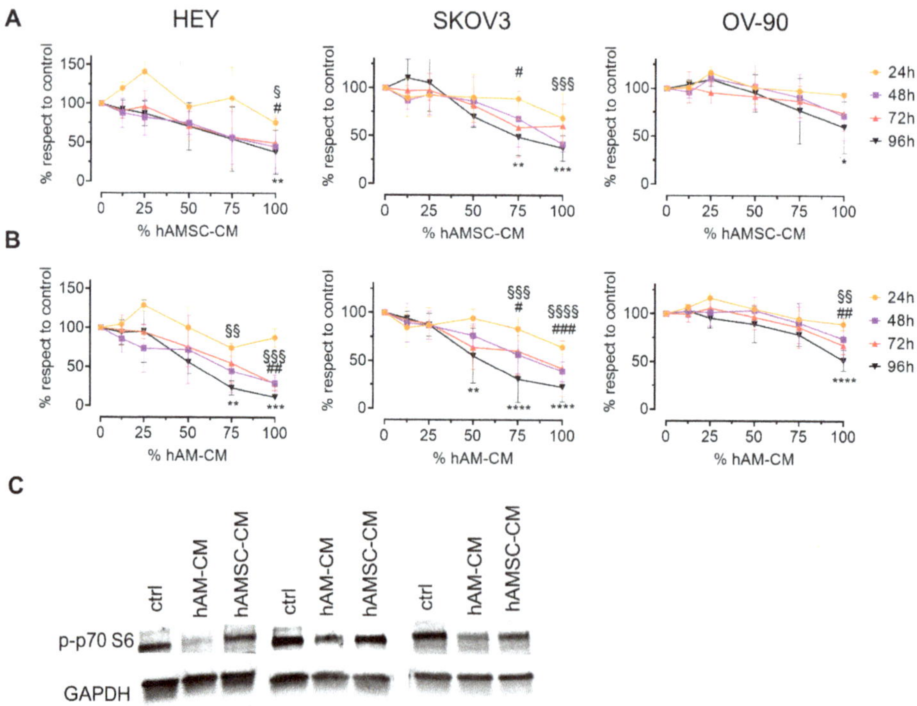


**Figure 1.** hAMSC-CM and hAM-CM inhibit ovarian cancer cell proliferation. HEY, SKOV3, and OV-90 cell lines were treated with differing concentrations of hAMSC-CM (**A**) or hAM-CM (**B**) (12.5%, 25%, 50%, 75%, and 100%) for 24, 48, 72, and 96 h. Cell viability was assessed using the CyQUANT

assay, $n = 3$–5. Results are expressed as a percentage relative to untreated controls at each time point (orange: 24 h; purple: 48 h; red: 72 h; black: 96 h). Data are presented as mean ± SD, with significance levels indicated (for 48 h: § $p < 0.05$, §§ $p < 0.01$, §§§ $p < 0.001$, §§§§ $p < 0.0001$; for 72 h: # $p < 0.05$, ## $p < 0.01$, ### $p < 0.001$; for 96 h: * $p < 0.05$, ** $p < 0.01$, *** $p < 0.001$, **** $p < 0.0001$). (**C**) Western blot for p-p70 S6 were performed on protein lysates of HEY, SKOV3 and OV-90 treated with 75% CM for 24 h.

Accordingly, in clonogenic assays, both CM types significantly reduced colony formation and size in all cell lines, with hAM-CM exhibiting the strongest effect (Figure 2A). To assess apoptosis, we analyzed treated cells via flow cytometry at 48 h. hAM-CM significantly induced apoptosis in HEY and OV-90 cells, while hAMSC-CM showed a less pronounced, non-significant effect. SKOV3 cells, lacking functional p53, showed no increase in apoptosis under either treatment (Figure 2B). These findings demonstrate that both hAMSC-CM and hAM-CM reduce cell viability in a dose-dependent manner, disrupt clonogenic potential, and induce apoptosis in a cell dependent manner.

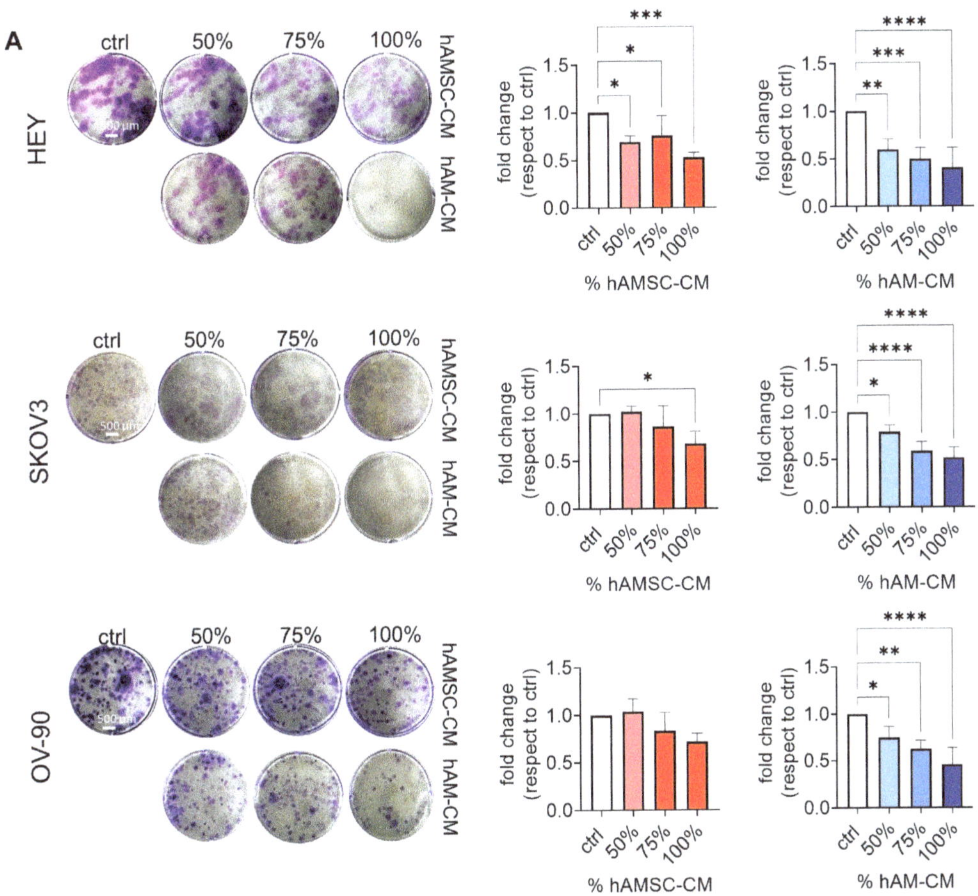


**Figure 2.** *Cont.*

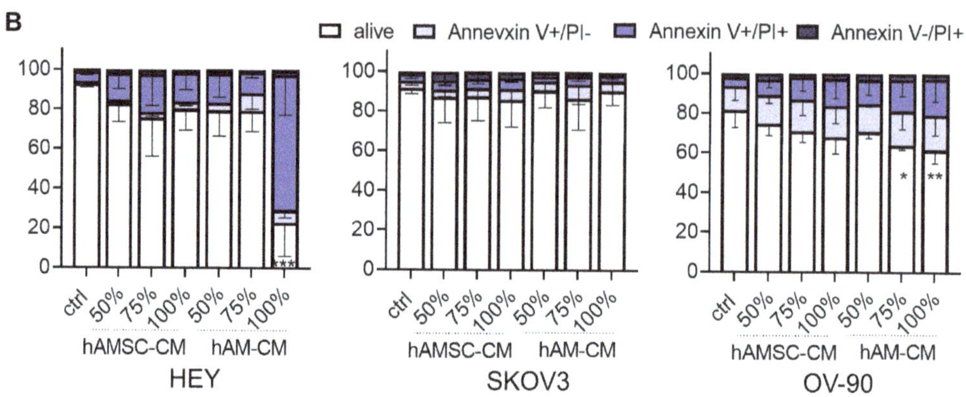


**Figure 2.** hAMSC-CM and hAM-CM affect ovarian cancer cell colony formation and apoptosis. (**A**) Colony formation assays for HEY, SKOV3, and OV-90 cell lines treated with 50%, 75%, and 100% CM. Representative images of stained colonies are shown (**left** panel, scale bar 500 µm), with quantification of colony formation expressed as fold change relative to controls (**right** panel, red: hAMSC-CM, blue: hAM-CM), $n$ = 3–4. (**B**) Apoptosis analysis of HEY, SKOV3, and OV-90 cell lines treated with 50%, 75%, and 100% CM for 48 h. Apoptosis was detected by Annexin V/PI staining and quantified using flow cytometry. Results are shown as percentages of apoptotic cells. $n$ = 3–4. Data are presented as mean ± SD, with significance levels indicated (* $p < 0.05$, ** $p < 0.01$, *** $p < 0.001$, **** $p < 0.0001$).

### 3.2. *hAMSC-CM and hAM-CM Differentially Affect 3D Spheroid Proliferation*

Ovarian cancer metastasizes in part through spheroid formation and peritoneal dissemination. To explore the impact of CM on tumor cells, we assessed its effects on 3D aggregates, known as spheroids. The three tumor cell lines exhibited distinct spheroid morphologies. On the first day of formation, HEY cells formed compact, rounded spheroids, OV-90 cells formed rounded but less compact spheroids, and SKOV3 cells formed spheroids that were both less compact and less rounded. Spheroids were treated with 75% CM for six days, and their areas were measured on days 1, 3, and 6. The cell lines displayed differential responses to CM treatment. Both hAMSC-CM and hAM-CM significantly reduced the spheroid area of HEY and SKOV3 starting on day 3 (Figure 3A,B). Notably, SKOV3 spheroids exhibited a more compact morphology following CM treatment. In contrast, OV-90 spheroids treated with CM maintained the same area as the control group (Figure 3C).

ATP content, an indicator of cell viability [27], was measured in spheroids after six days of treatment with hAMSC-CM and hAM-CM. ATP levels were normalized to the control spheroids. Remarkably, in all cell lines, both hAMSC-CM and hAM-CM treatments significantly reduced ATP content (Figure 3D–F).

To further investigate, we evaluated spheroid formation and growth when hAMSC-CM and hAM-CM were added directly during spheroid generation. After one day of treatment, HEY and OV-90 spheroids appeared less aggregated in the presence of either CM, resulting in a larger apparent area compared to the control. By day 6, however, the spheroid area of HEY—and to a lesser extent, SKOV3 and OV-90—was reduced following CM treatment (Figure 4A–C). Additionally, ATP content in all cell lines was significantly reduced in the presence of CM, mirroring the results observed when CM was added after spheroid formation (Figure 4D–F).

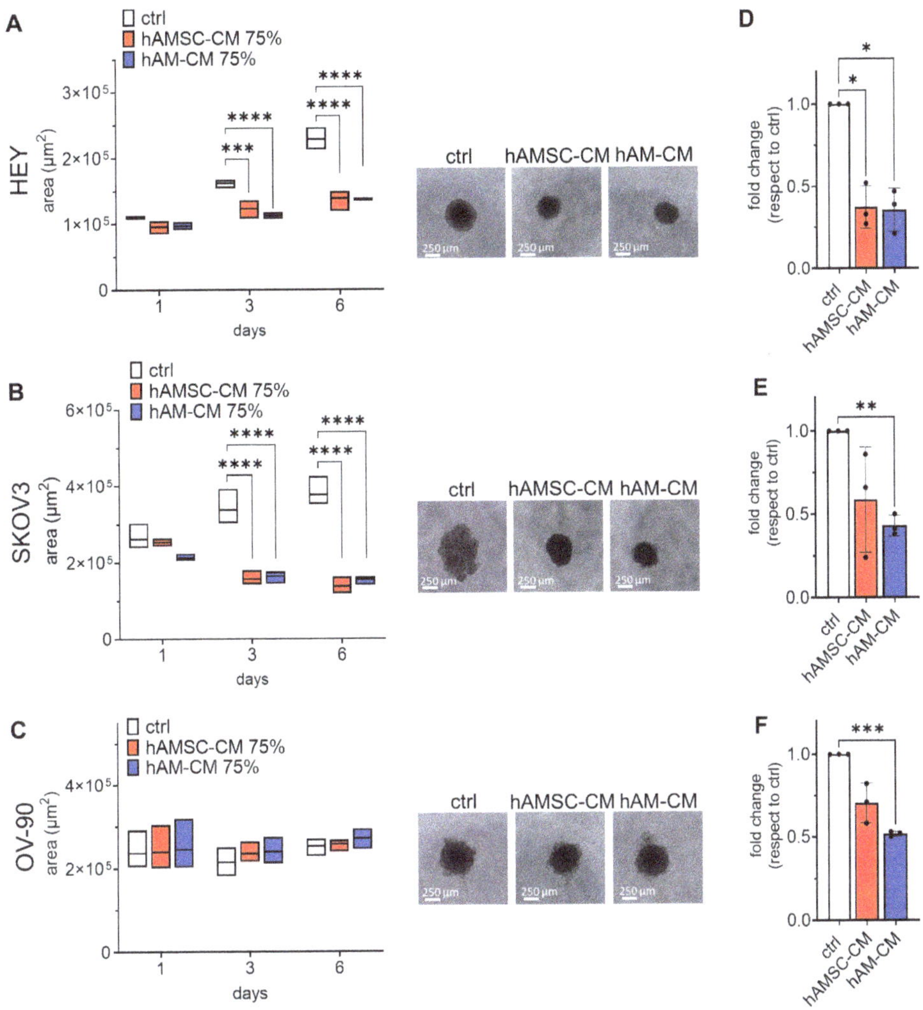


**Figure 3.** hAMSC-CM and hAM-CM reduce ovarian cancer spheroid growth and ATP content. Spheroids from HEY (**A**), SKOV3 (**B**), and OV-90 (**C**) cell lines were treated with 75% CM for six days. Spheroid areas were measured at days 1, 3, and 6 using ImageJ and expressed in μm$^2$ (white: control; red: hAMSC-CM; blue: hAM-CM). Representative micrographs of spheroids at day 6 are shown (right panel, scale bar 250 μm). (**D–F**) The ATP content of HEY, SKOV3, and OV-90 spheroids was measured after six days of treatment and expressed as fold change relative to untreated controls. Data are presented as mean ± SD. $n$ = 3. Significance levels are indicated (* $p < 0.05$, ** $p < 0.01$, *** $p < 0.001$, **** $p < 0.0001$).

In summary, these findings demonstrate that hAMSC-CM and hAM-CM decrease spheroid viability in a 3D model. This effect is observed in both pre-formed, treated with CM after 24 h of spheroid formation, and forming spheroids, where CM was added during the formation process, suggesting potential mechanisms of action on ovarian cancer cell aggregates.

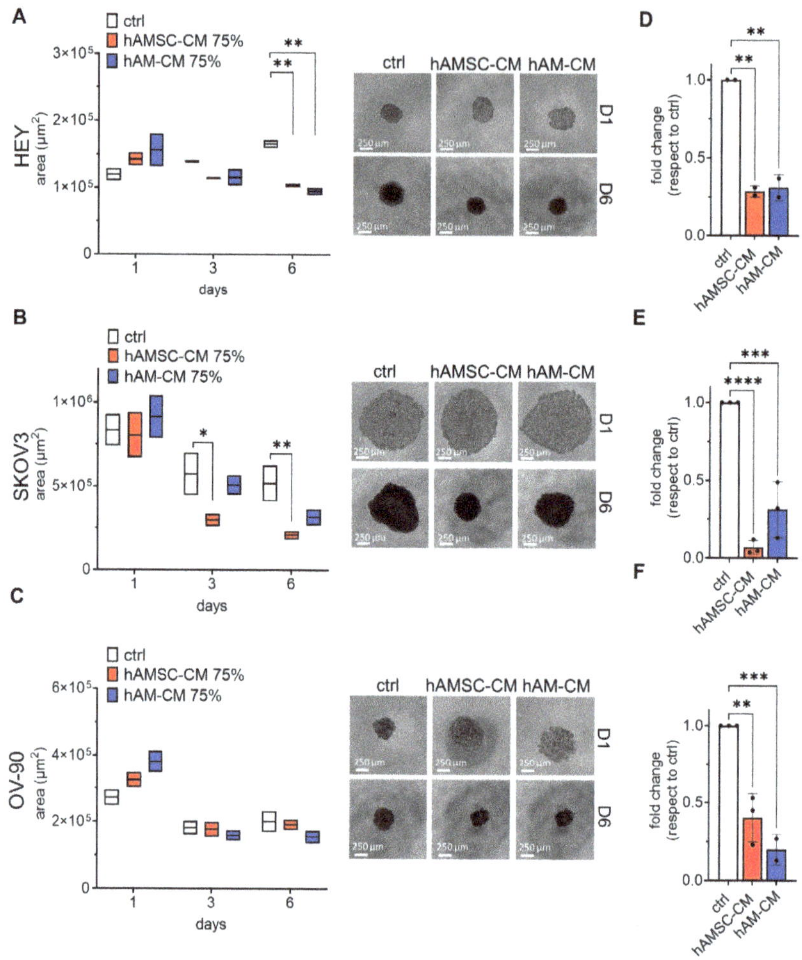


**Figure 4.** CM pretreatment affects spheroid growth and ATP content. Spheroids from HEY (**A**), SKOV3 (**B**), and OV-90 (**C**) cell lines were treated with 75% CM during formation and monitored for six days. Spheroid areas were measured at days 1, 3, and 6 using ImageJ and expressed in µm² (white: control; red: hAMSC-CM; blue: hAM-CM). Representative micrographs of spheroids at day 1 and day 6 are shown (right panel, scale bar 250 µm). (**D–F**) ATP content of HEY, SKOV3, and OV-90 spheroids was measured after six days of CM pretreatment and expressed as fold change relative to untreated controls. $n = 3$. Data are presented as mean ± SD, with significance levels indicated (* $p < 0.05$, ** $p < 0.01$, *** $p < 0.001$, **** $p < 0.0001$).

### 3.3. hAMSC-CM and hAM-CM Inhibit Ovarian Cancer Cell Migration

CM derived from hAM has been reported to inhibit bladder cancer cell migration [11], while CM from other MSC sources, such as Wharton's Jelly, has shown inhibitory effects on ovarian cancer cell migration [28]. Here, we examined how CM from hAMSC and hAM affects the migration of ovarian cancer cell lines. Using a wound-healing assay, we monitored the migratory ability of the cell lines in the presence of the two CM at 24 and 48 h. hAM-CM significantly inhibited the migration of all three cell lines in a dose-dependent manner. In contrast, hAMSC-CM reduced migration in HEY and OV-90 cells but had no effect on SKOV3 migration at 24 h. At 48 h, SKOV3 migration showed a slight, non-significant increase (Figure 5A–C). These findings were partially corroborated by single-cell migration assay (Figure 5D), where both CM reduced the total migration distance (path length) of HEY and OV-90 cells, while increasing SKOV3 migratory capacity. Interestingly, hAMSC-CM retained its inhibitory effects on HEY and OV-90 single-cell migration even after 24 h of pre-treatment, as shown in the transwell migration assay. Additionally, hAM-CM specifically inhibited HEY migration under these conditions (Figure S2). Collectively, these data suggest that hAMSC-CM and hAM-CM inhibit migration in both HEY and OV-90 cells, while having contrasting effects on SKOV3 migration, enhancing its single-cell and collective migration capacity.

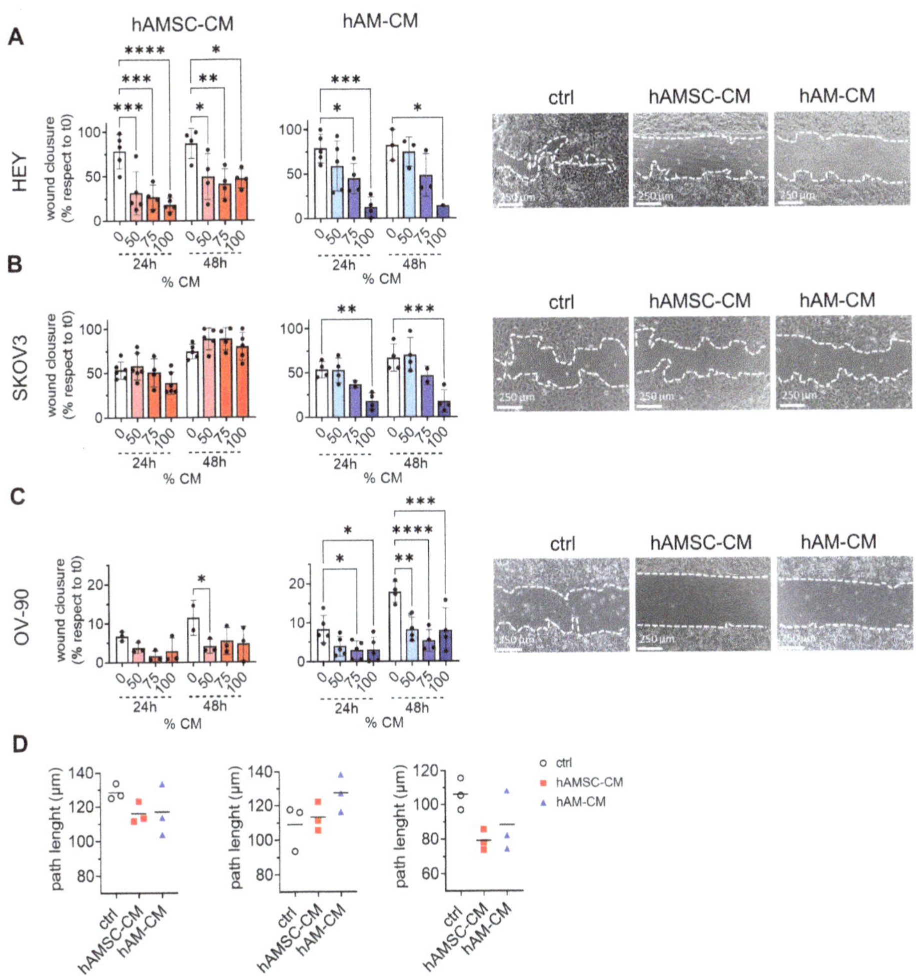


**Figure 5.** hAMSC-CM and hAM-CM inhibit ovarian cancer cell migration. Wound-healing assays were performed on monolayers of HEY (**A**), SKOV3 (**B**), and OV-90 (**C**) cells treated with 50%, 75%, and 100% CM. Wound closure was measured at 0, 24, and 48 h and expressed as the percentage of the initial wound area (white: control; red: hAMSC-CM; blue: hAM-CM). Representative micrographs of the wound area at 75% CM treatment are shown (right panel, scale bar 250 μm), with white dotted lines marking the wound boundaries. $n = 3$–5. Data are presented as mean ± SD (* $p < 0.05$, ** $p < 0.01$, *** $p < 0.001$, **** $p < 0.0001$). (**D**) Single-cell migration was performed on HEY, SKOV3, and OV-90 cells treated with 75% CM by time-lapse analysis. Each point is a replicate and refers to the mean of at least 30 cell paths for each condition.

### 3.4. hAMSC-CM and hAM-CM Affect Spheroid Invasion

In ovarian cancer, spheroids represent the minimal metastatic units capable of invading and implanting at distant sites. To investigate the impact of hAMSC-CM and hAM-CM on spheroid invasion, we evaluated the invasive ability of spheroids pre-treated with CM for 24 h within a surrounding matrix. HEY spheroids exhibited a strong invasive capacity, evident from 24 h onward. As shown in Figure 6A, spheroids pretreated with either hAMSC-CM or hAM-CM displayed a significantly reduced invasion area at both 24 and 48 h. SKOV3 spheroids, on the other hand, demonstrated a limited ability to invade the matrix, producing only a few protrusions from the spheroid core. Notably, after 48 h, treatment with either CM further inhibited their ability to form processes (Figure 6B). OV-90 spheroids also invaded the surrounding matrix, with a prominent invasion area observed on day 5. Interestingly, CM-pretreated OV-90 spheroids exhibited a smaller invasion area compared to the control group (Figure 6C). These findings suggest that both hAMSC-CM and hAM-CM effectively reduce the invasive capacity of ovarian cancer spheroids, impacting cell lines with varying invasive potentials.

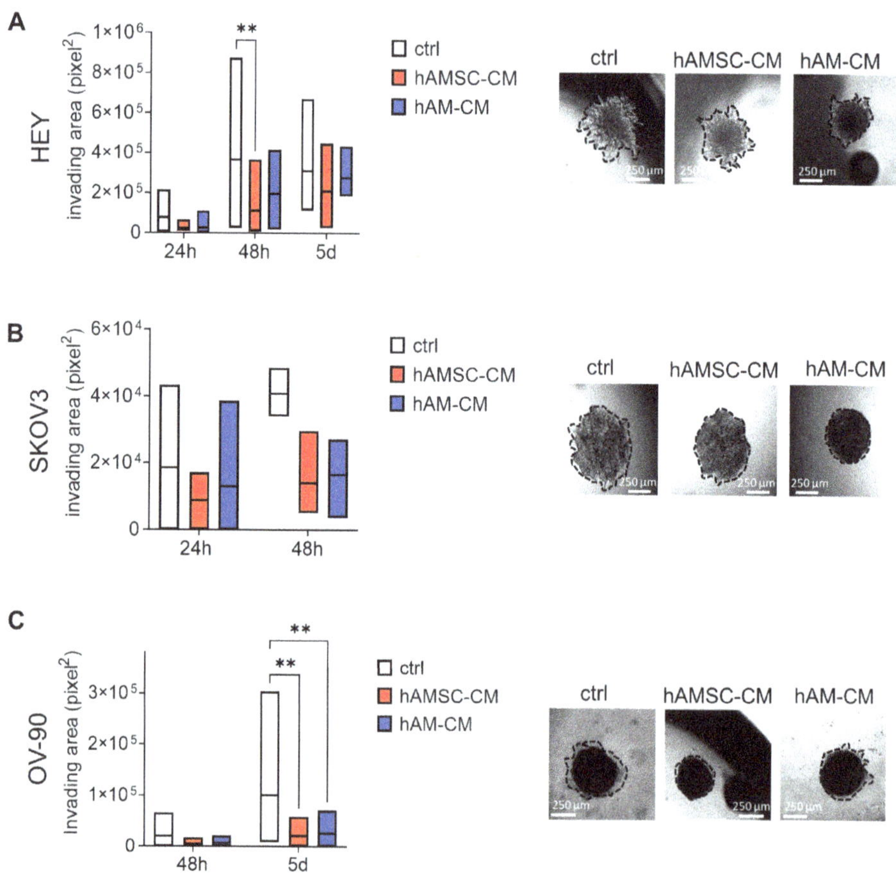


**Figure 6.** hAMSC-CM and hAM-CM inhibit spheroid invasion. Spheroids from HEY (**A**), SKOV3 (**B**), and OV-90 (**C**) cells were pretreated with 75% CM for 24 h and embedded in a Geltrex matrix. Invasion areas were measured after 24, 48, and 120 h and expressed in $\mu m^2$ (white: control; red: hAMSC-CM;

blue: hAM-CM). Representative micrographs of invading spheroids are shown (right panel, scale bar 250 µm), with invasion boundaries marked by black dotted lines. Data are presented as mean ± SD (** $p < 0.01$).

### *3.5. Effect of hAMSC-CM and hAM-CM in Combination with Paclitaxel on Ovarian Cancer Cell Lines in 2D and 3D*

To evaluate the potential enhanced therapeutic effect of hAMSC-CM and hAM-CM combined with paclitaxel in inhibiting ovarian cancer cell proliferation, combination treatments were conducted using both 2D and 3D models. These experiments included three ovarian cancer cell lines, with increasing concentrations of hAMSC-CM or hAM-CM and paclitaxel, to assess their combinatorial effects.

The combinatorial effects were analyzed using the ZIP reference model in SynergyFinder+ [29]. The results are shown in Figure S3 for the 2D model and Figure 7 for the 3D model. Positive deviations between observed and expected responses, indicative of synergy, are represented in red, while negative deviations, indicative of antagonism, are shown in green. The relative dose–response matrices are showed in Figures S4 and S5, showing the percentage of cell viability relative to controls.

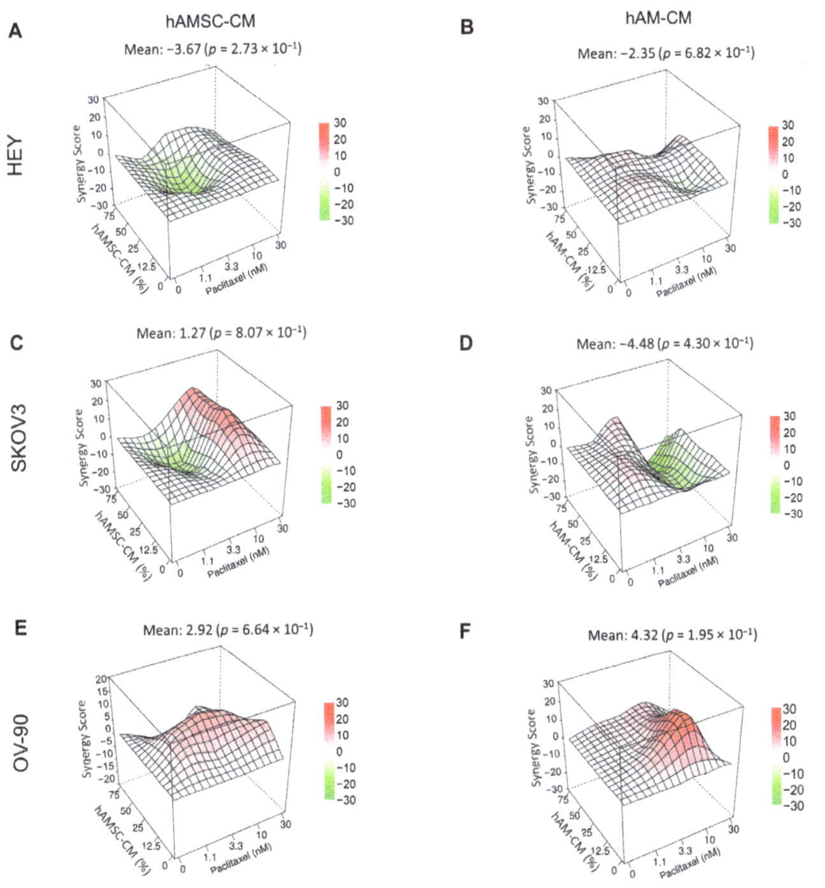


**Figure 7.** Synergistic effects of CM and paclitaxel on ovarian cancer spheroids in 3D. Spheroids from HEY (**A**,**B**), SKOV3 (**C**,**D**), and OV-90 (**E**,**F**) cells were treated with different concentrations of CM (12.5%, 25%, 50%, 75%) and paclitaxel (1.1, 3.3, 10, 30 nM) for 48 h. Viability was assessed using the

ATP-lite assay. Results are displayed as ZIP synergy maps and synergy scores for each combination and cell line are shown.

Both hAMSC-CM and hAM-CM demonstrated an enhanced therapeutic effect when combined with paclitaxel, particularly in the OV-90 cell line. This enhanced effect was observed consistently across both 2D and 3D models, underscoring the robust potential of these combinations to improve therapeutic outcomes. These findings suggest that hAMSC-CM and hAM-CM can amplify the efficacy of paclitaxel against ovarian cancer.

### *3.6. Effect of hAMSC-CM and hAM-CM in Combination with Paclitaxel in 3D Co-Culture Angiogenesis Model*

Angiogenesis is a hallmark of cancer, and it is responsible for tumor spread and metastasis in ovarian cancer by promoting new blood vessel formation. It is essential for tumor growth and development. To assess the effect of hAMSC-CM and hAM-CM on tumor angiogenesis, we used a 3D co-culture angiogenesis model. We evaluated the tubule-like endothelial structures by HUVECs on top of a layer of Geltrex after 24 h of co-culturing with ovarian cancer cell lines. The analysis of digital images of tube-like networks was carried out using ImageJ angiogenesis analyzer software. We measured the total segment length and number of isolated segments, two parameters with opposite trends when angiogenesis is inhibited. Specifically, a reduction in total segment length and an increase in the number of isolated segments indicate impaired angiogenesis. As shown in Figure 8, hAMSC-CM had no impact on angiognesesis, on the contrary, for all three ovarian cancer cell lines, hAM-CM impaired the formation of tube structures. Interestingly, angiogenesis was severely impaired when both hAMSC-CM and hAM-CM were combined with paclitaxel.

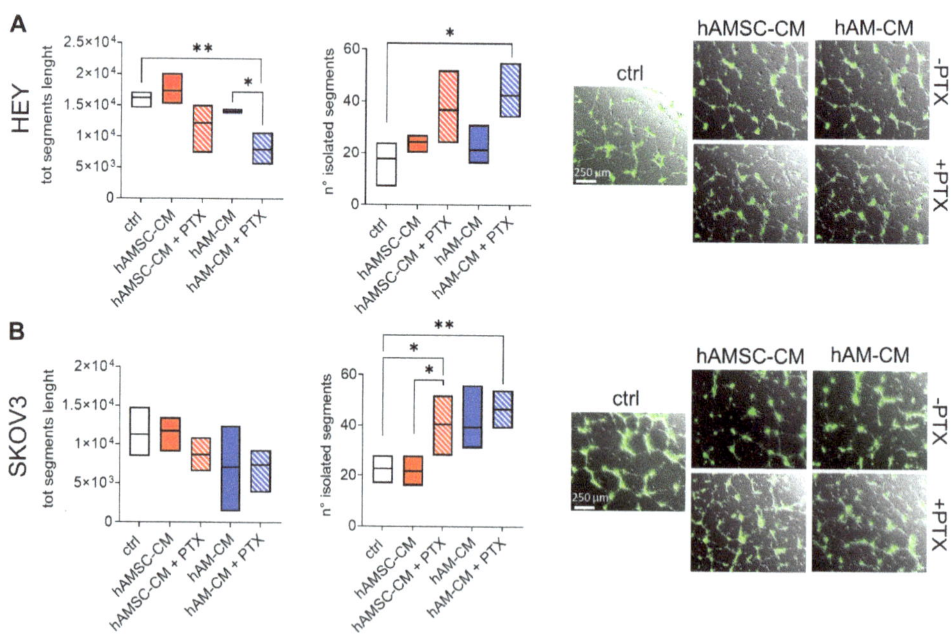


**Figure 8.** *Cont.*

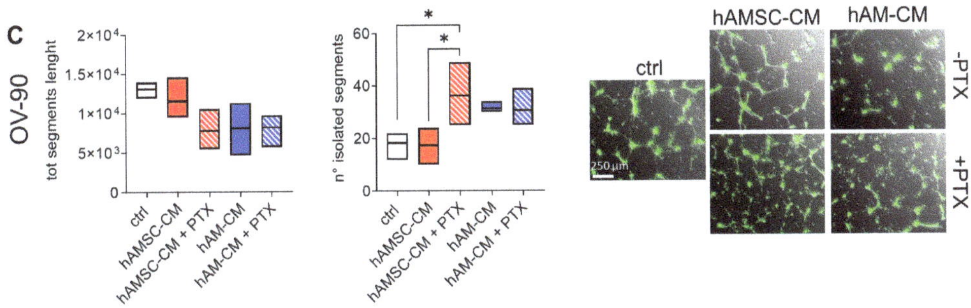


**Figure 8.** Effects of CM and paclitaxel in a co-culture angiogenesis model. Co-culture of HUVECs and ovarian cancer cell lines in a Geltrex sandwich. HUVEC were seeded on a Geltrex later for 4 h, then HEY (**A**), SKOV3 (**B**), OV-90 (**C**) with 50% hAMSC-CM or hAM-CM in the presence or absence of 10 nM paclitaxel (PTX) were seeded on the top. Tubule-like endothelial structures were analyzed after 24 h with the ImageJ Angiogenesis analyzer plugin. Data are expressed as total segment length and number of isolated segments. N = 3 (* $p < 0.05$; ** $p < 0.01$). On the right, representative micrographs of different treatments. Scale bar 250 µm.

## 4. Discussion

Ovarian cancer remains a formidable challenge in oncology, with high mortality rates due to late diagnosis, tumor recurrence, and resistance to conventional therapies. Despite advances in surgical techniques and the development of chemotherapeutics such as paclitaxel, the clinical outcomes for ovarian cancer patients remain suboptimal. This underscores a critical unmet need for innovative therapeutic approaches that target the biological underpinnings of tumor progression and metastatic dissemination. In this study, we explored the therapeutic potential of CM derived from hAMSC and intact hAM on ovarian cancer cell lines in both 2D and 3D models. These secretomes, enriched in bioactive molecules, offer a cell-free and scalable therapeutic strategy that could complement existing treatments. Our findings highlight the ability of these CM to inhibit multiple hallmarks of cancer progression, including cancer cell proliferation, migration, invasion, angiogenesis, and spheroid growth. Our results demonstrate that both hAMSC-CM and hAM-CM effectively inhibit ovarian cancer cell proliferation in a dose-dependent manner (Figure 1). Moreover, the combination of CM with paclitaxel enhanced the anti-tumor effects on proliferation in 2D cultures and spheroid growth.

Notably, hAM-CM consistently displayed stronger antiproliferative and pro-apoptotic effects compared to hAMSC-CM, likely reflecting the combined contributions of bioactive factors secreted by both stromal and epithelial cells within the amniotic membrane.

The differential response observed among the ovarian cancer cell lines—HEY, SKOV3, and OV-90—emphasizes the importance of tumor heterogeneity. HEY cells, which harbor wild-type p53, were the most sensitive to CM treatment, while OV-90 cells, characterized by a missense TP53 mutation, exhibited the least sensitivity. These findings are consistent with the notion that p53 status influences cellular responses to stress and therapeutic interventions [30,31]. Previous studies have reported similar antiproliferative effects of MSC-derived CM in various cancer types, attributed to the secretion of bioactive molecules, including cytokines, growth factors, and extracellular vesicles [10,32–35]. The stronger effects observed with hAM-CM may reflect the combined contributions of hAMSCs and hAECs, which are known to possess complementary anticancer properties [14,36–40].

In addition to reducing cell proliferation, hAM-CM significantly induced apoptosis in HEY and OV-90 cells, as evidenced by increased Annexin V/PI staining (Figure 2). In contrast, SKOV3 cells, which are p53-null, showed minimal apoptotic responses, further supporting the hypothesis that CM-induced apoptosis may depend, at least in part, on p53-mediated pathways. This mechanistic link between p53 status and CM efficacy highlights the potential for tailoring secretome-based therapies to the molecular characteristics of specific tumor subtypes [41].

Spheroids represent a more physiologically relevant model of tumor biology, closely mimicking the architecture and microenvironment of in vivo tumors [42]. Our study revealed that both hAMSC-CM and hAM-CM reduced spheroid growth and ATP content, indicating impaired viability (Figure 3). Interestingly, CM disrupted spheroid formation when introduced during aggregation (Figure 4), suggesting potential interference with cellular adhesion and extracellular matrix interactions [43,44]. These findings are particularly significant given the role of spheroids in ovarian cancer metastasis and chemoresistance [45]. The observed effects highlight the potential of hAMSC-CM and hAM-CM to target both established and forming tumor microenvironments.

Cancer metastasis is a major cause of mortality in ovarian cancer, with migration and invasion being critical steps in this process [46,47]. Both hAMSC-CM and hAM-CM inhibited the migratory capacity of HEY and OV-90 cells, as demonstrated in wound-healing, transwell migration, and single-cell motility assays (Figure 5). However, SKOV3 cells exhibited a unique response, with increased migration observed under certain conditions. This divergence may reflect differences in intrinsic cell motility mechanisms or interactions with CM components [11,48]. Additionally, the reduction in spheroid invasion (Figure 6) into the matrix after CM pretreatment underscores the potential of these secretomes to disrupt metastatic progression [49].

To further explore the therapeutic potential of CM, we investigated its combination with paclitaxel, a first-line chemotherapeutic agent in ovarian cancer treatment. The combination treatment demonstrated enhanced therapeutic effects in both 2D and 3D models (Figures S3 and 7), particularly in the OV-90 cell line. Using the ZIP reference model implemented in SynergyFinder+, we identified a significant interaction between CM and paclitaxel, with positive deviations indicative of synergy. This enhanced therapeutic effect may result from the complementary actions of paclitaxel, which disrupts microtubule dynamics and induces mitotic arrest [50,51], and the bioactive components of CM, which modulate key signaling pathways implicated in tumor survival, proliferation, and metastasis. Previous studies have linked CM-derived molecules to the inhibition of IL-6/JAK2/STAT3 and FAK/PI3K/Akt/mTOR pathways, providing potential mechanistic insights into the observed enhanced effect [9,11,52,53]. Paclitaxel has been reported to induce the upregulation of S6 as a compensatory adaptive response [54], and previous studies have shown that targeting p70 with specific inhibitors can enhance Paclitaxel efficacy in reducing cancer cell viability. While our interpretation remains speculative, the observed reduction in p-p70 S6 in our model may suggest a similar mechanism, potentially contributing to the enhanced effect of Paclitaxel. Notably, hAMSC can be loaded with paclitaxel and the drug released from hAMSC is able to inhibit pancreatic cancer cell line proliferation in vitro [55]. Interestingly, not only does the released paclitaxel impact proliferation but also hAMSC are able to inhibit tumor cell proliferation per se under specific culture conditions in vitro.

The mechanisms underlying the anticancer effects of hAMSC-CM and hAM-CM are likely multifactorial, involving the secretion of bioactive molecules that modulate cell signaling, immune responses, and the tumor microenvironment [19,56,57]. While our study establishes the therapeutic potential of these CM, further research is needed to elucidate the specific components responsible for their effects. Proteomic and transcriptomic analyses of CM could provide valuable insights into its active constituents and mechanisms of action. Additionally, in vivo studies are essential to validate the efficacy and safety of CM-based therapies and to assess their potential for clinical translation. Additional experiments are required to gain a deeper understanding of the mechanisms by which the amniotic membrane influences cancer dynamics, and to clarify its potential as an adjuvant therapeutic strategy for targeting tumor cells. Interestingly, we observed that hAM-CM alone is able to affect capillary-like structure formation, while hAMSC-CM had no effect (Figure 8). The combination with paclitaxel enhanced the effect, suggesting that the combinatorial approach, especially for hAM-CM, could have an impact also on the tumor microenvironment, which plays a pivotal role in tumor growth and dissemination. These findings prompt us to further investigate this aspect in different experimental models to better elucidate the impact of CM on tumor angiogenesis. Given the dual role of tumor vasculature in both sustaining tumor progression and modulating drug delivery, it will be crucial to assess not only the inhibition of angiogenesis but also the potential ability of CM to normalize the vasculature.

In conclusion, this study demonstrates that hAMSC-CM and hAM-CM exhibit potent antitumor activity against ovarian cancer by targeting critical processes in tumor progression, including proliferation, migration, invasion, and spheroid growth. The consistent enhanced effect observed across multiple experimental conditions highlights the potential of CM as an adjuvant therapy to improve clinical outcomes while potentially reducing the toxicities associated with high-dose chemotherapy. These findings position the CM as a promising, cell-free therapeutic strategy in the fight against ovarian cancer, warranting further investigation in preclinical and clinical settings.

**Supplementary Materials:** The following supporting information can be downloaded at: https://www.mdpi.com/article/10.3390/pharmaceutics17040420/s1, Figure S1: Effect of CM from normal dermal fibroblasts on ovarian cancer cell proliferation; Figure S2: Effect of hAMSC-CM and hAM-CM on ovarian cancer cell migration in transwell; Figure S3: Synergistic effects of CM and paclitaxel on ovarian cancer cell lines in 2D; Figure S4: Synergistic effects of CM and paclitaxel on ovarian cancer cell lines in 2D-Dose response matrix; Figure S5: Synergistic effects of CM and paclitaxel on ovarian cancer spheroids in 3D-Dose response matrix.

**Author Contributions:** Conceptualization, P.C. and O.P.; investigation, P.C., P.B.S., E.S., S.F., E.G. and A.P. (Alice Paini); methodology: P.C., S.F., E.G. and A.P. (Alice Paini); formal analysis, P.C., E.S. and P.B.S.; data curation: P.C., P.B.S. and E.S.; resources: O.P.; writing—original draft preparation, P.C., A.R.S., F.R.S. and A.P. (Andrea Papait); visualization: PC; writing—review and editing, P.C., E.S., P.B.S., S.F., E.G., A.P. (Alice Paini), A.R.S., F.R.S., A.P. (Andrea Papait) and O.P.; supervision, A.R.S.; funding acquisition, O.P. All authors have read and agreed to the published version of the manuscript.

**Funding:** This work was supported by Fondazione Alessandra Bono ONLUS, Brescia, Italy; Fondazione Poliambulanza Istituto Ospedaliero, Brescia, Italy; Università Cattolica del Sacro Cuore, Linea D1 (O.P.); the Italian Ministry of Research and University (MUR, 5x1000), and Contributi per il funzionamento degli Enti privati che svolgono attività di ricerca—C.E.P.R.

**Institutional Review Board Statement:** The study adhered to the principles of the Declaration of Helsinki, and informed consent was obtained following the guidelines outlined by the Brescia Provincial Ethics Committee (number NP 2243, 19 January 2016).

**Informed Consent Statement:** Informed consent was obtained from all subjects involved in the study.

**Data Availability Statement:** The original contributions presented in this study are included in the article/supplementary material. Further inquiries can be directed to the corresponding author.

**Acknowledgments:** The authors thank the physicians and midwives of the Department of Obstetrics and Gynecology of Fondazione Poliambulanza, Brescia, Italy, and all of the mothers who donated placenta.

**Conflicts of Interest:** The authors declare no conflicts of interest.

## References


1. Bray, F.; Laversanne, M.; Sung, H.; Ferlay, J.; Siegel, R.L.; Soerjomataram, I.; Jemal, A. Global cancer statistics 2022: GLOBOCAN estimates of incidence and mortality worldwide for 36 cancers in 185 countries. *CA Cancer J. Clin.* **2024**, *74*, 229–263. [CrossRef]
2. Armstrong, D.K.; Alvarez, R.D.; Bakkum-Gamez, J.N.; Barroilhet, L.; Behbakht, K.; Berchuck, A.; Berek, J.S.; Chen, L.M.; Cristea, M.; DeRosa, M.; et al. NCCN Guidelines Insights: Ovarian Cancer, Version 1.2019. *J. Natl. Compr. Cancer Netw.* **2019**, *17*, 896–909. [CrossRef]
3. Zhu, L.; Chen, L. Progress in research on paclitaxel and tumor immunotherapy. *Cell. Mol. Biol. Lett.* **2019**, *24*, 40. [CrossRef]
4. Cancer Stat Facts: Ovarian Cancer. Available online: https://seer.cancer.gov/statfacts/html/ovary.html (accessed on 20 January 2025).
5. Slama, Y.; Ah-Pine, F.; Khettab, M.; Arcambal, A.; Begue, M.; Dutheil, F.; Gasque, P. The Dual Role of Mesenchymal Stem Cells in Cancer Pathophysiology: Pro-Tumorigenic Effects versus Therapeutic Potential. *Int. J. Mol. Sci.* **2023**, *24*, 3511. [CrossRef] [PubMed]
6. Zhao, R.; Chen, X.; Song, H.; Bie, Q.; Zhang, B. Dual Role of MSC-Derived Exosomes in Tumor Development. *Stem Cells Int.* **2020**, *2020*, 8844730. [CrossRef]
7. Liang, W.; Chen, X.; Zhang, S.; Fang, J.; Chen, M.; Xu, Y. Mesenchymal stem cells as a double-edged sword in tumor growth: Focusing on MSC-derived cytokines. *Cell. Mol. Biol. Lett.* **2021**, *26*, 3. [CrossRef]
8. Papait, A.; Stefani, F.R.; Cargnoni, A.; Magatti, M.; Parolini, O.; Silini, A.R. The Multifaceted Roles of MSCs in the Tumor Microenvironment: Interactions with Immune Cells and Exploitation for Therapy. *Front. Cell Dev. Biol.* **2020**, *8*, 447. [CrossRef]
9. Wang, M.; Zhang, Y.; Liu, M.; Jia, Y.; He, J.; Xu, X.; Shi, H.; Zhang, J.; Liu, Y. Inhibition of STAT3 signaling as critical molecular event in HUC-MSCs suppressed Glioblastoma Cells. *J. Cancer* **2023**, *14*, 611–627. [CrossRef]
10. Aslam, N.; Abusharieh, E.; Abuarqoub, D.; Alhattab, D.; Jafar, H.; Alshaer, W.; Masad, R.J.; Awidi, A.S. An In Vitro Comparison of Anti-Tumoral Potential of Wharton's Jelly and Bone Marrow Mesenchymal Stem Cells Exhibited by Cell Cycle Arrest in Glioma Cells (U87MG). *Pathol. Oncol. Res.* **2021**, *27*, 584710. [CrossRef]
11. Janev, A.; Ramuta, T.Z.; Jerman, U.D.; Obradovic, H.; Kamensek, U.; Cemazar, M.; Kreft, M.E. Human amniotic membrane inhibits migration and invasion of muscle-invasive bladder cancer urothelial cells by downregulating the FAK/PI3K/Akt/mTOR signalling pathway. *Sci. Rep.* **2023**, *13*, 19227. [CrossRef]
12. Dominici, M.; Le Blanc, K.; Mueller, I.; Slaper-Cortenbach, I.; Marini, F.; Krause, D.; Deans, R.; Keating, A.; Prockop, D.; Horwitz, E. Minimal criteria for defining multipotent mesenchymal stromal cells. The International Society for Cellular Therapy position statement. *Cytotherapy* **2006**, *8*, 315–317. [CrossRef] [PubMed]
13. Parolini, O.; Alviano, F.; Bagnara, G.P.; Bilic, G.; Buhring, H.J.; Evangelista, M.; Hennerbichler, S.; Liu, B.; Magatti, M.; Mao, N.; et al. Concise review: Isolation and characterization of cells from human term placenta: Outcome of the first international Workshop on Placenta Derived Stem Cells. *Stem Cells* **2008**, *26*, 300–311. [CrossRef]
14. Alidoust Saharkhiz Lahiji, M.; Safari, F. Potential therapeutic effects of hAMSCs secretome on Panc1 pancreatic cancer cells through downregulation of SgK269, E-cadherin, vimentin, and snail expression. *Biologicals* **2022**, *76*, 24–30. [CrossRef]
15. Bu, S.; Zhang, Q.; Wang, Q.; Lai, D. Human amniotic epithelial cells inhibit growth of epithelial ovarian cancer cells via TGF-beta1-mediated cell cycle arrest. *Int. J. Oncol.* **2017**, *51*, 1405–1414. [CrossRef]
16. Riedel, R.; Perez-Perez, A.; Carmona-Fernandez, A.; Jaime, M.; Casale, R.; Duenas, J.L.; Guadix, P.; Sanchez-Margalet, V.; Varone, C.L.; Maymo, J.L. Human amniotic membrane conditioned medium inhibits proliferation and modulates related microRNAs expression in hepatocarcinoma cells. *Sci. Rep.* **2019**, *9*, 14193. [CrossRef] [PubMed]
17. Magatti, M.; De Munari, S.; Vertua, E.; Parolini, O. Amniotic membrane-derived cells inhibit proliferation of cancer cell lines by inducing cell cycle arrest. *J. Cell. Mol. Med.* **2012**, *16*, 2208–2218. [CrossRef]
18. Ramuta, T.Z.; Jerman, U.D.; Tratnjek, L.; Janev, A.; Magatti, M.; Vertua, E.; Bonassi Signoroni, P.; Silini, A.R.; Parolini, O.; Kreft, M.E. The Cells and Extracellular Matrix of Human Amniotic Membrane Hinder the Growth and Invasive Potential of Bladder Urothelial Cancer Cells. *Front. Bioeng. Biotechnol.* **2020**, *8*, 554530. [CrossRef]
19. Papait, A.; Ragni, E.; Cargnoni, A.; Vertua, E.; Romele, P.; Masserdotti, A.; Perucca Orfei, C.; Signoroni, P.B.; Magatti, M.; Silini, A.R.; et al. Comparison of EV-free fraction, EVs, and total secretome of amniotic mesenchymal stromal cells for their immunomodulatory potential: A translational perspective. *Front. Immunol.* **2022**, *13*, 960909. [CrossRef] [PubMed]
20. Ragni, E.; Papait, A.; Perucca Orfei, C.; Silini, A.R.; Colombini, A.; Vigano, M.; Libonati, F.; Parolini, O.; de Girolamo, L. Amniotic membrane-mesenchymal stromal cells secreted factors and extracellular vesicle-miRNAs: Anti-inflammatory and regenerative features for musculoskeletal tissues. *Stem Cells Transl. Med.* **2021**, *10*, 1044–1062. [CrossRef]
21. Buick, R.N.; Pullano, R.; Trent, J.M. Comparative properties of five human ovarian adenocarcinoma cell lines. *Cancer Res.* **1985**, *45*, 3668–3676.
22. Magatti, M.; Pianta, S.; Silini, A.; Parolini, O. Isolation, Culture, and Phenotypic Characterization of Mesenchymal Stromal Cells from the Amniotic Membrane of the Human Term Placenta. *Methods Mol. Biol.* **2016**, *1416*, 233–244. [CrossRef] [PubMed]

23. Rossi, D.; Pianta, S.; Magatti, M.; Sedlmayr, P.; Parolini, O. Characterization of the conditioned medium from amniotic membrane cells: Prostaglandins as key effectors of its immunomodulatory activity. *PLoS ONE* **2012**, *7*, e46956. [CrossRef]
24. Lim, G.J.; Kang, S.J.; Lee, J.Y. Novel invasion indices quantify the feed-forward facilitation of tumor invasion by macrophages. *Sci. Rep.* **2020**, *10*, 718. [CrossRef]
25. Wan, X.; Bovornchutichai, P.; Cui, Z.; O'Neill, E.; Ye, H. Morphological analysis of human umbilical vein endothelial cells co-cultured with ovarian cancer cells in 3D: An oncogenic angiogenesis assay. *PLoS ONE* **2017**, *12*, e0180296. [CrossRef]
26. Carpentier, G.M.M.; Courty, J.; Cascone, I. Angiogenesis Analyzer for ImageJ. In Proceedings of the 4th ImageJ User and Developer Conference proceeding, Luxembourg, 24–26 October 2012; pp. 198–201.
27. Ng, T.Y.; Ngan, H.Y.; Cheng, D.K.; Wong, L.C. Clinical applicability of the ATP cell viability assay as a predictor of chemoresponse in platinum-resistant epithelial ovarian cancer using nonsurgical tumor cell samples. *Gynecol. Oncol.* **2000**, *76*, 405–408. [CrossRef]
28. Kalamegam, G.; Sait, K.H.W.; Ahmed, F.; Kadam, R.; Pushparaj, P.N.; Anfinan, N.; Rasool, M.; Jamal, M.S.; Abu-Elmagd, M.; Al-Qahtani, M. Human Wharton's Jelly Stem Cell (hWJSC) Extracts Inhibit Ovarian Cancer Cell Lines OVCAR3 and SKOV3 in vitro by Inducing Cell Cycle Arrest and Apoptosis. *Front. Oncol.* **2018**, *8*, 592. [CrossRef]
29. Zheng, S.; Wang, W.; Aldahdooh, J.; Malyutina, A.; Shadbahr, T.; Tanoli, Z.; Pessia, A.; Tang, J. SynergyFinder Plus: Toward Better Interpretation and Annotation of Drug Combination Screening Datasets. *Genom. Proteom. Bioinform.* **2022**, *20*, 587–596. [CrossRef]
30. Wallis, B.; Bowman, K.R.; Lu, P.; Lim, C.S. The Challenges and Prospects of p53-Based Therapies in Ovarian Cancer. *Biomolecules* **2023**, *13*, 159. [CrossRef]
31. Mullany, L.K.; Wong, K.K.; Marciano, D.C.; Katsonis, P.; King-Crane, E.R.; Ren, Y.A.; Lichtarge, O.; Richards, J.S. Specific TP53 Mutants Overrepresented in Ovarian Cancer Impact CNV, TP53 Activity, Responses to Nutlin-3a, and Cell Survival. *Neoplasia* **2015**, *17*, 789–803. [CrossRef]
32. Shojaei, S.; Moradi-Chaleshtori, M.; Paryan, M.; Koochaki, A.; Sharifi, K.; Mohammadi-Yeganeh, S. Mesenchymal stem cell-derived exosomes enriched with miR-218 reduce the epithelial-mesenchymal transition and angiogenesis in triple-negative breast cancer cells. *Eur. J. Med. Res.* **2023**, *28*, 516. [CrossRef]
33. Li, X.; Liu, L.L.; Yao, J.L.; Wang, K.; Ai, H. Human Umbilical Cord Mesenchymal Stem Cell-Derived Extracellular Vesicles Inhibit Endometrial Cancer Cell Proliferation and Migration through Delivery of Exogenous miR-302a. *Stem Cells Int.* **2019**, *2019*, 8108576. [CrossRef]
34. Reza, A.; Choi, Y.J.; Yasuda, H.; Kim, J.H. Human adipose mesenchymal stem cell-derived exosomal-miRNAs are critical factors for inducing anti-proliferation signalling to A2780 and SKOV-3 ovarian cancer cells. *Sci. Rep.* **2016**, *6*, 38498. [CrossRef] [PubMed]
35. Kalamegam, G.; Sait, K.H.W.; Anfinan, N.; Kadam, R.; Ahmed, F.; Rasool, M.; Naseer, M.I.; Pushparaj, P.N.; Al-Qahtani, M. Cytokines secreted by human Wharton's jelly stem cells inhibit the proliferation of ovarian cancer (OVCAR3) cells in vitro. *Oncol. Lett.* **2019**, *17*, 4521–4531. [CrossRef]
36. Rahimi Lifshagerd, M.; Safari, F. Therapeutic effects of hAMSCs secretome on proliferation of MDA-MB-231 breast cancer cells by the cell cycle arrest in G1/S phase. *Clin. Transl. Oncol.* **2023**, *25*, 1702–1709. [CrossRef] [PubMed]
37. Liu, Q.W.; Li, J.Y.; Zhang, X.C.; Liu, Y.; Liu, Q.Y.; Xiao, L.; Zhang, W.J.; Wu, H.Y.; Deng, K.Y.; Xin, H.B. Human amniotic mesenchymal stem cells inhibit hepatocellular carcinoma in tumour-bearing mice. *J. Cell. Mol. Med.* **2020**, *24*, 10525–10541. [CrossRef] [PubMed]
38. Rolfo, A.; Giuffrida, D.; Giuffrida, M.C.; Todros, T.; Calogero, A.E. New perspectives for prostate cancer treatment: In vitro inhibition of LNCaP and PC3 cell proliferation by amnion-derived mesenchymal stromal cells conditioned media. *Aging Male* **2014**, *17*, 94–101. [CrossRef]
39. Pashaei-Asl, R.; Pashaiasl, M.; Ebrahimie, E.; Lale Ataei, M.; Paknejad, M. Apoptotic effects of human amniotic fluid mesenchymal stem cells conditioned medium on human MCF-7 breast cancer cell line. *Bioimpacts* **2023**, *13*, 191–206. [CrossRef]
40. Bolouri, M.R.; Ghods, R.; Zarnani, K.; Vafaei, S.; Falak, R.; Zarnani, A.H. Human amniotic epithelial cells exert anti-cancer effects through secretion of immunomodulatory small extracellular vesicles (sEV). *Cancer Cell Int.* **2022**, *22*, 329. [CrossRef]
41. Palmirotta, R.; Silvestris, E.; D'Oronzo, S.; Cardascia, A.; Silvestris, F. Ovarian cancer: Novel molecular aspects for clinical assessment. *Crit. Rev. Oncol. Hematol.* **2017**, *117*, 12–29. [CrossRef]
42. Florkemeier, I.; Antons, L.K.; Weimer, J.P.; Hedemann, N.; Rogmans, C.; Kruger, S.; Scherliess, R.; Dempfle, A.; Arnold, N.; Maass, N.; et al. Multicellular ovarian cancer spheroids: Novel 3D model to mimic tumour complexity. *Sci. Rep.* **2024**, *14*, 23526. [CrossRef]
43. Moss, N.M.; Barbolina, M.V.; Liu, Y.; Sun, L.; Munshi, H.G.; Stack, M.S. Ovarian cancer cell detachment and multicellular aggregate formation are regulated by membrane type 1 matrix metalloproteinase: A potential role in I.p. metastatic dissemination. *Cancer Res.* **2009**, *69*, 7121–7129. [CrossRef] [PubMed]
44. Usui, A.; Ko, S.Y.; Barengo, N.; Naora, H. P-cadherin promotes ovarian cancer dissemination through tumor cell aggregation and tumor-peritoneum interactions. *Mol. Cancer Res.* **2014**, *12*, 504–513. [CrossRef] [PubMed]
45. Swierczewska, M.; Sterzynska, K.; Rucinski, M.; Andrzejewska, M.; Nowicki, M.; Januchowski, R. The response and resistance to drugs in ovarian cancer cell lines in 2D monolayers and 3D spheroids. *Biomed. Pharmacother.* **2023**, *165*, 115152. [CrossRef]

46. Sliwa, A.; Szczerba, A.; Pieta, P.P.; Bialas, P.; Lorek, J.; Nowak-Markwitz, E.; Jankowska, A. A Recipe for Successful Metastasis: Transition and Migratory Modes of Ovarian Cancer Cells. *Cancers* **2024**, *16*, 783. [CrossRef]
47. Moffitt, L.; Karimnia, N.; Stephens, A.; Bilandzic, M. Therapeutic Targeting of Collective Invasion in Ovarian Cancer. *Int. J. Mol. Sci.* **2019**, *20*, 1466. [CrossRef] [PubMed]
48. Suresh, M.; Bhat, R. Ovarian cancer cells exhibit diverse migration strategies on stiff collagenous substrata. *Biophys. J.* **2024**, *123*, 4009–4021. [CrossRef] [PubMed]
49. Safari, F.; Shakery, T.; Sayadamin, N. Evaluating the effect of secretome of human amniotic mesenchymal stromal cells on apoptosis induction and epithelial-mesenchymal transition inhibition in LNCaP prostate cancer cells based on 2D and 3D cell culture models. *Cell Biochem. Funct.* **2021**, *39*, 813–820. [CrossRef]
50. Weaver, B.A. How Taxol/paclitaxel kills cancer cells. *Mol. Biol. Cell* **2014**, *25*, 2677–2681. [CrossRef]
51. Mosca, L.; Ilari, A.; Fazi, F.; Assaraf, Y.G.; Colotti, G. Taxanes in cancer treatment: Activity, chemoresistance and its overcoming. *Drug Resist. Updat.* **2021**, *54*, 100742. [CrossRef]
52. Jantalika, T.; Manochantr, S.; Kheolamai, P.; Tantikanlayaporn, D.; Saijuntha, W.; Pinlaor, S.; Chairoungdua, A.; Paraoan, L.; Tantrawatpan, C. Human chorion-derived mesenchymal stem cells suppress JAK2/STAT3 signaling and induce apoptosis of cholangiocarcinoma cell lines. *Sci. Rep.* **2022**, *12*, 11341. [CrossRef]
53. Salkin, H.; Satir-Basaran, G.; Korkmaz, S.; Burcin Gonen, Z.; Erdem Basaran, K. Mesenchymal stem cell-derived conditioned medium and Methysergide give rise to crosstalk inhibition of 5-HT2A and 5-HT7 receptors in neuroblastoma cells. *Brain Res.* **2023**, *1808*, 148354. [CrossRef] [PubMed]
54. Choi, J.I.; Park, S.H.; Lee, H.J.; Lee, D.W.; Lee, H.N. Inhibition of Phospho-S6 Kinase, a Protein Involved in the Compensatory Adaptive Response, Increases the Efficacy of Paclitaxel in Reducing the Viability of Matrix-Attached Ovarian Cancer Cells. *PLoS ONE* **2016**, *11*, e0155052. [CrossRef] [PubMed]
55. Bonomi, A.; Silini, A.; Vertua, E.; Signoroni, P.B.; Cocce, V.; Cavicchini, L.; Sisto, F.; Alessandri, G.; Pessina, A.; Parolini, O. Human amniotic mesenchymal stromal cells (hAMSCs) as potential vehicles for drug delivery in cancer therapy: An in vitro study. *Stem Cell Res. Ther.* **2015**, *6*, 155. [CrossRef] [PubMed]
56. Muntiu, A.; Papait, A.; Vincenzoni, F.; Rossetti, D.V.; Romele, P.; Cargnoni, A.; Silini, A.; Parolini, O.; Desiderio, C. Proteomic analysis of the human amniotic mesenchymal stromal cell secretome by integrated approaches via filter-aided sample preparation. *J. Proteom.* **2025**, *310*, 105339. [CrossRef]
57. Marassi, V.; La Rocca, G.; Placci, A.; Muntiu, A.; Vincenzoni, F.; Vitali, A.; Desiderio, C.; Maraldi, T.; Beretti, F.; Russo, E.; et al. Native characterization and QC profiling of human amniotic mesenchymal stromal cell vesicular fractions for secretome-based therapy. *Talanta* **2024**, *276*, 126216. [CrossRef]

MDPI AG
Grosspeteranlage 5
4052 Basel
Switzerland
Tel.: +41 61 683 77 34

*Pharmaceutics* Editorial Office
E-mail: pharmaceutics@mdpi.com
www.mdpi.com/journal/pharmaceutics

www.ingramcontent.com/pod-product-compliance
Lightning Source LLC
Chambersburg PA
CBHW040820250926
51850CB00007BA/1220
* 9 7 8 3 7 2 5 8 4 9 4 5 1 *